W9-BDR-424

Raising Parents

Raising Parents
Attachment, parenting and child safety

Patricia McKinsey Crittenden

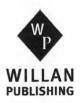

WILLAN
PUBLISHING

Published by

Willan Publishing
Culmcott House
Mill Street, Uffculme
Cullompton, Devon
EX15 3AT, UK
Tel: +44(0)1884 840337
Fax: +44(0)1884 840251
e-mail: info@willanpublishing.co.uk
website: www.willanpublishing.co.uk

Published simultaneously in the USA and Canada by

Willan Publishing
c/o ISBS, 920 NE 58th Ave, Suite 300,
Portland, Oregon 97213-3786, USA
Tel: +001(0)503 287 3093
Fax: +001(0)503 280 8832
e-mail: info@isbs.com
website: www.isbs.com

© Patricia M. Crittenden 2008

The rights of Patricia M. Crittenden to be identified as the author of this book have been asserted
by her in accordance with the Copyright, Designs and Patents Act of 1988.

All rights reserved; no part of this publication may be reproduced, stored in a retrieval system, or
transmitted in any form or by any means, electronic, mechanical, photocopying, recording or otherwise
without the prior written permission of the Publishers or a licence permitting copying in the UK issued
by the Copyright Licensing Agency Ltd, Saffron House, 6–10 Kirby Street, London EC1N 8TS.

First published 2008

Reprinted 2009

ISBN   978-1-84392-498-2 paperback
       978-1-84392-499-9 hardback

British Library Cataloguing-in-Publication Data

A catalogue record for this book is available from the British Library.

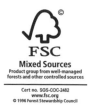

FSC
Mixed Sources
Product group from well-managed
forests and other controlled sources

Cert no. SGS-COC-2482
www.fsc.org
© 1996 Forest Stewardship Council

Project managed by Deer Park Productions, Tavistock, Devon
Typeset by GCS, Leighton Buzzard, Bedfordshire
Printed and bound by T.J. International Ltd, Padstow, Cornwall

Contents

Part 3   An Integrative Approach to Treatment

Acknowledgements

A book such as this requires the effort of many people and I am very appreciative to them all for making this volume possible. Andrea Landini has helped me from the beginning, reading each chapter in its earliest form while keeping my spirits up and my efforts focused through the long and intense period of writing that followed. Simon Wilkinson also has read every word and contributed greatly to my understanding of the genetic, neurological and somatic issues as well as many other issues.

A number of other people have been invaluable sources of ideas, information, and advice, especially Michael Rutter and Silvio Lenzi (structuring of the theory), Graham Towl, Clark Baim and Marcus Erooga (forensic issues), and Kim Barthel and Kasia Kozlowska (neurology). Gordon Sommerville, Robert Lee, Rudi Dallos, Mary Heller, Øyvind Urnes, Siri Gullestad, Steve Farnfield, Chris Purnell, Andy Slukin, Jennie Noll, Augusto Zagmutt and Gunhild Kulbotten have all added to my clinical awareness with ideas and cases.

In addition, several people have helped to free my time for this by filling in on urgent tasks; without their help, I would still be hoping to find the time to write. Therefore I'm grateful to Andrea Landini, Bente Nilsen, Valerie Ahl, Nicola Sahhar and Laura Fossi.

A special word is needed for the parents and children whose experience is represented here; each has been generous enough to allow me and those who work with me to share their experience in order to help others through what we have learned. Without their generosity in the face of their personal adversity, this book could not exist. I hope I have understood and related their experiences with both insight and compassion.

Finally, I am grateful to my husband and daughter who have each supported me and accepted my hours and hours – and hours! – of sitting behind my computer. They trusted that this was a worthwhile task and I appreciate what it costs to let one's wife or mother put so much energy into one task.

Preface

Every book has a special reason to be written. This is my first book and, although I had expected to write a general book on a new theory of human adaptation, this book on parents is really more fitting. Its roots lie in 40 years of working with parents and of being a parent, both a parent of my own child and a foster parent to another woman's children. It lies in my now distant experience as a child. Summer begins today and today I begin full-time duty as a grandparent to my nine-year-old granddaughter who is visiting us. The roles of child and parent define us and define our progress through life. This book is about how we learn to be a parent.

When I began teaching school, back in the 1960s, I worked with children from very poor families. Bubbling, bright, eager-eyed children who dragged into school tired, poorly fed, ill-kempt, and sometimes ill. They came to school every day, especially if they were sick. In school, there were two regular meals and a snack. There was a rest period. It was warm. And everything was orderly and organized around their needs. Their mothers pushed them out the door in the morning and they came to school, thirsty for life.

Back then, I got angry with their mothers, thinking that at least they could bathe and feed their children. At least, they could put them to bed in time for a full night's sleep. No matter if they didn't read to their children or count or give them the advantages of a middle class home. I, as a teacher, could correct that. But their children's bodies weren't ready – and why didn't their mothers see to that?!!! A few years later, I began working with mothers who abused and neglected their babies. You'd expect that I'd really harden in my accusations, but it didn't happen that way. Instead, I listened to them and I learned.

It was the fault of the men! The men who dropped into their lives, lived in their houses, drank their money, loved their bodies, slapped them around, and left them soon enough – left them with yet another child to care for. It was the men! Fix men and society would care for its children.

Some people can learn from books. I, it seems, learn from living. My next job was running a parent support center in a public housing project. Now

I was with these families every day and often into the night. I taught the women, gathered up the children, had coffee sitting on the front stoops, and I met the men. I watched them arrive with the blush of new romance, saw them settle in with the carefulness of being in someone else's home and the increasing casualness as it became their own. Then I heard the raised voices and saw the sullen looks on the women's faces. By the time I saw the occasional black eye, the man had slipped from sight. Not gone yet, but the direction was becoming clear. As he disappeared, the professionals began showing up. People like me, but, unlike me, they didn't spend so many hours right there in the neighborhood.

Before they left, I had gotten to know these men. Two anecdotes from when I was doing research, will show what I learned. Seventeen-year-old Kantisha and her boyfriend Jefferson came in for our Parents Interview. Kantisha held their newborn closely in her arms, but everything about her, her eyes, her shoulders, the lean of her body, was oriented toward Jefferson. The room, for Kantisha, was defined by the space between herself and her man.

Jefferson? His world was big. His body was open: legs spread wide, arms stretched out as he gesticulated, and his eyes? His eyes were not contained by his girlfriend and their child. His eyes drifted over all of the room and had the look of someone seeing far beyond the room. As Kantisha's world was defining itself by two attachments, to her baby and her man, Jefferson's world was just opening up. On the cusp of adulthood, he was expecting many things and was not ready to be tied down just yet. What did he think of Kantisha and the baby? He loved them! But his eyes were not confined to the little circle of his new family.

The second anecdote occurred in the same room in response to the same interview. Margaret came in with five squabbling children and the current boyfriend. There was a heaviness to her body, a weariness as she settled her children near the toys and slumped into her chair at the round table in the middle of the room. Driscoll and I sat so as to make a triangle with Margaret around the table. Margaret was half-oriented to me and half to the children. Her back was partially toward Driscoll and one shoulder was up, almost as if pushing him, *and all he stood for*, away. It was a frail line of defense against all the hurt and suffering brought by the men who had preceded him.

As they spoke, answering my questions about their childhood and parenthood, Margaret's face and posture became sultry. She wanted Driscoll; she no longer believed men could be had. She invited – and she feared; she no longer made a place for him in her world that, visually, was defined by the children and me, *the professional*. Margaret was older, wiser now, and sadder. She no longer expected what Kantisha had assumed.

Driscoll was older too, in his early thirties. He had assorted children, here and there, scattered in other women's homes. It's a good gene-survival strategy, but it didn't look like it comforted Driscoll. He leaned into the triangle of the three of us. His arms were stretched out toward Margaret.

His voice lacked authority; it was softer and carried a tone of pleading, of loneliness. Would he hurt the children, as Margaret feared? No! He loved little children, he wanted to stay and raise them … He was so gentle, like a supplicant, so tender, almost romantic as he described the role he wanted to play in this family.

Margaret wasn't having it. Dreams and life were different things. Men always came this way, then they drank the money for the children, yelled at her, beat her, and left, leaving a new baby behind. She wasn't buying into his dreams anymore. She needed him. A woman needed a man. But she would keep him outside the circle of her attachments.

That was when I understood. Timing can be cruel. Kantisha was too young, but biology made her ready. Jefferson wasn't ready. But by his thirties, he would have lived in many homes and left all his children behind. He would be alone. At 34, Driscoll was ready for a home. He was applying for the job of husband and father. With no qualifications except hope and a bit of hard-earned wisdom. Margaret couldn't believe in him. She had learned too, the hard way.

I also had learned. I began to see the big forces of society quite differently from the rhetoric of political movements, the civil rights and women's movements. For all the efforts of women to improve their place in the social order, it seemed to me that it is men in troubled families who have no home. They drift from family to family, first because they imagine more and then because they discover they lost too much.

In between, between that first baby and the jumble of children to come, the professionals show up. We become the missing parent – and we can't fill the role. Something very important has gone awry and we, the professionals, seem unable to correct it. Indeed, our best efforts often only record, and possibly assist, the death of a family.

My other perspective on parents is more personal. I was a foster mother. I went in with hope and the confidence that I could do what the biological mother could not. Through me and my husband, two children would be given a chance to find a better future. Maybe we were a bit like Kantisha at the beginning?

As our two years passed, my ideas about raising children became much more complex – and realistic. Like every parent, I learned over night what no non-parent believes: being a parent gives you a completely different perspective, one that you didn't have – and couldn't have – before being responsible for children. Professionals don't like hearing that and the non-parents deny its truth. Given the high proportion of professionals who are neither parents, nor spouses, nor even have a partner, maybe the lessons of parenting as it is lived (as opposed to how it should be lived) need to be articulated.

What did I learn from being a foster parent (that I relearned as a parent)? That loving children and intending well isn't enough. That once children's behavior becomes troubled, it has effects on the parent that the parent probably won't know how to handle.

For example, at three years of age, DeeDee, our oldest foster child, had experienced physical abuse and neglect, hunger, medical neglect, and abandonment. She had lived in a car for months and been dropped for weeks at a time in strangers' homes. She had seen men hit and hurt her mother. She had learned to care for Tina, her toddler sister, as if *she* were the mother.

When DeeDee came to us, I misunderstood her sudden affection to me, *a complete stranger*, and thought (foolish me!) that her false positive affect was true acceptance of me. How hungry was I for this love? (Are other foster parents similarly eager to be loved by children?)

Then when she defended her role as protector of her younger sister, I was confused. I became resentful and frustrated when she continued to horde food in her closet, even after more than a year of predictable meals and an always full fridge. The first blush of false love wore off into mutual doubt and disappointment.

Slowly, I was becoming a different sort of mother than I had expected to be. Looking into DeeDee's eyes, when I felt most distressed by her, I saw an image of myself as I didn't want to be.

Slowly I came to see how hurt children hurt the parents who care for them. Did it matter that I hadn't created DeeDee's problems, that I was innocent of her mother's inadequacies? It did not. I lived with the outcomes and was changed in ways I had not expected.

Toward the end of their stay with us, I finally dared to ask for help. (Why hadn't I asked earlier? I didn't want them taken away! I feared the social workers' power to remove the children I now loved. So I hid the problem until it was really out of control.) What did I want from the professionals? I wanted them to fix my child! She was broken. She couldn't get over her past. Here! Take her, fix her! Repair my dream.

Looking back now, I realize that I sounded like the many adoptive parents whose older or handicapped or formerly institutionalized children don't fit into their homes or fulfill their dreams. I didn't see myself as part of the problem and I wanted a quick solution, one that would restore my dreams.

By the time our foster children left to be adopted, I had a different perspective. I sympathized with their biological mother! I had a bit of understanding of how difficult it was to raise her children. That she had 'caused' the problem no longer made any difference. Now I knew that once the problem was there in the relationships, it was very difficult to correct.

I began to wish that, instead of fostering her children (and feeling in competition with her for her children), I had known *her* and fostered her. I wished I could have supported her to become a better mother.

Now, as a grandmother myself, I really wish that an older woman, one who could have been like a mother to DeeDee's mother, could have fostered their troubled family.

I know how the story ends. There will be a 'detachment' foster placement to prepare DeeDee and Tina for their adoptive home (to wash them clean of their attachment to us so they would be ready to be born freshly into their new family). Then three failed adoptive placements will come and more foster placements between each of those. At 14 and 15 years old, Tina and DeeDee (with their new names chosen by their adoptive parents) will be on the streets. Boys will become their attachment figures and the fathers of the babies that will be removed. When DeeDee finds me through her hospital records and calls to ask if I am her real mother and if I can help her with her troubled daughter, I will know that our plans for improving children's futures did not work out as we had intended.

In two decades of travel that followed my daughter's growing up, I've had the opportunity to try to understand thousands of lives in at least a score of countries. I have become immersed in the effects of mental illness on families.

One in five of us experiences mental illness at some point in our own lives and more of us have a family member who suffers intense psychological pain. When that person is a mother or father, the effects are more troubling than the direct and clear effects of abuse. It can be very difficult for the children of mentally ill parents to know what happened when they were growing up – far less to understand it. Telling the stories of our lives is crucial to understanding ourselves and understanding ourselves is crucial to our relationships, especially those with our children.

I came to know Jane personally through a colleague who cared very much for this extremely distressed young mother. As Jean began to come apart through cutting herself, abusing alcohol, and attacking her husband, my friend asked if I would give her an Adult Attachment Interview (AAI) to see if it could point them in a new direction. Jean was willing, but hesitant. It was an awful time in her life and, although no one knew it yet, it was going to get worse. Jean was just weeks from another near-fatal suicide attempt and then the struggle to be admitted to hospital for long enough for her to feel safe and begin the process of change.

During her interview, Jean spoke slowly and quietly. Her voice was filled with withheld pain; often she was silent. My job was to listen and wait, to tolerate hearing the suffering that weighed her down until she wasn't sure she could go on. It was a moving experience for us both. In the fury of her drunken outbursts, Jean had been seen as manipulative and in need of learning to inhibit her anger. Her interview suggested the opposite. Jean used a compulsively inhibitory strategy that dipped into depression and exploded occasionally with rage and fear.

I've seen this many times. The danger of treating compulsive individuals as if they were willfully acting out is a major theme in this book. When we misunderstand parents' outbursts, we sometimes offer harmful treatments. Jean was using every resource there was, but it wasn't helping. In fact, things were getting worse. For a summer, my friend and I struggled to help both Jean and an unwilling service system to change in ways that would help her.

A year later, my friend's letter to me told a story of hope – and the process of finding hope – that we hardly dared to imagine during that terrible summer.

Hello Pat

I found your talk about compulsions fascinating and have found myself thinking a lot about Jean and the interview. Jean was heavily medicated when you interviewed her and I'm sure this changed the way she was. There was only one point in the interview where I thought she came close to having an intrusion of anger whereas this had been frequent before she was medicated. On the other hand, she seemed to recall events she had not talked about before. She was amazed by what she described as 'little neurons firing' in her head the day afterwards and things popping into her mind for a few more days.

One of these was of being with her dad when she was little and him comforting her. She recalled being stroked and held by him. This has been lovely because it's a very different part of her history, unlike anything she had recalled before and it has come up many times over the past year. When we talk about it, the effect is noticeable; she seems to feel comforted and settled.

This is what it is all about. Finding a way to be with someone that frees their mind to find a truth they can live with.

It's easy enough to say that you need to understand that your parents meant well and really loved you, that their own problems got in the way of their acting lovingly and protectively. But what really turned things around for Jean – and all of us Jeans – was finding the scraps of memory that permitted her to feel loved, however briefly. With that, we each can begin to change how we understand ourselves. Asking good questions and listening empathically enabled Jane to recall her deceased parents' love for her. This connected her to my friend and, ultimately, enabled her to make changes that helped her to become a better mother to her own small child.

Suffice it to say that being a parent and raising children looks different to me today than it did 40 years ago when I began as a young mother and professional working with families.

This volume tries to tell some of what I've learned about raising parents. It is an attempt to bridge the gaps between parent and child and parent and professional, always by keeping the experience of each world in mind.

This is a book about learning to understand, love, and forgive because, without these, we cannot raise anyone.

Patricia M. Crittenden
2008

*This book is dedicated to the memory of
my parents and my sisters*

Part 1

Growing Up

Chapter 1

Yesterday's children: Today's mothers and fathers

This is a book about parents. It is intended for professionals who work with children or adults who were harmed as children. The parents in question are those who endanger their children or whose children may endanger themselves or others. It is important to consider the functioning and needs of these parents because our treatment systems are organized almost entirely around the needs of children and funded almost exclusively to offer services for children or for parents about children. Yet sometimes children's needs would be met best by meeting their parents' personal needs. Even then, however, direct service to adults around the adults' issues is often impossible to provide.

Nevertheless, children rarely live better than their parents. If the parent suffers, so will the child. One need only see how poorly children fare in foster care to see the truth of this. Foster children are 3–6 times more likely to experience emotional, behavioral, and developmental disorders than children not in care (Dubowitz 1990; Garwood and Close 2001). Youth aging out of foster care less often complete high school (52 per cent), are often emotionally disturbed (38 per cent), more often use illegal drugs (50 per cent), and are more often involved with the legal system (25 per cent, Vandivere et al. 2003). Children with long and multiple placements were more likely than other children to experience problems such as unemployment and homelessness (Courtney and Piliavin 1998).

Foster care is an attempt to free children from the limitations of their parents and enable them to develop more advantageously. But this outcome is rarely achieved. To the contrary, children in care seem to carry the risks of their biological parents, the risks associated with changing families, and any risks associated with the recipient parents. Avoiding this sort of outcome is very important, and we can best avoid it by helping children's biological parents to become more adequate parents.

Understanding and helping troubled parents to become secure and balanced people is crucial – for the parents themselves, for their children, and for society at large. This book is a guide to understanding parents as people who have children – as opposed to seeing them as existing solely in terms of their ability to fulfill their children's needs.

An anecdote can suggest how the change in perspective might change what we see – and how we respond.

Talisha,[1] her mother, and her 6-year-old daughter were in my office for evaluation following a complaint to child protection that Talisha often hit her daughter abusively. Usually, this story would be told from her daughter's perspective, with discussion of the bruises, her mother's sullen withdrawal and refusal to admit to the abuse, the daughter's vigilant looks of concern to her mother, and the grandmother's report of Talisha's excessive punishment of her daughter.

Instead, one comment from Talisha lets us see a different perspective. When being asked yet again about the bruise and whether she had inflicted it, Talisha looked with resentful eyes toward her own mother and blurted out, *'Yes, I did it! But nobody came to help me when she did the same thing to me! I don't understand why it's abuse when I do it and just punishment when she did it.'* Then, turning to me, Talisha said softly, *'I love my daughter just as much as she loves me. I don't see what I did wrong.'* And Talisha cried.

Raising children

Raising our children is the most important and complex task in our lives, and yet, as many have pointed out, we receive little or no formal training for this role. Instead, parents are assumed to inherently 'know' what to do.

How do parents know what to do and how did they get that information?

This book considers the process by which this inherent, implicit knowledge comes to be. However, because it is quite clear that not all parents raise their children the same way, understanding individual differences in what parents do is crucial. Some of the differences are cultural while others are specific to families and yet others to individual parents. This book explores both the universal processes by which parenting knowledge is acquired and also individual differences in the specific information that is acquired. The focus is on those parents who find it difficult to keep their children safe and comfortable.

Knowledge, however, is a complex concept. Sometimes we do what we 'know' we shouldn't do. That is, there can be a difference between what parents think they should do and what they actually do. To address this discrepancy, we need to think of knowledge as having several forms such that what parents know explicitly and in general may not be the same as what they know how to do or how they feel. This book addresses different ways of knowing what to do and the reasons why one sort of knowledge might influence behavior more than another sort.

Put another way, this book explores how parenting develops in terms of what information is brought to bear on the task, when and how that information was generated, how we employ the information, and which aspects of the task have priority when not all can be managed or when success is at risk. Doing so highlights the importance of protection and preparation for reproduction as essential and universal components of parenting. These are precisely the functions that are distorted in cases of risk, i.e., cases of child maltreatment and parental mental illness.

Individual differences in how parents raise children

Everyone has seen parents treating their children in unacceptable ways and wondered why they did that. Everyone has been horrified at the 'inhumanity' of parents whose extreme abuse and neglect of their children have garnered media attention, and wondered how they could do those things. Each of us who is a parent has, on occasion, acted in ways that appalled us – and we wonder, even now, why we did that.

> Luke's arm was broken. No one knew how it had happened and Luke at 19 months couldn't tell. He simply curled up tightly in the hospital crib, not talking or walking. He wouldn't look at his parents when they came to visit. He seemed grossly neglected and abused, and the hospital staff were anxious to help him, believing that no child should have to live like this.

> On a crowded aeroplane, a family – mother, father, and 3-year-old boy – squeezed into the aisle and waited to disembark. The boy hung limply on his mother's arm – while she tried to gather her bags. She tried to pull him up to stand; he protested and slumped to the floor among the feet and bags. His father barked, 'Nick! Stop that! Stand up! Help your mother!' and, with raised hand, he threatened Nick with a slap. Nick ignored this, while his mother pleaded, 'Nick, please stand up like a nice boy. If you stand nicely while they open the door, I'll give you a piece of candy when we are off.' Nick only whined, cried, and kicked harder. The father looked away, the mother scanned her audience of other passengers apologetically. Nick began screaming.

> Nancy was failing in school. Everyone knew she was bright, but she didn't pay attention and she couldn't get her assignments done. The zeros and failing grades piled up. One evening her mother sat with her and together they got every single division problem done, correctly. Her mother used positive reinforcement throughout, then praised her for the completed assignment and pointed out how today she would surprise the teacher by having everything ready. The next morning, walking to school, Nancy threw the homework in the neighbor's trash can.

David cowered under his covers in bed, but the sounds of his father's accusations, his mother's pleas, and the thuds and howls kept coming. Then a door slammed and it was over. The next day, as he did every day, David left home as early as possible and wandered as far away as he could. Away from the sounds of families, away from the taunts of other children, away from anything familiar and anyone who would know him. He reached a seedy part of town where no one questioned him and no one knew or cared who he was. Things seemed less intense, less accusing, safer. That's where the truant officer usually found him – when there was time to go looking for him.

At 16, Jackson was on probation for knifing his father; he was living in a homeless shelter and his girlfriend had dumped him. His mother? No one knew where she was; she'd taken off when he was about 10. Since then, he'd lived in all sorts of places. Today, like a lot of kids with a history of multiple placements and no viable current placement, he had dropped in unexpectedly on one of the professionals he used to know. She took time with him, but he wasn't on her client list and wouldn't be; he was now too old. Jackson was tough, charming, egotistical, and self-negating. He didn't have much to lose and, under his cool surface, a frightened little boy almost cried as he tried to find a guide to a life without committed people or a permanent home.

Parents do what they think is right. Only the most thoughtful of them are able to identify and think about the moments when what they did was, in their own eyes, the wrong thing to do.

Strangely, when parents do the right thing, no one wonders why. But the psychological processes that organize appropriate and inappropriate behavior are the same handful of mental processes that all humans have available. What differs is the context in which individuals, and *their* parents, learned to use those processes and, therefore, the learned organization of the processes. That is, humans learn, as they develop from infancy to adulthood, how to use their brains to organize their behavior (although, of course, this is often accomplished without conscious awareness). Differences in what they learn have immense implications for their children.

Why? This is the important issue. Parents who do 'the wrong thing' are like all of us. They began with the same genetically maturing brains that we all have. And all of us occasionally behave in ways that are dangerous to our children. Why? Why do we endanger the most treasured and loved thing in life – our children? Once we recognize that we (ordinary parents and professionals) aren't different in kind from parents who actually harm their children, then this question can elicit inquiry, not accusation. Maintaining curiosity throughout this volume will permit us to move beyond prescriptive, accusing answers that don't work to some fresh ideas that might work.

This book considers how parenting behavior is generated in terms of

1 what information is brought to bear on the task;
2 how it is given meaning;
3 which aspects of the task have priority when not all can be managed or when success is at risk.

These issues highlight the importance of protection and preparation for reproduction as essential and universal components of parenting. They also point to the paradox that these appear to be precisely the functions that are distorted in cases of risk, i.e., cases of child maltreatment and parental mental illness.

The problem of risky parenting

The scope

Most parents, while not being perfect, are in fact 'good enough' (Winnicott 1986). This volume is concerned with those parents who are not 'good enough' and who, therefore, need assistance from the professional community.

How many is that? Of course, there is no exact count, nor is there a line that divides adequate from inadequate parents. Nevertheless, there are some figures that suggest that the problem is quite substantial.

* Some 13–40 per cent of American children are maltreated during their childhood (Finkelhor *et al.* 2005; Goodman *et al.* 1998; Kessler *et al.* 1995). Egypt, South Korea, Ethiopia and China have higher rates (ranging from 22 per cent to 64 per cent). Italy has a lower rate (8 per cent) (World Health Organization 2002). These figures suggest that cultural factors, including support of vulnerable families, affect the safety of individual children.

* About 10 per cent of British children receive a mental health diagnosis (Meltzer *et al.* 2000) whereas 20 per cent of American children and adolescents experience a mental health problem in the course of a year (Foster *et al.* 2005). By the time a child is 10 years old, 8 per cent of married parents and 43 per cent of cohabiting parents will have split up; children not brought up with both parents have more educational problems, substance abuse and, later, debt and unemployment (Etherton *et al.* 2007; Wilson and Oswald 2005).

* About 2.5 million Americans are exposed to potentially traumatizing experiences each year (Perry, Conroy and Ravitz 1991).

* Almost 20 per cent of crimes in Germany are committed by juveniles, and the rate is rising each year; 22 per cent of crimes against juveniles and

children cause some type of physical damage (Federal Criminal Police Office 2004). Some 9 per cent of American children admit to assaulting someone with the intent of hurting them and 16 per cent admit to having carried a gun (Snyder and Sickmund 2006);

• About 13 per cent of Australian children and 7 per cent of American children live in foster care (Australian Institute of Health and Welfare 2004; US Department of Health and Human Services (US DHHS) 2005; US Census Bureau 2007). About 5.5 per cent of English children are in care, with 17 per cent of these in group or residential placements (England National Statistics 2006).

These are not mutually exclusive groups, and not all children in them experience inadequate parental care, but these data suggest that a quarter or more of all children (in economically advantaged countries) could benefit from more appropriate parental care.

Conversely, when these children become parents themselves, they are at risk of mistreating their children. Most studies suggest a rate of maltreatment by maltreated parents of about 30 per cent (Bender and Lösel 2005; Buchanan 1996; Kaufmann and Zigler 1987; Oliver 1993). Similarly, about 26 per cent of abuse victims become criminals in adolescence (Widom 1989).

If one considers only the effects of dangerously inappropriate parental behavior, one might think the parents are misinformed (and, therefore, in need of information and education) or malicious (and, therefore, in need of a judicial response). But if one considers the developmental process through which adults have learned to make meaning and organize their behavior, other explanations become possible. In particular, overzealous attempts at reversal and correction of childhood experience (i.e., overcompensation) and overapplication of learned safety measures (i.e., compulsion) are frequently observed among well-meaning, but endangering parents. In addition, many troubled parents feel *themselves* to be unsafe or uncomforted and act so as to protect or comfort themselves. This book focuses on these explanations in the expectation that they can lead to more effective treatments.

To follow the developmental process of making meanings that organize behavior requires that one note both (1) the distortions of information that functioned self-protectively for the parents when they were children, and (2) the maturation-induced changes, especially sexual motivations, that were applied to childhood representations. It is proposed here that dangerous parental behavior can be seen as having comprehensible and self-protective roots in adults' early development and that this development is a continuing process. That is, development is not determined at some early stage (Bowlby 1969/1983), but instead continues throughout life, with each new accomplishment being built on the base of the past. Nor is development linear. Each successive period of childhood has both the advantage of greater maturity and the disadvantage of new, stage-salient threats. In addition, unexpected events intervene. For example, a special teacher, a divorce, an accident or a premature death, or the arrival of an especially caring stepparent can all change the course of a child's development. As a consequence, what can be understood retrospectively cannot be predicted prospectively. Even siblings, who might appear to have the same developmental context, in fact experience their family very differently because they differ genetically, because they differ in such things as birth order and gender, and because each child fills a different role in the family, some roles boding better for the future than other roles.

Our interest in this book is in following the developmental pathways of those parents who harm their children. These parents constitute only a few of those who at some point in childhood were at risk of parenting problems. Central to this conceptualization is the notion that, without adequate reflective integration, (a) childhood strategies may be applied inappropriately to adult contexts, (b) errors of attribution and behavioral response may be carried forward without awareness, and (c) new distortions and errors may be added in response to newly maturing capacities (for example, reflective capacities that mature in adolescence may be distorted by preceding experience). This combination of contextual errors, implicitly maintained distortions, and newly acquired distortions can lead to inappropriate parental behavior that endangers children.

The advantages of taking such a complex view of inappropriate and dangerous parental behavior are that

1 professionals can develop understanding of and compassion for parents;
2 professionals can talk to parents in terms that are meaningful to parents, thereby increasing the probability of engaging the parents' cooperation;
3 parental change may become more likely.

Why understanding parents' experience is important.

Often we act as though simply becoming 18 or 21 years old or having a baby turned one into an adult. Of course, we know that this is not the case, but when one works in an evaluative, judgmental role, one can forget how development really occurs and focus instead on how parents should behave.

To suggest how unrealistic this is, let me relay a brief incident that occurred during a talk that I gave recently. The talk was to therapists who treat incarcerated or recently released sexual offenders. I was describing, as compassionately as possible, the developmental pathway of a typical incestuous sexual abuser. I had my audience with me, seeing how the baby, the boy, and the young adolescent were victimized in a series of ways. But when he became a young father and I described how he dressed, bathed, and comforted his preschool-aged daughter, the 'temperature' of the audience suddenly shot up. People got agitated, began interrupting me, and felt urgent distress. *'He's grooming her!' 'That's sexual abuse!'*

It took some time to cool the audience down a bit. Indeed, at the next break, more people came up to me than at any other point in my two days of presentation. *'Didn't I recognize …?'* *'How could I condone …?'* It was only when I asked, 'On which day does a victim of repeated abuse – who should be protected – become transformed into a perpetrator who should be punished?', that my audience paused. After some moments of silence, a hand went up. I nodded and a man responded, *'The day the report hits my desk'*.

That is the point. We, the professional community, turn victims into perpetrators – and we punish them accordingly. We strip a complex and painful situation of its complexity, reducing it to a simple, albeit unrealistic, dichotomy. Why? Because it makes our job easier. It is ironic that the Western community has risen up in unison to protest the punishment of a Saudi Arabian woman for being raped and accusing the men who harmed her, when we routinely punish those victimized parents who have not discovered the miracle of remaking themselves when sexual desire and biology transformed them into parents.

One thesis of this book is that understanding human development accurately and dealing realistically with the complex reality that some parents are both victims and perpetrators of maltreatment may be essential to helping both the parents and their children. Part of that process may be looking at the dichotomizing and distorting function of the language we use. 'Groom', 'abuse', 'molest', and other such words portray only part of the complex experience. When we use such terms, we can easily lose access to the actual experience and to alternative ways of representing it and attributing meaning to it. That is, our choice of terminology may function like a self-fulfilling prophesy: what we name may become what we see.

Sexual abuse of children, particularly one's own children, provides a clear example of how dynamic-maturational model (DMM) theory might change our perspective in ways that could improve both treatment and prevention. The process of changing perspective might, however, be a bit shocking in that it will involve finding the perspectives of vulnerable men in addition to retaining those of the harmed children and the community that seeks to protect them. In this volume, I want to capture both Talisha and her daughter's perspective, both that of a man who is sexually involved with his child and the child's, and both the perspective of a mother with periodic psychosis and that of her threatened child. To accomplish this, I will try to stay with behaviorally descriptive language, holding attributions of its meaning for later – and stating that they are attributions very explicitly.

I will hunt for accurate descriptive language that both parents and professionals can agree is accurate and avoid language that contains implicit accusations, prescriptive prohibitions, or assumptions about motivation. This precision is, I think, essential to enable us to understand how parents use information and what developmental experience has led to that learned psychological process. The purpose is to enable professionals to think differently about parents' behavior, especially when that behavior endangers children.

The dynamic-maturational model (DMM) of attachment and adaptation

The theory around which this book is organized is the DMM of attachment and adaptation (Crittenden 1992c, 1995, 1997, 2000a). It is based on Bowlby's theory (Bowlby 1969/1982, 1973, 1980), together with Ainsworth's empirical finding of individual differences in the organization of attachment relationships (Ainsworth 1979; Ainsworth and Wittig 1969; Ainsworth et al. 1978). In addition, however, following Bowlby's lead, several other major theories are integrated into the DMM, in particular Bronfrenbrenner's theory of social ecology (Bronfenbrenner 1979b). This addition creates a hierarchy of nested systems theories (from genetic systems to behavioral systems, to family and community systems, to political/cultural systems) through which to understand the many transactional influences upon individual behavior. In addition, the DMM takes up Bowlby's lead of considering attachment through information processing to consider the cognitive neurosciences and genetics as crucial to understanding both continuities and discontinuities in developmental pathways.

The role of danger

The DMM treats separation and loss, the focus of Bowlby and Ainsworth's work, as special categories of danger and proposes that danger is the primary organizer of human behavior. Further, the DMM returns to Bowlby's roots in psychoanalytic theory by treating sexual motivations as being as important as protective motivations. Together, staying safe and reproducing constitute the basic biological imperatives of any species. For humans, these result in three related, but sometimes competing, motivations: protecting the self, finding a sexual partner, and protecting one's progeny until their reproductive maturity.

Attachment as a dynamic, changing process

The words 'dynamic' and 'maturational' in the label for the DMM indicate a shift in emphasis from Bowlby and Ainsworth. The DMM is a life-span theory in which on-going maturation (as a genetic and epigenetic process) is in dynamic interaction with experience such that early experience influences later development, but does not determine it. Instead, maturation creates natural points of reorganization and experience provides both new opportunities to organize strategic responses and new information about the world and oneself. Further, in line with Erickson's thinking, the nature of threat (to survival and reproduction) changes as one becomes older and moves into larger and more complex contexts, e.g., elementary school, secondary school, work settings (Erikson 1950). This bidirectional transaction (Sameroff 1983, 2000) between self and context generates developmental 'pathways' as opposed to trajectories. The notion of pathways carries with it the idea of changing probabilities (as opposed to fixed predictions) regarding the future.

Relationships, strategies, and information processing

Attachment itself is seen as being central to one's safety across the life span and to one's reproductive opportunity in adulthood. Moreover, 'attachment' is defined as having three equally important aspects:

1 a unique, enduring, and affectively charged *relationship* (e.g., with one's mother, with one's spouse);
2 a *strategy* for protecting oneself (of which there are three basic strategies, Types A, B, and C, as identified by Ainsworth, and many substrategies, as described by the DMM;
3 the *pattern of information processing* that underlies the strategies.

Attachment relationships function in each person's zone of proximal development (Vygotsky 1978) to promote the individual's successful adaptation to the threatening and advantageous conditions of the context. Thus, attachment behavior (e.g., crying, reaching, etc.) and attachment strategies (organized functionally) are children's contribution to their own welfare in that they increase the probability of parents being protective at a moment when the child feels threatened.

An expanding array of strategies

Information processing becomes more complex as children mature and, when they are exposed to complex dangers, children develop more complex strategies than do infants. The array of possible strategies (still grouped under the rubric of Types A, B, and C) is defined by the information processing necessary to organize the strategies (see Figures 2.1, 2.2, 3.1, 3.2, 4.1). These strategies result from exposure to danger. Indeed, progressive exposure to threat, in each individual's zone of proximal development, is seen as necessary to long-term adaptation. Although (a) the nature of the threat, (b) the signals used to elicit caregiving, and (c) the self-protective strategies that are organized change in sophistication across the life span, the basic functions of turning to another person to support self-protection, reproduction, and protection of progeny do not change.

Information about safety and sexuality

As the brain matures, it becomes able to transform information in more complex ways, particularly temporally ordered information (called 'cognition' in the DMM) and information derived from the intensity of the sensory stimulation (called 'affect'). These two sources of information are transformed to generate predictions regarding safety and comfort and dispositional representations of how one might act so as to promote safety, comfort and (after puberty) sexual opportunity. The asymmetry of already-sexual parents raising not-yet-sexual children is used to discuss maladaptive sexual behavior. The similarity of basic arousal to sexual arousal and the high overlap of attachment and sexual behavior are used to explain, in part, the behavior of adults who direct sexual behavior toward children.

Strengths versus deficits

Most theories of psychopathology focus on deficits: bad genes, developmental anomalies, and untoward events. The default position in the DMM is that children have the normal complement of human genes, but have had to apply immature psychological processes to threats which they were unable to manage without the benefit of appropriate support. As a consequence, they did the best they could, given their maturity and context. This resulted in misperceptions, misattributions, and misdirected responses that have been carried forward and elaborated as the children developed. Framed this way, humans are seen to be trying to make meaning and construct solutions to their problems. The ability to find solutions is framed as a strength (not a deficit), again given the children's initial situation. Of course, there are cases of genetic anomaly and of physical insult (e.g., anoxia at birth); when these exist, they are addressed as limitations. Because such limitations are relatively rare in the population (compared with behavioral and psychological dysfunction), they do not constitute the default assumption of the DMM.

Adaptation

Throughout the life span, adaptation, i.e., staying alive and reproducing, is emphasized over security, with adaptation in adulthood being defined by (a) access to, and recognition in others of, all the behavioral self-protective strategies and (b) the ability to implement each in the context in which it is most likely to be adaptive without skewing the mind about what one is doing, nor becoming stuck in the strategy when it is no longer adaptive to use it. Maladaptation is the reverse; it is applying a strategy that was developed because it was adaptive in one context to contexts in which it is not adaptive, and being relatively unable to change that. Adaptation is deemed more important than security because people cannot always control whether they live in safe contexts, but they can become 'balanced' with regard to information processing and selection of strategy, and this, more than steady use of a secure strategy, promotes safety, comfort, and reproduction. In adulthood, adaptation requires that formerly secure children (Type B) 'earn' their balanced strategy by coming to understand danger, whereas formerly anxious children (Types A and C) must earn their balanced strategy by coming to understand safety and comfort.

13

Self-correction, resilience, and maladaptive parenting

In most cases, the developmental process, as an interaction between genetic, epigenetic, and contextual factors (Rutter 2006a), functions self-correctively, promoting resilience in the face of threat. In some cases, repeated exposure to unprotected and uncomforted threats beyond the individual's zone of proximal development results in accumulated risk that leaves the individual with maladaptive strategies in most, or even all, contexts. This volume is focused on those cases of limited adaptation or maladaptation in which the individuals are parents.

These ideas, as they relate to parenting, are developed in the chapters that follow.

Changing professionals' response

The ideas in this book lead to some recommendations for change in how we deliver mental health services. Compared with what we do now, these ideas are nothing less than revolutionary. Indeed, when I suggest these things to groups of professionals, they uniformly say that this is impossible, that they can't possibly do that because it isn't in the structure of the services, isn't how agencies work together, goes beyond their expertise, takes too long, and costs too much.

Yet, are these ideas really so revolutionary, so very impossible?

Recently, I was taking my daily morning walk when a neighbor joined me. How was I? What was I doing now? We chatted and I said I had ideas that could revolutionize how treatment was delivered. He asked what they were. I listed four or five. He stopped. He looked at me, mouth hanging open. *'Are you serious? Any fool knows that.'*

Of course, anyone knows what I told him – but not professionals. The whole service system is set up in contradiction to these simple, potentially helpful ideas. Why? Well, that's another story. The question is whether we can change *ourselves* enough to change the way hurt parents raise their children (cf. Thomas-Peter 2006 with regard to violent and sexual offenders). If we want to reduce child abuse and neglect; forestall rising rates of childhood autism, attention-deficit (hyperactivity) disorder (ADHD), and other childhood disorders; reduce delinquency and violent crime; increase marital and family harmony; and prevent serious psychological disorder, we must do business differently.

This book is for professionals. We are the most flexible link in the chain. If we can change how we do business, we might be able to reduce the human suffering that comes from being unsafe and uncomforted.

Note

1   A number of cases are described in this book. Those that I have seen privately have names and identifying details made anonymous, thus retaining the universal aspects of the case and modifying or eliminating the case-specific aspects. Where quoted dialogue is used, its structure is retained even if factual details are changed to retain anonymity. Public cases are identified accurately and referenced. For both sorts of cases, a distinction is made between the data of the case, which are accurate, and the interpretation of the meaning of the data – which is my own. The cases themselves are drawn from ten countries and four continents.

Chapter 2

Early childhood: Learning to be safe at home

Humans have an exceptionally long childhood and delayed puberty because it takes that long for them to learn to protect themselves and prepare to protect their children. The focus of Chapters 2 and 3 is how, during the 15–20 years of childhood, children learn to be parents. Again, the emphasis is on universal processes that are accomplished with individual differences and the implications of these differences for parental competence.

Human babies (except those with genetic anomalies or physical insults during gestation and birth) are born with the potential to adapt to almost any familial conditions. The immediate issue for babies is to adapt to their specific mother and family. That is, early in life, infants in interaction with their parents transform their universal potential into a specialist's competence. This chapter is about how infants become specialists in surviving – and thriving – in their families. As always in this volume, the focus is on those children for whom survival is most threatened.

Protection, danger, and attachment figures

Staying alive

Daniel Stern proposed that the essential task of parents is to keep their children alive (Stern 1985). That is surely true, but with it comes the equally important task of enabling children to protect themselves. This involves learning to recognize danger and respond self-protectively to it (Rutter 2006b). Accomplishing this requires that parents let children experience danger, both guiding them through it and discussing the experience with them. Without appropriate exposure to threat and danger, children might grow up naively thinking that life is safe and other people will protect them. Thinking that way can be very dangerous!

This creates tension between protection from danger and exposure to danger. Both are needed, but professionals tend to focus more on protection (or its absence), whereas parents are forced to adapt to an expanding range of threats because physical maturation repeatedly increases children's exposure. To reconcile protection with exposure, one needs Vygotsky's notion of a 'zone of proximal development' (ZPD) (Vygotsky 1978). The ZPD refers to the set of competencies that are emerging for a given individual at a specific moment in time. It reflects the unique variation in what each individual, of any age, is ready to learn next. That, of course, is constantly changing as skills are acquired (such that former threats are no longer threatening), new threats become salient, and maturation makes new competencies possible. Because maturation and learning constantly change children, parents' protective role also changes. That is, being a parent is no more static than is being a child. Both are processes of continuing adaptation and change (Sameroff and Chandler 1975; Sameroff 1983).

Parents function as attachment figures in children's ZPD. That is, the attachment function of parents is to protect and comfort children when children cannot do so themselves, to guide children to protect and comfort themselves as they become ready to learn new skills, and to let children take complete responsibility for themselves when they can do so competently. Put another way, the attachment function of parenting is always in dynamic interaction with children's development. Of all the roles that parents take (i.e., playmate, teacher, etc.), attachment is the one that is crucial to children's survival and, across generations, to the survival of our species. For this reason, attachment is central in cases of threat to children's adaptation or survival.

When attachment figures misjudge children's competencies and needs, they hamper children's development. This can be in the forms of offering children unnecessary assistance or failing to provide help that is needed – or both. For example, some parents are overly attentive and helpful, imagining threat to their children at every turn. They intrude by giving unneeded advice, assisting unnecessarily, doing the task themselves, or keeping their child out of potentially challenging situations. They take no chances – and their children fail to learn to adapt and also either begin to doubt themselves or become angry with their constricting parents. Other parents fail to foresee dangers, leaving their children to face threats that they are unprepared to manage. Others assign children responsibilities beyond their competencies, such as caring for younger siblings or, even worse, caring for a parent. Finally, some parents gauge their children's self-protective skills accurately, but fail to address their children's need for comfort. These children are safe, but uncomfortable. Failing to protect and comfort children appropriately almost always makes it harder for them to learn to predict, identify, and respond appropriately to threat.

A particular issue in infancy is learning to regulate arousal and attention, i.e., learning to regulate the body as well as the mind. Learning occurs throughout the body, some peripheral learning (both input sensation and output somatic functions) not being mediated by processes in the central nervous system; that is, not all peripheral processing reaches the brain. Peripheral learning is implicit and leads to change in several bodily systems,

17

some of which, such as the immune system, use the same transmitters as the central nervous system. Implicit peripheral learning can be conditioned by feedback (as described by learning theory) from the environment in a transactional process that affects development by adapting individuals to perceive and respond to their unique developmental context.

In most cases, the developmental context is normative; that is, it promotes survival. Such contexts support development well enough that we notice few if any differences in somatic functioning among individuals and, therefore, these distal and implicit processes pass unnoticed (they do not come to our awareness). It is when the context is sufficiently atypical to threaten survival that peripheral adaptations may become apparent. When the adaptations are very great, we may see the effects either in somatic functioning or in more centralized learning, or both. Often the somatic effects are visible in the unwell appearance of distressed individuals.

Development in infancy may be particularly vulnerable to extreme variations in contextual input both because early organization is taking place and because a greater proportion of the total organization is peripheral and none of it is conscious (cf. Godfrey 2006). This may help to account for the severe and not fully reversible effects of institutionalization (Rutter 2006d), the failure to grow of some children in extremely stressed families (e.g., nonorganic failure to thrive, Crittenden 1987), or possibly even asthma, conditions indicating poor sensory integration, and the aversion to touch of some infants.

The need for a comprehensive theory

There are many theories about how children develop, but none is focused precisely on the central issue of staying safe and becoming able to raise one's own children safely. In this chapter and the next, I outline a comprehensive theory of attachment and adaptation that combines and integrates aspects of other major theories around empirical information regarding the developmental process of staying safe and preparing to raise one's children.[1]

It is important to note that theory always runs ahead of empirical data. Theory tries to paint the full picture where data establish small points of empirical certainty. Like a connect-the-dots drawing, theory connects the data points to reveal a picture. How does the theorist know what's in the blank space? In the case of the dynamic-maturational model (DMM) (Crittenden 1995, 2000b, 2006), clinical case experience, one person and one family at a time, suggests how the whole might look. Empirical data, clinical cases, and reflective integration are the ingredients that make theory.

This makes theory a bit bold and prone to error. On the other hand, the picture suggests which crucial points of data are needed, thus guiding empirical research in potentially useful directions. When the new data arrive, theory drops the data point into the picture – and reconnects the dots. The picture always changes in a dynamic interaction of ideas, clinical case experience, and empirical data.

The DMM applies Bowlby's *process* of combining theories to his *idea* of organization around protection from danger (Bowlby 1969/83). Although attachment theory retains and adapts psychoanalytic theory's concepts of 'defense mechanisms' (that is, psychological processes for transforming and distorting information) and 'inner psychic processes' (including implicit processes of which we are unaware) to organize behavior, it changes Freud's excessive emphasis on drives and sexuality.

Sexuality seems so conspicuously absent from attachment theory that one might quip that, to Bowlby, mothers were sexless protectors (but how did they ever become mothers!) whereas, to Freud, babies responded with sexual feelings and drives (even before puberty created the capacity for sexual responses!). This comparison highlights the problem of thinking about sex and children at one time. The two seem so incompatible that adults are almost forced to distort the situation (by desexualizing mothers or sexualizing children) to make reality palatable. The truth, however, is that mothers and fathers are sexual and sexually responsive, whereas infants and young children can elicit sexual feelings in adults, but they themselves are not yet sexual. To reflect the developmental process accurately, theory must address the asymmetries in self-protective competence and sexual response.

The DMM is based in both biology and behavior. Biology creates the need for behavior to accomplish the physical functions of survival and reproduction. The means are centered in the brain because the brain connects the self (both physically and psychologically) to its context. The connection occurs neurologically, neurons receiving information in the form of sensory stimulation, processing it psychologically, and then using the output to organize behavior. This chapter is about that process. The chapter is crucial to anyone who wishes to change another person's behavior because what must be changed is the information processing that culminates in behavior.

Two types of information are crucial to protection and reproduction: the sequential order in which the stimulation is perceived and the intensity of the stimulation. The *sequence* of neuronal activation is processed through the cerebellum and leads to information about temporal contingencies. This information is used to organize sensorimotor responses. This is learning theory, and it produces *cognitive* information to regulate behavior (Ornstein and Thompson 1984; Thompson 1991). The *intensity* of neuronal activation is processed through the limbic structures and, when intensity exceeds a genetically defined threshold, it leads to activation of the autonomic nervous system, i.e., bodily changes in heart rate, breathing, circulation, sweating, etc. (LeDoux 1994, 1995; MacLean 1990). These prepare the body to fight, flee, or freeze (Schore 1994; Selye 1976). Because these effects are felt somatically, this form of transformed information is tied to feelings and is labeled *affect*.

To summarize, the DMM proposes two essential functions of parenting: protection and reproduction. That is, not only must parents themselves stay safe and reproduce, but they also must protect their children (at least until they reach reproductive maturity), help them to learn to protect themselves, and prepare them to select safe reproductive partners. They accomplish these by using cognitive and affective information to identify threat and to organize self-protective and child-protective strategies. The nature of these strategies is described next.

Developmental pathways

Children mature continuously, but unevenly. The unevenness is created by periods of rapid neurological change, together with major changes in the contexts in which children live. When development progresses well, the new possibilities of maturation are applied to the new demands of daily life such that, with attachment figures' support in the ever-changing ZPD, new competencies are learned. This prepares the child for the next period of change.

On the other hand, if the competencies are not attained on schedule, the parent must adapt to the child's actual ZPD. When this does not happen because parents are limited or because the demands of the context are excessive, children must fend for themselves. However, having an incomplete understanding of the situation, they are forced to take shortcuts. The shortcuts usually (a) take the most salient information and exaggerate it to make it appear more predictable than it really is and (b) omit from further processing the least clear information. For example, when the parents' behavior is difficult to predict, children may rely almost exclusively on displaying their feelings in ways that demand attention. Alternatively, when showing negative feelings results in being rebuked or ignored, children may inhibit display of their feelings, and rely almost exclusively on the predictable effect of being pleasant. When these sorts of reductionistic shortcuts are taken, children's developmental pathways diverge from those of more fortunate children.

The result is individual differences in the effects of the universal processes of transforming stimulation into cognitive and affective information on development. Using attachment terminology, these are labeled:

1 Type B: balanced use of both cognition and affect;
2 Type A: shortcuts that rely on exaggerated cognitive predictability and ignore (inhibit) negative affect;
3 Type C: shortcuts that rely on exaggerated negative affect and ignore cognitive unpredictability.

Infancy (birth to 1–2 years)

Strategies
Infants need to learn to regulate their own arousal so as to spend less time sleeping (low arousal) or crying (high arousal) and more time alert and

attentive (moderate arousal). This is accomplished partly through parents' predictable responses (cognition) to infants' distress signals (affect) (Yerkes and Dodson 1908). When parents' response is quick, predictable, and comforting, infants learn to make meaning of both the comforting actions of their parents and the sequence of events that leads to feeling comfortable again; that is, crying leads to parents' coming, which leads to feeling good. Such infants become aroused, they signal, and then their arousal drops in anticipation of the response.

All babies feel distressed when their parents fail to respond predictably or comfortingly. The distress is experienced as desire for comfort, anger, and fear. These normal negative feelings, however, motivate incompatible behavior. Desire for comfort motivates approach with signals of affection, i.e., attachment behavior. Anger motivates approach with aggression. And fear motivates escape behavior. Infants differ, however, in how they manage these feelings.

Parents who predictably

1 fail to respond to infants' distress (e.g., lack of response);
2 respond with anger or irritation (punitive response);
3 respond with false-positive cheerfulness, i.e., laughing at the crying baby (incongruent response)

tend to have babies who organize by a Type A strategy of hiding their negative feelings. They inhibit the display of negative affect (specifically, A1–2; see Figure 2.1).

On the other hand, parents who respond unpredictably, but are comforting at least some of the time, tend to have babies who cry more and display more somatic distress (C1–2; see Figure 2.1). These babies feel and display mixed negative feelings of desire for comfort, anger, and fear. This mixed display confuses their parents who become less sure about how to comfort their baby.

Both adaptations (inhibition and exaggeration of negative affect) mislead parents about their infant's actual state (see Figure 2.1).

The anxious patterns of attachment (i.e., Types A and C) are often thought of as undesirable, and interventions have been developed to promote secure (Type B) attachment. I think that misses the point. Anxious attachment is the infant's strategy for eliciting needed caregiving from the parent and for reducing possible rejection or harm. Anxious attachment is *good*; it is the child's contribution to his or her own survival.

Anxious attachment is not the problem; danger is the problem, and that is what we, as professionals, should focus on. Change the danger, not the child. Create an environment in which infants and children do not need to feel anxious and do not need the A and C strategies, and attachment will take care of itself. How do we do this? Through parents. Parents should comfort and protect their children from external danger and should not be

A Dynamic-Maturational Model of Patterns
of Attachment in Infancy

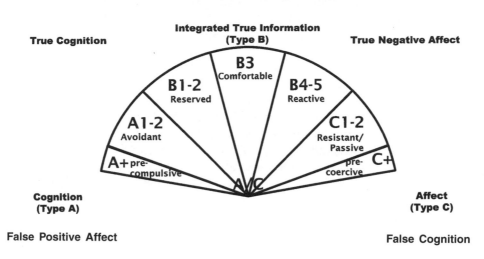

Copyright: Patricia M. Crittenden, 2001

Figure 2.1 The infant patterns of attachment

themselves the source of the danger. If parents are insufficiently protective, this book addresses their needs.

Affect and cognition

One might think that moderate arousal is best and that humans should seek to maintain a moderate homeostasis. A more complex perspective, based on the notion that changes in arousal are necessary and protective, is presented here. High arousal is adaptive when there is threat because it heightens perception (for identifying potential danger); prepares the body to fight, flee, or freeze; and signals to others that one needs help. It even improves resistance to infection and promotes healing, so long as it does not last too long. Low arousal is adaptive when there is little or no threat. It reverses the effects of high arousal, enabling the body to relax and restore its resources. Moderate arousal promotes attention and learning.

If one considers the opposite process, the importance of change in arousal becomes immediately apparent. What would happen if, in the face of danger, one's arousal dropped and one became sleepy? What if there were no evidence of danger and yet arousal remained high? This, of course, is an 'anxiety disorder'. It rarely kills, but it surely is uncomfortable. Finally, a steady state of moderate arousal, even under safe conditions, could feel as though one was out of synchrony with one's context; this might be why psychotropic medication is often resisted and discontinued as soon as patients feel better.

The points are that changes in arousal serve a self-protective function and this function is realized in interaction with the context. The desirable condition of arousal, therefore, is flexibility tied to variation in the context.

The basis for knowing whether high arousal is warranted or not is not in the aroused feeling itself. The needed information lies in previously experienced outcomes, in the cognitive contingencies associated in the past with conditions like the present ones. Because cognition and affect are processed differently in the brain, cognition and affect provide different predictions from the same stimulation. When used together and *integrated*, they provide the best representation of the meaning of the current context for the self and, therefore, the best basis for organizing one's response.

Infants are able to use only very simple forms of affect and cognition and to generate correspondingly limited behavioral responses. This leaves them very dependent upon their parents to perceive what they cannot, to derive meanings that they cannot, and to organize protective responses that they cannot. Nevertheless, by about 1 year of age, infants have the full repertoire of attachment behaviors (see Table 2.2, column 1) and organize these in three basic attachment strategies (see Figure 2.1; Ainsworth 1979). This and the following chapters follows the development of self-protective behavior, i.e., attachment strategies, from their simple organization in infancy to the complexity of adulthood that is needed for successful child-rearing.

Opportunity for adaptation

First-time parents know very little about raising babies and, as the slogan points out, babies don't come with directions. But they do come with innate signal systems. They signal how they feel and their signals change when their feelings change; moreover, the fit between signals and arousal (internal state) improves when infants experience sensitive responses. When parents perceive the effect of their responses, they learn what works with their baby – and their baby refines the signals. Parent and infant begin a dynamic process of communication and adjustment around the infant's safety and comfort. Of course, not all parents are able to perceive with equal clarity, or to respond in equally protective and comforting ways. Understanding these less adept parents is what this book is about.

At the same time, however, infants differ in (a) how sensitive they are to changes in parental behavior and their own internal state and (b) how robust their responses are when they do perceive change. These characteristics are 'temperament', and, although all humans have these characteristics, we vary genetically in their display. When a sensitive parent has a baby who is moderate on both temperament characteristics, dynamic communication and adaptation between parent and infant easily become attuned. Affect and cognition work to keep the dyad in harmony and the baby safe and comfortable. Not surprisingly, when babies are happy, parents feel good about themselves and about their babies. Without regard to the extent of parent or infant contribution to this outcome, the result is secure and balanced Type B attachment.

After Nancy (the girl who threw her homework away) got into treatment, her therapist wondered how things had started out. Discussions with her parents produced only the information that everything was fine until Nancy went to school. A look at the family's photographs seemed to support that notion. Nancy was a clear-eyed, bright, and happy child whose body seemed relaxed and whose range of activities seemed quite normal. Her parents were possibly a bit unsure of themselves and quiet, but, really, nothing stood out. Nancy seemed to have managed infancy and early childhood in her family just fine.

Nevertheless, as we will see in the next chapter, problems lay ahead. Looking back, the questions to ask are how her parents handled her negative affect. Were they more comfortable with her tears and fears than with her anger? Did she learn to avoid direct refusals and instead display uncertainty, incompetence, or fearfulness – all as a way to avoid confrontation without complying either? Were both she and her parents unaware of her anger? If so, this will bode poorly for both the regimentation of school and also peer relationships.

Problems

Problems develop when either the parent perceives and responds in insensitive ways or the infant signals and responds in incomprehensible ways. The result is a mismatch characterized by dyssynchrony and experienced as distress. Regardless of the contributors to this condition, parents who cannot establish a harmonious relationship that enables their infant to be safe and feel comfortable initiate a developmental pathway that obscures the situation. To cope with insufficient safety, infants usually organize a Type A strategy that inhibits the display of negative affect. To cope with feeling anxious about parent unpredictability, infants usually organize a Type C strategy that exaggerates negative affect. Both distort communication to achieve the immediate (short-term) goal of being safer or feeling more comfortable. Ironically, the short-term adaptation creates a long-term risk of reliance on distortions of cognition and arousal/affect to regulate relationships. In other words, short-term adaptations, especially those made early in life, can backfire at later ages. Maturation, however, provides potential turning points.

Risk

The riskiest period is around birth when the parent either finds a satisfying synchrony with the infant or fails to, after which the infant's attempts to accommodate the parent may mislead the parent about the infant's actual state. That is, infants who adopt a Type A response may mislead their parents into thinking they are OK – when they are actually uncomfortable. Infants who adopt a Type C strategy may mislead their parent into thinking they are either very distressed or exaggerating distress in order to control the parent – when, in fact, they are somewhat distressed. These misperceptions affect parental behavior which, in turn, may force the baby to accommodate further, thus, keeping the dyad out of balance.

The riskiest conditions are when parents are so unresponsive (i.e., unaroused and inattentive) that they fail to protect the infant (neglect) or so angrily aroused and excessively attentive to detail that they attack the infant (abuse) – or both. The reasons for such behavior are myriad and form the basis for Part 2 of this book.

Preschool years (approximately 2–5 years of age)

The preoperational shift and coy behavior

Beginning at about 18 months of age, infants' brains begin to mature more rapidly such that, by about 2 years of age, toddlers are able to walk, run, climb, talk meaningfully with other people, and use new displays of affect, specifically coy behavior (Hinde 1982) and false-positive affect. Coy behavior is a powerful set of co-occurring signals that terminate others' aggression and elicit their nurturance. Coy signals establish a dominance hierarchy in which the aggressive person is dominant and the coy person is submissive. Coy signals are the opposite of aggressive signals (see Table 2.1).

All people face conflict at one time or another and everyone loses sometimes. A way to end the conflict without getting hurt is needed. Communication and negotiation can accomplish this, but in early childhood, verbal skills are very limited. Children need a way to disarm parental aggression, especially when they first gain the ability to act independently of their parents. Toddlerhood is when children need effective, nonverbal ways of managing parent–child conflict.

Some coy behaviors function to terminate the other individual's aggression; these include displaying the neck and belly, both of which are so vulnerable that, if attacked there, the wounds could lead to death. Displaying the neck and belly, i.e., making oneself vulnerable to destruction, clarifies a dominance hierarchy. A third part of the body functions similarly. The genitalia are very sensitive; attack on the genitals would be exceedingly painful and could destroy one's reproductive potential. In extreme cases, display of the unprotected genitals can signal the end of the dispute through submission. In other primates, rear-facing exposure of the anus and genitals, i.e., pseudocopulation, signals self-protective submission (de Waal 2000; Feldman 1994; Hinde 1982; Issa and Edwards 2006).

Other coy behaviors elicit nurturance; this is essential when the victor (in this case a parent) is crucial for the survival of the submissive individual (in this case a toddler). Signals like a partially open mouth, a pigeon-toed stance, and a broken ankle stance all attract parental nurturance by making the child appear weak, handicapped, or hurt. Victims claim the right of the vanquished to be protected by the victor. Displays of the genitals can function this way as well.

That might seem far removed from childhood, and in most cases it is. But cases of extreme failure to perceive danger can elicit genital signaling even in preschool-aged children.

Table 2.1 Coy and aggressive signals

Coy signals	Aggressive signals
Unprotected display of the neck, belly, and genitals	Protected neck, belly, and genitals
Stance with belly protruding	Stance with weight solid over legs
Lifting of clothing as if to reveal belly, e.g., lifting skirt in a curtsey	Top pulled down, covering belly
Half-smile with teeth covered	Lips drawn back with teeth bared
Sideways 'coy' glance out the side of the eyes	Hard, direct, and threatening stares
Chin down and to the side	Chin thrust forward aggressively
Head cocked sideways or bowed down	Head upright, straight, and strong
Hands up and open (no-weapons position) or in praying position	Hands fisted in raised, threatening-to-hit position
Toes and knees together (knock-kneed and pigeon-toed)	Legs in straight, stiff position and ready to kick

For example, a depressed mother, using a Type A strategy of inhibiting negative affect, might watch her children, but fail to respond to their needs for protection. In a videotaped sequence, one expressionless mother sat very still at one end of the family sofa. Her two-year-old began jumping toward her across the length of the sofa. Even when Jenny signaled that she would leap and raised the hem of her dress in a fragment of the disarming belly-display gesture, her mother made no anticipatory gestures, neither forbidding the jumping, nor preparing to catch Jenny. Instead, she sat stiffly immobile. Jenny jumped! Her mother barely took hold of her and showed no affect. Jenny rolled over, briefly displaying her underpants. Then she scrambled up on the armrest to jump again, lifted her skirt further, shouted ... and her mother did nothing. Jenny jumped, then crawled back to the armrest displaying her rear.

What was this? Just a child's lack of modesty? Or something more?

Jenny's brother rushed in, stood on the armrest and prepared a huge jump that threatened to crush both his mother and Jenny – who had scrambled into her mother's lap. As he jumped, every audience to whom I have shown the interaction gasps audibly. Jenny's mother does not respond at all; she neither forbids the dangerous jump, nor prepares to protect her daughter. No one is hurt – but this is only because the boy is skilled and careful. He then leaps back onto the armrest. From there he takes a huge leap off the sofa. Audiences gasp; the mother is immobile and silent. Jenny returns to her spot and jumps several more times, raising the hem of her skirt, shouting more loudly each time, and increasing the exposure of her bottom, in both prostrate and supine positions. In the final jump, she first shows her rear pointedly to her mother, then flips over, lifting her legs high and waving them to her mother. Who remains impassive and immobile.

What do these apparently sexualized signals mean? Both children act out their need for protection by taking risks. Their mother fails to respond and protect. Jenny, I think, uses a very strong signal of submission to assert her right to be the protected one, to get so low hierarchically, relative to her mother, that her mother must assume a dominant and protective role. Such signals can be seen in many mammals and all the great apes (Hinde 1982). This apparently sexual signal is not about sex (and Jenny has had no form of sexual contact). It is the use of a submissive signal to elicit protection.

Ironically, coy signals are a subtle form of control, one that allows victors to feel unchallenged and in control while in fact their behavior is regulated by the victim. This subtle shift in power is inherently deceptive. Coy behavior hides aggressive intent and, when victims act aggressively, it is usually through deception, the weapon of choice among those who feel weak.

It is crucial to recognize that deception is inherent in coy behavior. When one loses a conflict, one submits, but the anger that fueled the fight both disappears from view and increases in resentful intensity. The anger is no longer visible, but it remains out of sight where it cannot easily be resolved. Similarly, nurturance-eliciting signals are misleading: one does have teeth behind the half-smile, one isn't crippled or hurt, etc. Even the hands-up, no-weapons signal is false. The weapons are not rocks, bats, or guns; instead deception itself becomes the weapon. The attack can come in an unexpected moment and in an unexpected way that leaves the dominant member of the struggle (the parent in this case) feeling helpless and hurt. Thus, preschool children use signals that mislead observers regarding what they will do; this is *false cognition*.

It should be clarified, however, that preschool-aged children are not capable of intentional deception. Their behavior has strong innate characteristics, is used by all children, is adaptive for everyone some of the time, and is carried out without conscious awareness. The children merely use a behavior that functions to meet their immediate needs, given their parents' behavior.

The preoperational shift and the splitting of incompatible affects
The second change in affect that occurs during the preoperational shift is the ability to inhibit display of a truly felt feeling while displaying an

incompatible feeling. Both the Type A and Type C strategies employ this new potential. In Type A, where negative affects have not been displayed, preschool-aged children are now able to display *false positive affect*. This enables them to avoid punishment or rejection (by inhibition of negative affect) and also elicit caregiving or approval (for displaying positive affect, albeit false positive affect). It is misleading, but the deception improves children's relationships with their attachment figures. This same skill is employed in the Type C coercive strategy when children inhibit some of their negative feelings while exaggerating the display of incompatible feelings – and then alternate the displays. This is described more fully below.

Strategies

With coy behavior and the ability to split the display of affect that one feels while displaying a different affect, more sophisticated strategies can be organized. These enable children to fit the characteristics of their families more precisely than did the infant strategies. The most important of the new strategies is the Type C coercive strategy. The coercive strategy works best with unpredictable parents, that is, with the majority of human parents who are more or less unpredictable. The strategy involves splitting the display of mixed negative feelings such that one feeling is visible and exaggerated to make it seem absolute while display of incompatible feelings is inhibited.

For example, anger is displayed strongly while fear and desire for comfort (which are felt) are not displayed (the display is inhibited.) The display of anger attracts the parent's attention. The parent responds by either fighting or placating. If the parent placates, the child discards all peace offerings, changing the demand continually and thus retaining the unpredictable parent's attention. Eventually, however, the parent almost certainly will become frustrated and angry. When the parent responds to the child's angry display with greater anger and threats, such that the child judges that he or she will lose the battle and might be punished, the child changes the display, hiding the anger and displaying fear and desire for comfort. The parent feels ashamed of frightening the child. She offers comfort. The child acts infantile; he can't do anything, help, help! For as long as the parent comforts and placates, the child will act weak and submissive – claiming the right of the vanquished to be protected by the victor. At some point, however, the parent will see the deception and demand angrily, 'Stop it.' 'Cut it out!' And the battle is on. The child flashes a bit of anger, the parent reconsiders … off they go in an interminable struggle that effectively changes the probabilities of the parent's behavior without resolving the problems of the child's safety and comfort. Indeed, the strategy is based upon using heightened display of anxiety to elicit attention. If the children permitted themselves to be satisfied, their arousal would lower, their parent would attend to other things, and the state of not knowing whether or when the parent would become available to protect the child would be reinstated.

Nick, from Chapter 1, is an example of a coercive child. A serious concern is that he will discover how to pit his parents' two different approaches against one another, thus causing dissension within their marriage. If that occurs, the contingencies will become more complex (so Nick may need to heighten his attempts to get contingency even more), and his parents' unhappiness may sap some of their parenting attention away from him, redirecting it to themselves and their need to feel better both individually and as a couple. Although neither of his parents is extreme, Nick's behavior and their lack of unity could create escalating problems for everyone. Either the mother's tenderness or the father's firmness could function adequately, but the struggle between the parents cannot work for anyone, least of all Nick. An important point is that, as Nick's behavior escalates and each parent's approach fails, his parents may begin to feel bad about themselves. Parents who feel that their best efforts are insufficient and that their child doesn't love and respect them become less able to be competent parents. Instead, they may withdraw from a painful relationship or flounder, trying out different responses, thus increasing their unpredictability. A plan that they shared and implemented consistently could easily turn this situation around (cf. Rolls 2007).

The structure of the coercive strategy allows us to cluster children using the Type C strategy into four groups: angry, but not overwhelmingly so (C1), disarming, but not overwhelmingly so (C2), angry beyond reason and hardly able to shift to disarming behavior when necessary (C3), and so disarming that the child feigns helplessness and almost lacks the potential to display anger when it is needed (C4) (see Figure 2.2).

Finally, the A1 and A2 strategies of infancy remain, but when they do not function to reduce the threat of attack or abandonment, the child may organize a compulsive Type A strategy. Compulsive caregiving (A3) uses inhibition of negative affect together with false positive affect and entertaining or caregiving behavior to draw parents who are too distant, depressed, or preoccupied closer – where they might perceive threats to their child and respond with protection or comfort. Compulsive attention (A3–; the minus sign (–) signifies less than the full A3 strategy) is a milder form of compulsive caregiving in which inordinate approving attention is needed by the parent from the child, but not caregiving. Compulsive compliance (A4) and compulsive performance (A4–) use inhibition of negative affect together with false compliant or performing behavior to elicit approval and attention from otherwise threatening, demanding, and punitive parents (see Figure 2.2).

New opportunities for adaptation
Newly maturing skills create the possibility of change in the parent–child relationship. Some children using a Type A strategy find that coy behavior (that is not alternated with aggression) reduces the threat from their parents by clarifying that the child accepts parental authority. In other cases, coy behavior elicits needed caregiving from parents. When parents respond to children's coy signals with more appropriate behavior, the dyad may settle into a mildly stressed relationship that nevertheless increases the child's

A Dynamic-Maturational Model of Patterns of Attachment in the Preschool Years

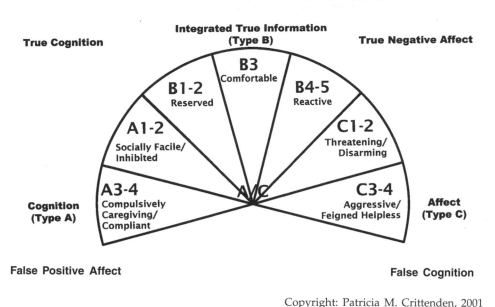

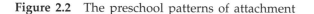

Copyright: Patricia M. Crittenden, 2001

Figure 2.2 The preschool patterns of attachment

safety. When the Type A strategies function well, generating more positive attention and less threat from the parent, they stabilize the dyad, leading to a mildly anxious, fairly structured relationship that keeps the child safe and defines ways of obtaining approval and attention. Moreover, the beginning of productive verbal communication may enable explicit statement of parental rules and child needs, thus opening the way to a secure relationship, albeit one marked by emotional reserve.

In Type C dyads, mild use of coercion by the child may be just enough to engage the parent more fully. This, too, can stabilize the dyad. Reorganization toward Type B may occur when the toddler's coy and threatening signals clarify to the parent how the child feels, permitting the parent to make better predictions about what will protect and comfort the child. When language use increases, as it will by about 2½ years of age, some of the acted-out struggle may be managed verbally, permitting the dyad to form a predictable and comforting relationship.

The point is that maturation creates opportunities for change. The change may be toward security and balance, stabilization in a non-B pattern, or greater distortion (Rutter 2004). Greater distortion is the focus of this volume, but it should not be forgotten that maturation simply creates an innately occurring dynamic moment in development, one that can move forward without change or result in change toward either balance or greater distortion. In all cases, the outcome will reflect the strategy that keeps the child as safe and comfortable as possible, given the context and parents' behavior.

Problems

Problems develop when parents of children using the compulsive Type A strategies (compulsive attention, caregiving, compliance, and performance) fail to respond to the strategy and continue to be unavailable or threatening. Such children may become depressed or very anxious – or both. They may become at risk of somatic disorders, disorders of arousal, and, possibly, unexpected breaks of their strategy in which the inhibited affects are displayed strongly, intrusively, and without interpersonal regulation.

Among children using a Type C strategy, the greatest risks are that the parent will actively deceive the child or, more confusingly, try to protect the child from negative aspects of the parent's life that affect the parent and motivate the behavior with the child. For example, a mother who is upset about a dispute with her husband may try to hide both her distress and the dispute from her child. Nevertheless, she is likely to be less sensitive to her child, and the child won't be able to understand why. In both cases, young children will find it extremely difficult to understand what causes what in their relationships. This will raise their anxiety greatly and make them angry. Lacking a clear focus for their anger, they may heighten their attempts to wrest contingency from their parents. Extreme behavior, including various forms of risk-taking (both active and passive), become possible.

Risk

The riskiest period is around 18 months when the new skills are coming into place. This includes locomotion. Toddlers can run into danger without being able to anticipate it. This forces parents to take an often-resented dominant position to protect toddlers by establishing safety rules. This is the point at which a change in developmental pathway is most likely, with newly acquired competencies clarifying the dyadic communication or obscuring it further. If it is obscured further, the direction can be either toward compulsive Type A strategies or obsessive Type C strategies. Of course, in many cases, the pathway from infancy is unchanged and simply carried forward into the preschool years in a more sophisticated form that incorporates the child's new skills.

The riskiest conditions occur when even the new strategies (A3–4, C3–4) fail to protect children or when they elicit inappropriate responses in adults. For example, when caring for a depressed mother doesn't draw her psychologically closer to her child, the risk is greater than when the strategy functions to make the mother more aware and available. Similarly, when rigid obedience to a demanding father doesn't elicit approval, the risk of both physical abuse of the child and psychological disorder in the child is increased.

On the other side of the model (i.e., Type C), some parents are both unpredictable and unable to tolerate challenges to their authority. When parents respond with excessive aggression themselves, children may be physically abused. Rates of both child abuse and accidental injury are exceptionally high for preschool-aged children. The highest rate of child abuse is from birth to 3 years of age. More than 80 per cent of all children who die as a result of abuse are less than 4 years old; 79 per cent of all abuse is committed by parents (US DHHS 2006a). The rate of accidental injuries goes up by about 24 per cent from infancy to preschool age (Freid *et al.* 1998).

> Luke, the toddler from Chapter 1 who had an unexplained broken arm, was placed in a foster home. According to a later psychiatric report, he suffered from post-traumatic stress disorder (PTSD) tied to his father; he became upset, couldn't sleep, cried, wet the bed, and acted fearful before and after contact. In fact, the services had come to focus on the father as the probable abuser. This, however, only made things worse because he was hesitant to talk and distant. He admitted nothing, with both parents saying that for the two days after the injury and before going to the hospital, they were unaware of any injury.
>
> The professionals were uniform in their concern that a man who did not admit to abusing his child could not be trusted to care for his child. At 3 years of age, Luke was being considered for adoption by his foster family. His parents opposed this, asking for an outside evaluation, particularly of Luke's attachment to his father.
>
> The outcome was startling. First, all four parental adults were given Adult Attachment Interviews (AAIs). In addition, Luke participated in a 'Strange Situation' (the 'gold standard' assessment of attachment) (Ainsworth *et al.* 1978) with both his father and, a month later at a different location, his foster mother. The results were striking. With his father, Luke was comfortable and attached in a relationship that looked secure, albeit not very intense. With his foster mother, Luke was actively angry and rejecting, even though his foster mother almost begged Luke to stay close to her. During the separations from his father, Luke had remained calm and, when alone, had gone to the door, and then welcomed him with a smile and climbed onto his knee briefly. With his foster mother, Luke had ignored repeated goodbyes, played happily while alone, and refused to acknowledge his mother's returns. His foster mother had found it very difficult to leave and had cried outside the playroom during the second departure.
>
> On the AAI, Luke's father was found to be reorganizing his strategy from a probable compulsively self-reliant strategy (A6; see Chapter 3) to a simple A1. More informative were the traumas he had experienced as a child. He had been both abused harshly and repeatedly and also neglected. In mid-adolescence, he had left home and had lived alone without any close relationships, traveling from place to place for his work. During the AAI, he spoke thoughtfully and with feeling about his painful childhood and his father's demands that he perform perfectly

and the sudden and extreme punishment when he broke a rule. Luke's foster mother, on the other hand, was assigned to a compulsive caregiving (A3) strategy. She cried throughout her interview. Her own mother had been blind and had needed care from her. Eventually, the foster mother had had to drop out of high school to care for her mother, who then died when the foster mother was about 20.

The outcome of the full set of attachment assessments was the hypothesis that Luke's father had broken his arm as he pedalled his tricycle down the driveway toward the street, ignoring his shouts of 'Stop!' He had probably grabbed the boy, both out of fear that he would be hit by an oncoming car and in a flashback of fear of disobeying his father. His AAI suggested that he was becoming aware of the impact of his childhood abuse and would be able to regulate himself better in the future. In addition, however, Luke's 'PTSD' symptoms appeared to be an artifact of his foster mother's fear of losing Luke to his biological parents. Two processes appeared to be at work. First, the foster mother was so vigilant to threat that she misattributed threatening meaning to Luke's behavior. Second, when his foster mother acted fearful, Luke's behavior deteriorated.

The court returned Luke to his parents and five siblings, all of whom were doing well and none of whom had been maltreated. Psychological treatment was recommended for the foster mother, whose effort had brought her unexpected suffering, but the state accepted no responsibility for her psychological welfare.

The important points from this history are that:

1 Childhood experience affected both the father's and foster mother's parental behavior in ways that affected Luke.

2 The father's silence was not a crafty attempt to avoid discovery, but rather part of his Type A strategy of keeping to himself, combined with dismissal from recall of his own abuse.

3 The diagnosis of PTSD was made on the basis of reports from the foster mother, who, like most of us, was unable to see how she had created these effects herself.

4 Luke's attachment strategy was different with his father and his foster mother, thus, showing clearly that attachment is a *dyadic* feature, not a personal characteristic.

5 This sort of injury was tied to Luke's developmental state in toddlerhood and unlikely to be a continuing risk once Luke could predict dangerous outcomes and use language effectively.

Finally, it might be worth pointing out that Luke's father tried to reverse his parents' too intrusive strategy by being more distant whereas his foster mother sought to complete her interrupted caregiving of her mother by adopting Luke. In both cases, a past adaptation was being applied maladaptively in adulthood.

Other parents fail to protect children who use the disarming side of the coercive strategy; the risks for C4 children include failure to develop self-protective skills, eliciting bullying, isolation from family and peers, and eliciting sexual abuse (from either family or nonfamily). The last of these can occur when children signal desire for comfort and contact too strongly and widely.

The riskiest condition of all is having parents who combine two or more of the risky conditions (Crittenden *et al.* 1991).

> David, the child in Chapter 1 who witnessed repeated spousal violence, had parents who combined risk conditions. His father displayed the angry side of the Type C strategy and did so with dangerous aggression against David's primary attachment figure, his mother. His mother displayed a submissive devotion to her violent husband and gave that relationship priority over protection of her son. David's efforts to protect her (a caregiving strategy) elicited both psychological abuse (taunting and mocking) and occasionally physical threats from his father. Moreover, his mother was unappreciative such that his caregiving did not make her more protective or comforting of him.

It is easy to see that these parents were not competent, and it is easy to judge them. However, as a colleague of mine said, as soon as he reads the AAIs of parents whom he finds obstructive of their child's treatment, he suddenly finds compassion for them (an absolute essential to working effectively with anyone) and also that their behavior has a basis in their experience (S. Wilkinson, personal communication, 22 April 2006.) Unlocking parents' childhood history, with a focus on their needs as individuals as opposed to seeing them as tools for their child's treatment, can clear the way for parents to orchestrate their own process of change. This, in turn, frees their child to change.

Unfortunately, David, as in most cases of domestic violence, did not cause enough trouble to bring him to professional attention. Because there was no treatment for him and his family in early childhood, the issue becomes how he will manage at older ages and how the accumulation of these yet-to-be-had experiences will affect him when he becomes a father.

There are conditions, however, where these strategies are not sufficiently protective. Most involve problems that will not become apparent until the school years or adolescence, leaving us to fill in the gaps from what we learn later. An incident that Jackson (from Chapter 1) related when he was 16 gives a sense of his early experience.

Jackson recalled a night when his family and relatives were present in the living room and everyone was upset. At bedtime, he had wanted to stay up with the adults. So instead of going to bed, he said that he had resisted. In the end, he was in bed – in a hospital bed. This was dropped into the story like a slap in the face, a joke on himself, but also on us who hadn't expected it. Jackson returned to the plot. He had teased his father, who chased him upstairs. They ran up and down the stairs, up and down and up and down. Once in the bedroom, Jackson said he had hidden behind the dresser. His father came and 'lifted' him and 'placed' him on the bed. Then Jackson stepped away from his story again, describing his huge father and the unevenness of a fight between an attacking 3-year-old and a man, as if the child had had the upper hand. Then we plunge back into the story with fragmented speech about pain and being set down 'feather-light' and 'your' arm. Jackson became clear again with the explanation that it only broke because it was in the wrong position (not because his father had grabbed him roughly and thrown him hard ... no, that's our conclusion). Jackson described how his arm went through the springs, twisted, and snapped. 'My arm's gone into the springs!' Jackson, at 16 years old, cries this out, like a child in pain. Then he returned to telling the story. He said it felt like being stabbed a thousand times. When his father pulled it out, he could see that it hung at the wrong angle. While saying this, Jackson held his arm up crookedly to demonstrate. He said that his father's face was white with fear and that he kept saying he was sorry. According to Jackson, it wasn't his father's fault; it was his own because he should have gone to bed properly. He said he kept screaming and screaming and screaming. Even in the hospital. Suddenly, Jackson switched again, taking the adults' perspective and describing how upset they were. He concluded by saying his father still feels guilty.

The way Jackson told this story is outstanding for the shifts among Jackson speaking as if it were happening now, the vivid images of pain and a huge man, the rational-sounding explanations that make no sense to an adult listener (Jackson was responsible for what must be considered, from our perspective, child abuse?), and the repetitions that rev the story up. The sudden switches leave the listener confused and alarmed. Possibly the strongest moment is when Jackson switched to the present tense and used direct speech to call for help – as if the emergency were happening now, at age 16 while he told the story.

This pattern of speech is indicative of unresolved trauma. Unresolved trauma means not only failing to understand what happened coherently, but also being unable to regulate strong, motivating feelings that are elicited by associated stimuli in the present. That is, recall of such past experiences can irrationally motivate behavior in the present. Most worrisome in Jackson's case is the range of perspectives that he takes, any one of which could motivate his behavior. This creates great uncertainty. Will he attack? Seek caregiving? Offer caregiving to someone dangerous? Our understanding of the combination of events and the incomplete and still active processing of the events suggests that tipping off recall of this trauma could endanger both other people and Jackson himself.

Although much risk associated with coy signals is not discovered until the school years, there is one major exception. Coy behavior connects the protective and comforting functions of attachment with its reproductive functions. Sexuality overlaps in both function and form with protection and comfort. Specifically, both attachment and sexuality function to bring individuals together and to maintain closeness with enduring affectional bonds. Further, both use the same behaviors to accomplish this: smiling, calling, extended eye contact, touching, caressing, holding, embracing, kissing, etc. Only genital contact is largely limited to the sexual/reproductive function (see Table 2.2).

To understand parents' contribution to sexual abuse of young children, it is necessary to think about strategies that will be introduced in Chapter 3. It should be noted, however, that it is in the preschool years that rates of sexual abuse rise from negligible (in infancy) to concerning (US DHHS 2007). Children's unwitting contribution may be the use of coy behavior and the children who use it most intensively are children using the compulsive A strategies (compulsive attention, caregiving, compliance, and performance) and, within Type C, feigned helplessness. These children not only use coy signals frequently and intensively, but they also are more in need of support from adults than other children. That is, the children are seeking attention from adults and using signals that both function to attract attention and also can be misunderstood by adult viewers as being flirtatious. It should not be surprising that photographs of sexually abused and missing children

Table 2.2 Attachment behavior and sexual behavior

Attachment behavior	Sexual behavior
Holding	Holding
Gazing	Gazing
Sucking	Sucking
Reaching	Reaching
Touching	Touching
Caressing	Caressing
Kissing	Kissing
Following	Following
	Genital contact

often reveal the children to be exceptionally attractive in coy or 'sexual' ways (e.g., JonBenet Ramsey and Madeleine McCann).

Parenting and protection at home

The strategies developed by the end of the preschool years (by about age 5) constitute the strategies used by most people of any age, including most parents. In most cases, they are sufficient to keep children reasonably safe and comfortable at home such that intervention is not mandatory – even though it might be helpful in some cases.

Although the Type A and Type C strategies are not ideal, they function well enough to nudge parents in a more protective and comforting direction. Moreover, these strategies are rarely associated with ongoing and repeated endangerment of children. That is, by the end of the preschool years, most children are ready to face the world outside their home.

The next chapter focuses on (a) the new abilities that allow children to expand their strategic functioning to contexts such as the neighborhood and school and (b) the new and more complex strategies that more mature children can organize. The children who need these strategies the most are those who face more enduring and complex risk.

Note

1 Because it is not central to the issue of why parents behave as they do, the roots of this theory are not described. But the ideas offered here come from ethology, psychoanalytic theory, behavioral learning theory, family systems theory, social ecology, Gestalt theory, Piagetian theory, evolutionary theory, the cognitive neurosciences, and others.

Chapter 3

Going to school: Coping with a complex world

Between the ages of 5 and 7 years, almost all cultures send their children to community settings for large parts of the day. In Western cultures, this is school. This change in context is a powerful influence on children's development, bringing (a) greater personal freedom, (b) protection by nonfamilial adults who stand *in loco parentis*, but who lack an affective attachment to the child and have different expectations than the child's parents, and (c) substantial involvement with and influence from peers.

In the first 5 years of life, children became specialists in the problems experienced in their families and their families' ways of handling problems. This was essential for immediate, short-term survival. But to live successfully in the world at large, children need to recognize other problems and use other strategies. Development of self-protection in the school years and adolescence is about broadening children's experience and competence. Risk is increased when, instead, children continue to refine their family-based strategies and to apply them to contexts where they are not adaptive.

School-aged (approximately 6–12 years)

Developmentally, school-aged children are better able to protect themselves and regulate their own behavior than are younger children. Cortical maturation makes explicit reasoning about concrete situations possible. In terms of overall adaptation and preparation for later parenthood, maturation gives school-aged children the opportunity to understand the basis for their own behavior. Further, they can use emerging competencies to generate, practice, and use alternative strategies when reflection indicates that their behavior did not achieve the desired outcome.

Strategies

The new strategy that develops in the school years is the C5-6 punitive/seductive strategy (see Figure 3.1) that reflects an obsession with revenge

(C5) or rescue (C6).When simple threatening or feigned helpless behavior no longer attracts parental attention (because parents recognize that it is a bluff), children must raise the ante. In particular, they need to hide the bluff. The more mature cognitive abilities of school-aged children enable the shift to a deceptive strategy, i.e., C5-6. Of course, most Type C children do not need to make this shift, but many endangered children do. Children who come to professional attention are among those who do.

The C5–6 coercive strategy is based on children's incomplete understanding of why things happen the way they do and their pervasive sense of vulnerability in the face of this. Like all people who feel weak and have learned that directness will be used against them, school-aged children use deception to combat the unpredictability that they cannot understand.[1] Deception is a powerful strategy that misleads both others and the self regarding the child's motivations. The most obvious displays of the C5–6 deceptively coercive strategy are in bully–victim relationships and gang warfare, but there are many other forms of distress attributable to the C5–6 strategy.

The C5–6 strategy uses splitting of the display of incompatible negative affects and adds cognitive deception (i.e., intentional false cognition). The

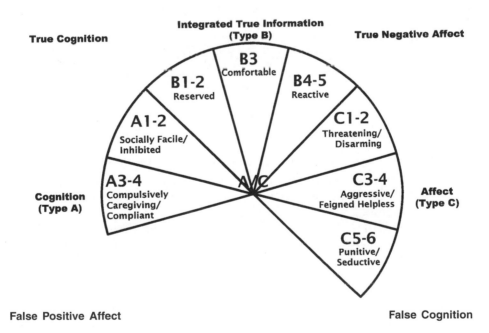

A Dynamic-Maturational Model of Patterns of Attachment in School Age

Integrated True Information (Type B)

True Cognition

True Negative Affect

B3 Comfortable

B1-2 Reserved

B4-5 Reactive

A1-2 Socially Facile/ Inhibited

C1-2 Threatening/ Disarming

A3-4 Compulsively Caregiving/ Compliant

A/C

C3-4 Aggressive/ Feigned Helpless

C5-6 Punitive/ Seductive

Cognition (Type A)

Affect (Type C)

False Positive Affect

False Cognition

Copyright: Patricia M. Crittenden, 2001

Figure 3.1 The school-aged patterns of attachment

focus of the strategy is not necessarily on the person who directly failed or offended the child. Instead, the focal figure may hold a role similar to that of the attachment figure and, thus, be overgeneralized by the child into bearing responsibility for the child's negative feelings. Unfortunately, the strategy is involving and misleading and can turn potentially balanced relationships into coercive relationships, thus coming to justify, in the minds of the coercive children, their feelings and actions.

The strategy is used aggressively against others when children feel that they have been treated unfairly, but cannot discover the reasons in ways that enable them to change the situation. When used aggressively, deception permits attacks in which the intended victim is unaware of the impending attack. This is both safer for the aggressor and more frightening for victims and people who imagine that they could become victims. That is, behavior typical of children using a punitively coercive strategy is taken quite seriously by adults and can result in substantial censure and punishment.

The strategy is used against the self, i.e., self-deception, when the child feels that the attachment figure is too weak to be attacked and too caring and available to justify destruction. When deception uses fear and desire for comfort, the child's anger isn't visible. Instead, children using the C6 strategy seem childlike and appealing. Instead of being direct about what they think, feel, or want, such children use their appealing appearance to try to get what they want obliquely; that is, they are seductive. When rescued, the children appear to bear only goodwill toward the rescuer even while harboring hidden resentment (anger) that they could not be direct about. Children using the C6 strategy will less often elicit criticism and punishment from adults than aggressive children. Nevertheless, there is a passively aggressive process that is not apparent to either party; enacted, it leaves self-created victims unsatisfied and rescuers angry. One reason for the endless need for rescue is the child's resentment for having to cripple themselves and then beg for care.

Opportunity

Entry to school and neighborhood relationships, combined with concrete logic, creates new opportunities. Almost all children are exposed to strategies not used by their family members. Learning how these strategies function can expand a child's range of adaptation.

Some troubled children cannot receive the support they need at home. They have a chance to find responsible and caring 'auxiliary' attachment figures at school or in their neighborhood. Such figures might be teachers, religious or club leaders, or the parent of a friend. These adults help the children to increase their range of adaptability by working in the child's ZPD to support conversion of nonverbal strategies to verbal ones that reflect both the child's context and his or her inner experience. Putting discrepancies in words can help to make integration possible. If there is someone to discuss how things go with the child in ways that increase the child's understanding, even a very troubled child may be able to learn integrative processes.

Reflective integration is a learned skill that becomes possible for the first time in the school years and then only in a limited way. The process involves being aware of one's various dispositional representations, particularly those that are in conflict, and being able to think about, i.e., reflect on, what the differences mean to oneself so as to make a judicious choice of what to do. Often this cannot be done in the moment – because thinking takes too long. Therefore, reflective integration includes reconsideration of past experiences in the hope of being able to apply what one learned to the future.

Learning to reflect and integrate is crucial because the successful use of any strategy requires knowing when to use and *not* use it; that is, the ability to accommodate change regardless of whether the change is induced by maturation, change in context, or change in the behavior of others is central to adaptation.

Integration is not possible before school age, but an interaction of neurological maturation and social circumstances makes this a central emergent task in the school years. That is, it is in the school years that cortical integrative processes become mature enough to be of practical import in daily life. At this point, the assistance of parents or of alternative attachment figures in activating and shaping emerging integrative abilities is quite important. The question, 'Why did you do that when you knew you shouldn't?', is one form of activating this function, but there are many daily opportunities for occasion-specific integration. Even if integrative processes can only be used in very limited circumstances, they are very valuable and can protect the child from entering a downward spiral of misinformation that can be difficult to reverse.

Problems

The central problem that prevents some school-age children from reorganizing their strategies is their inability to see clearly why things do not work out. Instead, not knowing what is wrong, they escalate their existing strategy. The lack of clarity can be because

1 the causes are too complex to be discerned or understood by school-aged children; e.g., the parents are deceptive;
2 the child is discouraged from looking or 'punished' psychologically for looking (Crittenden *et al.* 1994);
3 the causes are hidden or obscured, e.g., unspoken marital problems;
4 the causes are not tied to the child, so nothing the child would do could resolve the problem, as in parental mental health issues.

These may be the same reasons why professionals cannot easily get a handle on why school-aged children have problems. When professionals misunderstand the problems, they are unable to help children to clarify them. In this chapter, some possible hidden factors are described.

Some children using a Type A strategy apply their parent-pleasing compulsive strategy too broadly. For example, a caregiving child who was overly helpful to the teacher might be accepted by the teacher in this role and also be considered a 'teacher's pet' by peers. Children using compulsive performance might dazzle peers with their positive affect and excessive attention to pleasing their friends. Such children may become popular, but fail to develop either their own perspective or close peer relationships. As one father of a boy who died of binge drinking said, 'My son was a leader. He had to be out front. If everyone else was having four beers, he had to have six.' That's not leadership; that's walking backwards, looking at the followers to decide what to do. Similarly, excessively high-performing children might elicit high expectations from teachers, who then reinforce the importance of very high performance. In each case, the child's compulsive strategy from home is applied more broadly than necessary, but because it yields obvious benefits, the risks are rarely noticed, at least not in the school years.

Similarly, children who find reasons to remain home from school may feel that they must monitor conditions at home to keep their parent(s) safe (probably a A3 compulsive caregiving strategy) (Bowlby 1973). Quiet, submissive children with low arousal who have no friends may also be at substantial risk; queries should be made about their unsupervised time because they may be in dangerous places (a compulsive A strategy that is not resolving the child's problems). More than children with friends, they may be at risk of bullying by older children and sexual abuse by both older children and adults.

> By school-age, David was a withdrawn, fearful boy who readily attracted taunting from his peers. He stayed away from home and school and any place where he could be mocked or bullied. This left him lonely and on the fringes of childhood society. He might have attracted an adult male who might have sexually abused him in exchange for attention and affection. But that didn't happen. Instead David occasionally hung out with other rejected boys, but never the rough ones. His parents remained caught up in their problems: his father drank like crazy, beat his mother, and mocked David for being a mama's boy. David dreamed of growing up and going away. Still professionals were unaware of David because he caused no trouble.

Among children with a Type A strategy, worrisome behavior includes agitation and hyperactivity that expresses the child's concern about doing the right thing. Although it can be quite irritating to adults, this agitation is the opposite of Type C children's agitated challenges to authority. This is a reminder that symptom behaviors do not always indicate the nature of the problem.

A particular concern is children who do not respond to pain or who are concerned about their parents' state when they (the children) are in pain.

Some children who use a Type A strategy display chronic somatic problems that lack evidence of medical origin (tics, gastrointestinal disorders, auto-immune disorders; see Kozlowska *et al.* 2007). In many cases, these children have visible signs of distress, e.g., tics, but fail to complain about pain (Wilkinson 2003). However, physical and psychological pain share overlapping patterns of brain activation (Mee *et al.* 2006) and perception of pain involves a dynamic process that is influenced by the effects of past experience (Melzack *et al.* 2001). These findings suggest that too great psychological inhibition or, conversely, too intense focus on something other than the harm to the self might result in lack of perception of physical pain or even in the painful event being the signal of desired outcomes and, therefore, not perceived as pain.

If there is no physical symptom and the child is excessively good and quiet, and displays false positive behavior, there may be risk of unexpected breakdowns, marked by inexplicable outbursts of violence, fear, or sexual displays (i.e., psychotic-like behavior). When misunderstood (as being 'acting out' or coercively Type C behavior) or mismanaged (by responding so as to increase the child's inhibition of the outbursts), this organization can lead to disastrous consequences.

Darren is typical of children in child protection care for long periods. The details of the problems vary from family to family, but the situation of numerous intractable problems and a service system that lacks appropriate services is typical.

> Darren and his younger sister were removed from their parents when Darren was 3 years old. His mother was mentally retarded and his father was alcoholic. The family broke up following an incident of domestic violence that resulted in a call to the police. At that time, his mother was institutionalized, Darren and his sister were placed in foster care, and his father disappeared. Soon after, the placement broke down because Darren was disruptive and uncontrollable, but his quieter sister stayed with the foster parents.
>
> By 8 years of age, Darren had had several foster families and now was making the rounds of the group homes. In the group homes, Darren had a rotating team of workers. That is, he was not abandoned, but, at the same time, he had no one. Even his dog, whose arrival had comforted him somewhat, was taken away when he forgot to feed her.
>
> His mother's condition was deteriorating and she could no longer recognize or speak to him when he visited her. Until he was 8, no one had explained her medical situation to Darren; this left him feeling personally rejected by both his mother and all the foster mothers. When he was finally told, at age 8, that his mother was very ill, he was less distressed by her behavior (being able to assign it properly to its cause and not to himself). His closest relationship was with his sister. Since kindergarten, Darren had not completed a single full week of school and had been suspended for outbursts. In the last year alone,

he had changed primary worker, group home, staff, and school – and been suspended from school. To prevent Darren from getting upset (extremely upset!), he was not told when workers were changing jobs – and, thus, leaving him. They just never showed up again.

Darren is easily mistaken for a coercive, defiant child. For example, at the beginning of the School-Aged Assessment of Attachment (SAA) (Crittenden 1997–2005), when asked to say his name, Darren said, *'Owww, I don't want to do it'*. Then in response to a series of requests and encouraging statements from the interviewer around providing his name and putting on the lapel microphone, Darren said, *'I don't like doin' that stuff.'* [interviewer's responses are omitted] *'But I don't like doin' that stuff.'* [...] *'Um ... ah ... like um ... like testing, testing stuff.'* [...] *'Hook it to what?'* [...] *'Why?'* [...] *'How do I use it?'* [...] *'Am I the first to use it?'* [...] *'Can you just say why we needed to come here?'* To this, the interviewer said they were working with someone overseas and Darren replied, *'We've got friends overseas'*. Then: *'Really? What are interviews?'* *'But don't don't you's know that or but because I think you should know that because you's are ok aw you's worked with kids before.'*

Darren then goes on to complete the SAA, having difficulties in only a few spots. This beginning, however, is very important to understand. On the surface, it looks challenging; some professionals might feel threatened and wonder whether Darren was going to be defiant. Discourse analysis reveals that Darren can't or won't say his name and that he asks about every step of the interview. On the other hand, he seems quite familiar with testing (albeit distressed, as marked by the repetition), he is eager to discover whether he is unique (the first to use the 'mic'), he speaks like a professional ('Can you just say why...'), and allies himself with the professional (*'we* needed' ... and having 'friends overseas'). Finally, we see how dysfluent he becomes over the idea that professionals (the people who are raising him) might not know about kids.

The remainder of the SAA consists of seven picture (story) cards, each showing a common sort of threat to school-aged children. Like other children, Darren is asked to generate an imagined story about the boy on the card, and then to recall and tell a similar story about himself.

On the very first story card (boy going out alone), Darren asked whether he was doing it without permission and then immediately said, *'But um I went out eh alone without permission'*. Asked to tell that story, he said, *'I don't really remem remember bad stuff that I do'*. In the end, Darren could not tell this story, and instead he focused on what he and the interviewer were doing. Indeed, he attended to her every move with great care: *'And what's that for? What is it doing? ... You're taping everything I say.'* In what follows, Darren is absolutely factual and will hazard no guesses: *'I don't know because he [the team leader] didn't tell me.'* Later he said: *'I don't like making up stories.'*

Not knowing is thematic for Darren. So is not knowing about his body, which, in fact, is quite reactive during the SAA:

> So did anything happen, did anybody find out you'd done that or not?
> *Well, um he rung the police, but um they didn't come cos I settled down then after that.*
> And so were you a bit unsettled?
> *Uh hum, because I had a bad day at school.*
> So when you say unsettled like, what happens to you when you are unsettled?
> *Um ah I don't know.*
> You're not sure, so do your legs or arms get agitated or do you get a bit yucky inside or ...?
> ... ——
> Do you know what happens?
> *No.*
> No? OK, that's all right.

We notice that Darren uses borrowed adult/professional language to describe himself and his reasons for behaving as he does. That is, adults talk about 'settling down' and 'having a bad day'; children rarely do. Darren speaks like an adult, a professional adult.

There are two story cards that produce material that can help us to understand Darren. One is the 'moving house' card.

> Can I just ask you, in the place you are in now, who is the person who you can talk to if you feel sad?
> *Um that's a hard question.*
> Is it, so is there anybody you can talk to?
> *Well, I don't really have a choice cos there is only one, there is only one worker at the, at the house where I live.*
> OK and what is their name?
> *Well, do you want to know all of their names?*
> Yeah.
> *Do you want to um know the team leader's first?*
> Yeah.
> *Um his name is Peter ... Peter Dryton and this one is Jamal and there is another one called Tracey and Saun.*
> And who is the one you feel most comfortable talking to like if you're feeling a bit yucky?
> *Um I ... I've never really thought of that.*
> So do you talk to any of them or not really?
> *Well, I talked to Saun last night because um ... I'm afraid of the dark and had a blackout because I forced a piece of bread into a toaster and um and*

then um the toaster was about to catch on fire so the switch in the garage just quickly turned off automatically.

And what was that like when the blackout happened?

Like I couldn't see a thing and I um I quickly ran out the back because that's where Saun was, he was having a cigarette and then I asked him what happened and he said and I think he said I don't know. Then he wanted to go out the front the front um to open the door but I ... I said no because I'm afraid I'm afraid of the dark and then um I said um that I wanna go out the um the um I wanna go out the fence ... like there's a um like like the fence can open.

And what happened?

Like he said um he kept on saying to um ... go through the front door then he um decided um to go ... to the ... to go to the um ... back gate.

And so how did it end?

It ended good.

So what happened?

Um then we went then um cos I thought there was um the the switch with the that controls the lights, yeah, um he thought it was out out the front, but it was in the garage.

And did he know that you were so scared?

Um yeah, because I was like this; I was goin' like this.

So you were breathing like crazy?

Yeah.

OK and how did you manage your fear?

Um I had a um had another piece of toast which I made sure that um it went in it it just slipped in because I don't want it to happen again.

And did he help you at all in managing your fear, what did he do?

Um while I was eating my toast um he um had a talk.

And what did he say or what did he do?

Um I can't remember what he said.

Did it make you feel any different?

Uh hum.

Yeah so how did it make you feel after you had a talk?

Feel good.

This story is interesting for both its content and the form of the discourse. In the content, we learn that Darren is afraid of the dark, doesn't imagine that talking to adults could help, and understands the issue of staff shortages. All of these are unfortunate – for a boy's healthy development. The form, however, has much more information. First, Darren is excessively careful to determine what the interviewer wants so that he can comply. When he gets upset, parents and professionals alike forget how hard Darren tries to please them and be a good boy. His sentences are structured cognitively with 'then' and 'because (cos)'. Affect, on the other hand, is stated semantically (I'm afraid of the dark) and displayed somatically (rapid breathing). Then, while Darren ate his toast, 'he um had a talk'. How can one person have a 'talk' while the other eats? One is left wondering whether a conversation, for Darren, is a professional explaining or lecturing.

The other interesting section is in response to the 'father leaving' card.

What's it like, can you tell me what it's like seeing your mom? Is it hard, is it good, do you look forward to it, you don't look forward to it?
To me that's a personal question.
Aw haw OK and it's a bit hard to talk about?
Welllll, no … it's easy to talk about it, but that's personal to me.
Yeah that's OK. So have you got any story you can tell me?
Well, I've got one, I think, to tell you um I'll leave now.
You'd like to leave now, can we finish the other pictures?
Is there much pictures?
There's two.
OK.

In this excerpt, we see both his attempt to protect himself from the impending disaster and then an intrusion of forbidden negative affect almost enacted – and just saved by the attentive and aware interviewer. Talking (thinking even) about his mother is too much for Darren. He's ready to bolt. A full intrusion doesn't occur during the SAA, again because of the interviewer's awareness of this process, recognition of when it is in process, and ability to soothe and protect Darren so that he can continue to be a good boy. This is a point when an unaware professional might conclude that Darren was being rude and possibly defiant. Instead, he may have been trying to prevent an affective explosion by tucking the arousing ideas away in his 'personal' life.

Darren used a Type A strategy – as do most children in care, especially those with multiple moves. In fact, he was not only compulsively compliant (A4), and a bit socially promiscuous (A5), but he was also beginning to use an externally assembled strategy (A8) in which he let professionals define what he experienced and how he spoke about it. In addition, he had unresolved traumas around moving and separation. He also had signs of depression. The latter were tied in the discourse specifically to his not knowing about himself, his family, or what would happen to any of them. He spoke about himself as if he were an object that was picked up and dropped off, here and there. He spoke with sighs and an almost inaudible voice, until those moments when feelings were too nearly accessed – and then negative affect intruded, generating one of those disastrous moments. The outcome was that his extreme effort to please adults escaped notice altogether and he became defined by the inexplicable disruptions. These, in turn, ensured that his life would have no permanence or predictability.

His treatment in all settings had been highly behavioral: posted lists of specified behavioral goals and consequences. Often the treatment was aimed at reducing Darren's explosive behavior by increasing his inhibition, e.g., anger control. Given Darren's existing Type A strategy, this was probably the opposite of what Darren needed in order to reduce the number of intense and unregulated intrusions. Rather than needing to control his feelings, Darren needed to be protected from the threatening changes of home and family that elicited them.

Given his current situation, Darren probably needed the possibility of expressing his anger (at his loss of family and the capricious behavior of the treatment system), fear (of being abandoned altogether), and desire for comfort (that had never been fulfilled, except partially by his puppy). Stability of home and caregivers was probably the single most needed component of a treatment plan, and it was the one thing the state could not provide.

The horrible irony is that everyone was insisting that Darren behave predictably and rationally when the basics necessary to maintain children's lives – home and caregivers – were not stable, predictable, or rational. Nor were there any consequences when professionals could not provide the required stability. That is, the state imposed a standard on Darren that it could not meet itself. Darren's family was responsible for his needing alternate care; after that, most of his problems were iatrogenic, that is, caused by the nature of the care he received.

Children using a Type C strategy face a different problem. Their strategy is to draw attention to themselves by irritating or frightening adults enough to change the adults' behavior. If that has functioned even intermittently, the child is likely to use it more extensively. The risk is that doing so will create a context outside the home that maintains the strategy (as is true for all strategies). For example, a coercive child might so frustrate a teacher that their relationship would come to mirror the child's relationships at home. Such children create a niche that then traps them in a distorted strategy.

Nancy's problems became apparent in her first year of school. Her initial enthusiasm soon gave way to boredom and daydreaming. As more work was required, Nancy did less. Her grades were poor, but mostly from undone work rather than poor performance. Nevertheless, her coy shyness pleased her teachers and each vowed to be the one who would break though the invisible barriers that held Nancy back. Eventually, however, each teacher lost hope. It was as if Nancy somehow had tricked them, leaving them feeling bad about themselves – and angry with her. Day after day, teachers kept her in from recess to finish her work while the other children played. Nancy sat and sat; she didn't complain – and she didn't work. Instead, she got used to being cast out. Soon she had fewer friends in the neighborhood and spent more time alone.

Nancy's problems were spreading; it wasn't just her grades that suffered. Now it was all her relationships – with parents, teachers, and peers. There were lots of parent–teacher meetings and the adults made lots of plans and promises. But Nancy didn't change. Referrals began. The school psychologist sat in the classroom to observe Nancy. What he saw was striking.

Nancy sat slumped, quiet, and daydreaming off to the side of the room. No one seemed to notice her, not even the teacher. On the other side, Tommy was whispering to the boys near him, surreptitiously throwing spitballs, and otherwise entertaining a whole group of kids. The teacher reprimanded Tommy again and again. He answered with a charming, *'Yes, ma'am!'*, then turned to his friends, smirking and wisecracking. The teacher was boiling. She threatened, *'If you don't stop playing, I'll move you!'* Tommy carried on as if she wasn't there. The battle was on and the teacher couldn't afford to lose. She moved Tommy – to the seat behind Nancy. Tommy pulled her pigtails. She slumped further down. He began kicking under her seat. He pulled her pigtails some more. She didn't giggle, she didn't turn around, she didn't disrupt the teacher, and the teacher was happy to be teaching again.

Where were her parents in all this? Worried. They tried everything: being strict, being sympathetic, setting standards with consequences and then dropping them when it became clear that they could take everything away, but Nancy wouldn't change. Together they trooped off to treatment, but very quickly the psychologist dismissed them all. He saw no problems: healthy and bright child, cooperative, caring parents. He recommended that Nancy get to work.

But Nancy was failing in school year after year and, although we could say it was self-induced, she wasn't learning what the other children had learned. 'Feigned helplessness' (C4) was becoming genuine lack of skill.

What was going on? Nancy was bright, her parents were caring, concerned and involved. Isn't that how it should be? Two things stand out immediately. One is Nancy's strength in pursuing her self-destructive strategy in the face of all the concerned adults. She looked weak and vulnerable and perceived herself to be weak and vulnerable, but, goodness!, she was resolute. Without intention, or even awareness of the frustration she caused, she was taking her parents, teachers, the principal, and psychologists down with her! Everyone was experiencing the frustration that she felt and, in the end, everyone sought what she had come to seek: just to be left alone. Send her to another class (which one teacher asked), to another school (which the principal recommended), or out of therapy. No one likes failure! Indeed, one of the strongest unintended effects of being helpless and seducing others to assist without success is that the child shares the despair. Nancy's parents didn't leave, but, feeling that she could only make things worse, her mother stopped trying to help; when 'help' only harms and no one knows what to do, she stopped 'helping'.

From our perspective, we must ask, what did Nancy want? Moreover, for a helpless-looking little girl, she had powerful effects; maybe the appearance wasn't the reality? If it wasn't and she was creating powerful effects with her strategy, how could she be helped to perceive and regulate those effects so as to have the outcomes she sought?

The other surprising aspect of the story is the role of the teacher in defining for Tommy and Nancy their roles of bully (C3–5) and victim (C4–6). Without awareness and for her own ease of managing a class, the teacher helped Tommy and Nancy to assume maladaptive roles. This is an unintended iatrogenic effect, but of course, it isn't the entire story. Tommy clearly acted as a bully, but Nancy was a complicitous victim, neither protecting herself, nor protesting to others.

Finally, it is worth noting that all of the professional focus was on the here and now. The school's goal was to get Nancy to do her schoolwork. The questions and observations about her family had to do with whether the parents supported education, whether they had a clean, safe, and stable home, and whether there were problems such as violence. All seemed fine. Yet, clearly, it was not fine. Something was missing from view and no one knew what to look for. (Good theory points to the spots where information is needed.)

Children like Nancy cause less trouble and are referred for evaluation and treatment less often than children like Tommy. I use Nancy as an example because her situation clarifies that the information we have isn't sufficient to resolve the problem. That is true for the 'Tommies' as well, but their acting-out behavior gives a focus to treatment that creates the appearance of effectiveness – even when outcome measures and the need in adolescence for police involvement suggest otherwise.

Some children distort the best-friend relationship by creating bully–victim relationships organized around a dominance-submission strategy. Dominance gives the bully the victim's loyalty and submission gives the victim the bully's protection from outsiders' aggression. Other coercive children attract a peer group of similar children, thus forming gangs that provide the defense that the children feel they need while exacting revenge for felt injustices. However, both the defense and revenge are misdirected and can lead to police involvement.

Another group of children remains locked in a distorted parent–child triangle in which the child is unable to see the factors that motivate adult behavior (often parental conflict or past unresolved trauma). These children appear to be at risk of substance abuse, eating disorders, schizophrenia and other self-harming disorders (Bell and Bell 1979; Guerin et al. 1987; Khashan et al. 2008). This is particularly likely if direct communication of negative feelings and thoughts is not welcome at home, either because it challenges parents too much or because it makes the parents feel like failures. Both parental responses are, of course, distorted, but many parents feel these ways. When that happens, it can force children into nonverbal sorts of communication (e.g., eating disorders) or solutions that block the problem from awareness (e.g., substance abuse). It should be kept in mind, however, that these sorts of serious disorders are almost certainly multiply caused, with causal factors including, in unknown proportions, genetic, biochemical, prenatal, environmental, and familial factors (Rutter 2002, 2006a). It is the latter that are considered here.

Finally, some children face threats that have nothing to do with them. When there is domestic violence, addiction, or other adult-focused threats, children's strategies may be irrelevant to adults' behavior. In some cases, this results in children being taken into care, and that can have negative effects of its own.

By 8 years of age, Jackson was in psychiatric care for chaotic and destructive behavior, including bullying, violent outbursts and defiance of adults. He was diagnosed with ADHD and medicated. Soon, however, he was dabbling in drugs of his own choosing, with addiction only a few years ahead. He and his siblings were placed in care when he was 10. Although this was his first official placement, they had been cared for, from time to time, by both sets of grandparents.

The child-protection placement followed spousal violence ('*Blood was everywhere, on my father's hands, on my mother's face, on the walls*'). The fight was over his mother's cheating. Then she fled to her lover, abandoning her children to their violent and alcoholic father, who was unable to manage them alone (he abused them and threw them out). Then Child Protection stepped in. In describing this, Jackson's speech changed completely from his discussion of his broken arm. He became animated and angry, even shouting that he '*hates, hates, and hates*' his mother – ever since she cheated on his dad. Prior to this, he said, he had loved her the most. Now, he said, his feelings had '*completely switched*'. When asked about his mother leaving, he could only say that '*everything changed*'.

To explain his mother's leaving and his violent father caring for him and his siblings, Jackson tries almost every available strategy, both Type A and Type C strategies; that is, Jackson uses an A/C strategy). He exonerates his mother, but does so by addressing a different kind of abandonment (her turning her attention from him to younger siblings, as each was born) than the one that most hurt him, her abandoning all the children for her lover ('*They always leave you for babies; it is natural for moms*'). We, of course, read between the lines, seeing what he could not say and understanding how much it still hurts. He idealizes his father (*he gave us everything, tons of money, hundreds, even thousands, at Christmas*). All of this is Type A. But he also blames them each bitterly, leaving no space for reasons or extenuating circumstances, using Type C strategies. Most of all, however, he struggles around his own role, being at times a frightened child fighting to be cared for in a world of crazy, mad adults. Alternatively, he is grandiose in his forgiveness and unquenchable in his wrath. In the end, however, he seems to hold himself to blame: if he weren't so bad, if he hadn't told his father ... He preserves some shred of perceived control over a dangerously out-of-control situation by making himself responsible for the downfall of the adults, the breakup of the household and the displacement of his siblings.

We know almost nothing about Jackson's early years because he had not come to professional attention yet and there are no adults available to provide a history: his father is hostile, his mother has fled, and his grandmothers are both dead. Consequently, his developmental beginnings can be known only through his recall and that is limited by his immaturity at the time of the events and the lack of an attachment figure to help him expand his understanding.

Nor do we have direct observational evidence of his functioning in the school years, but the known facts are chilling: lack of a permanent home or caregiver, frequent violence and severe injuries (the arm was not a unique incident), abandonment by the less dangerous of his caregivers, and a need to idealize his violent father, who stayed, his only remaining parent.

How does a child manage his feelings when he must seek care from a dangerous father? What strategy makes that possible? And how does he manage his feelings of loss of his mother when the loss is actually abandonment? On top of that, Jackson believes that, because he told his father that his mother was cheating on him, he bears responsibility for the breakup of the household. How does a 10-year-old understand sexual matters between parents, especially deceptive sexuality? How does he understand his role in it, especially when his information comes secondhand through his older sister? Triangulation is always difficult for children; this extended and involving form of multiple triangles makes a young boy party to the destruction of his family. It also leaves him with no knowledgeable guides to what happened.

Being triangulated may lead to development of C5-6 strategies in children, with triangulation then being employed by the children themselves. Finally, if we consider (a) the range of feelings that Jackson must experience and the limited support he had for managing them (could you or I manage such events and the accompanying feelings? I am not confident that I could!) and (b) the models he would have for conflict resolution, we will not be surprised that his first foster placement failed – as did the placements, both familial and institutional, that followed it. Each change inflicted more psychological damage, each made Jackson more vulnerable while reducing the possibilities of his having protective and comforting caregivers, and each was followed by an increase in his violence and, with his increasing strength and body size, an increase in the damage he inflicted. Jackson, having been endangered and unprotected since birth, is becoming a source of danger.

Whether the strategy functions protectively or not, children whose effort goes into refining an already distorted strategy (rather than developing new strategies and understanding when to use them) limit their range of adaptation. This niche-picking maintains the pre-existing distortion and reduces the probability of reorganization.

Risk

The riskiest times are (a) the '5–7-year shift' when maturation is incomplete, but the change in context is underway, and (b) the onset of puberty in early adolescence. At-risk children tend to experience puberty sooner than children from more stable and supportive homes (Belsky and Draper 1987; Migliano *et al.* 2007). This can result in behavior that functions to elicit comfort, but appears sexual. Such sexualized attachment behavior can occur between peers or between an adult and a school-aged child. Most cases of 'sexual abuse' between children probably reflect confusion of attachment and sexual behavior around fulfilling the attachment functions of comfort and safety.

The riskiest conditions are when the basis for the child's problems is unclear or, being clear, cannot be resolved. Ironically, for their effort to please adults, children using the Type A strategy often succeed only in generating approval for being 'good' and rarely elicit the concern that they need.

School-age children know when what they do isn't working and they struggle to make things better. But if the problems are out of sight or too complex for them to understand, their effort will fail. When that happens, some become depressed, some isolate themselves, and some become resentful and vengeful. In the latter case, the solution is likely to be misdirected. This will lead to two errors: the distortions of affect and cognition that constitute the strategy and the focus of the strategy. Thus, as the distorted strategy becomes more refined, the focus of the strategy may become less precisely defined. For example, a boy using a threatening, Type C strategy with his parents may refine that to a C5 strategy, but apply it more widely as a bully. This has consequences for the next developmental step.

Professionals' roles

A particular difficulty for professional service providers is that the Type C child's accommodation to the parent actually improves the parent's behavior (making the parent appear less deviant) and concurrently makes the child appear extreme. This leads to the many parents who bring extremely disturbed children to clinicians for diagnosis. Why would the professional 'waste' time (and possibly generate offense) by assessing the parent's psychological state when it is so obviously the child who is abnormal? Indeed, if we used a symptom-based diagnostic evaluation, we often would find little or nothing. Only in cases where we have longitudinal information (e.g., interaction in infancy or 'Strange Situations' from 1–5 years of age, parents' AAIs) and view it through DMM theory do we see the developmental progression. It begins with (a) unpredictable parents of infants who, (b) in the preschool years, become extremely vigilant, excessively active, and risk-taking preschool-aged children whose parents are becoming both more attentive and also habituated to their behavior to (c) actively concerned parents of explicitly troubled school-aged children. By then, of course, many other factors are operating (e.g., lack of earlier learning, teachers' and peers' reactions, etc.) The combined complexity of (a) years of developmental history and (b) the nonfamilial influences in the school years makes it very difficult to pinpoint a cause of children's problems. This leaves professionals groping for explanations.

Biogenetic explanations are currently in vogue to explain the more troublesome disorders. Although genetic factors probably contribute to the form dysfunction takes and may contribute to the probability of dysfunction occurring in some form, there is little evidence that single genes or even clusters of genes can account for psychological and behavioral disorder (McGuire *et al.* 2007; Rutter 2006a). Further, even statistically significant genetic variation has not yet been shown to be clinically meaningful in either group or case studies (Couzin and Kaiser 2007; Rutter 2005).

A more circumspect approach is needed, one that applies the same standards for evidence of clinical utility as are required of psychological and behavioral explanations. It is unlikely that genes can account for the rapid increase in diagnosis of some disorders that are thought to be genetically based, e.g., ADHD, autism, bipolar disorder, and eating disorders (National Institutes of Health (NIH) Consensus Statement 1998; Weiss *et al.* 2008). A particularly provocative finding is that the pattern of cortical maturation of ADHD children is the same as for non-ADHD children, but delayed, reaching maturity at 10.5 years for ADHD children versus 7.5 years for non-ADHD children (Shaw *et al.* 2007). The delay was most prominent in the prefrontal areas associated with attention and motor control. Causes of the delay were not explored, but the findings are consistent with expectation, based on DMM theory, if the parents of the ADHD children were less predictable than those of the non-ADHD children. For these and other disorders, a more realistic hypothesis is that unique genetic variation interacts with universal genetic processes unfolding in a context of family-specific distress and cultural change (McGuire *et al.* 2007; Rutter 2005, 2006a). The cultural change may reflect either new child-rearing patterns (e.g., working mothers, high rates of early childcare, greater involvement of fathers, etc.) or more stringent standards regarding parenting or child behavior. Indeed, the change might be the health and social care industry itself seeking to expand its 'market share' of distress and problems of adaptation. If any of these causes has actually affected the rate of disorder, it would not be the first time that intentions to do good had untoward, iatrogenic effects.

Adolescence (puberty – 16 years)

Puberty, like the preoperational shift in the second year of life, is a period of biologically based maturation. Cognitively, adolescents become able to think abstractly and, thus, to reflect on both their own and others' behavior in generalized ways. The onset of sexual desire and behavior changes ... everything! It is like adding technicolor to a black-and-white world. The obvious effect is in peer relationships, but the effects of sexual hormones color every relationship and many, many other aspects of behavior and development.

It is important to recognize that feelings of anxious arousal and sexual arousal are quite similar and can be confused easily (see Table 3.1). The extensive overlap in function, behavior, and feeling between attachment and sexuality creates particular circumstances for families in which one or the other system malfunctions. Because one system can elicit or substitute for the other, the essential functions of protection and reproduction appear overdetermined to the point of being almost fail-safe processes. Thus, in families with attachment problems, sexuality may provide a pathway to achieving closeness and comfort.

Strategies

The new strategies in adolescence are compulsive promiscuity (A5) and compulsive self-reliance (A6). Both are possible outcomes of compulsive caregiving (A3) and compliance/performance (A4) failing to make the parent–child relationship workable.

Individuals using the compulsively promiscuous strategy (A5) still seek close relationships, but they seek them with not-yet-known people (strangers) because their experience with family relationships has been uniformly disappointing and often dangerous. Still, they believe that there is someone for them, someone they don't know yet. When the strategy is

Table 3.1 Parallel arousal systems

Autonomic arousal	Sexual arousal
Death	Death
Pain	Sexual pain
Fear	Sexual terror
Anger	Sexual aggression and submission
Desire for comfort	Romanticism
Comfort	Sexual satisfaction
Bored	Afterglow
Tired	Drowsiness
Sleep	Sleep
Depression	Numbness
Death	Death

only social, its dangers are limited, but when the promiscuity is sexual, the strategy carries risk of danger (including violence, venereal disease, and feelings of abandonment and worthlessness) to all parties. The extreme of the strategy is prostitution, the predictable exchange of services for money. Prostitution isn't just a way to earn money for women down on their luck (fast-food restaurants can serve that function); it is a way of life, a way of thinking and feeling – or more accurately of not feeling while acting out false sexual desire (see Figure 3.2).

Compulsive self-reliance (A6) reflects the opposite solution. Such individuals conclude that they are unfit for relationships, that the problem lies inherently with them. Some individuals using an A6 strategy can manage social relationships, but not intimate spousal or parent–child relationships. Others are isolated to the point of not being able to sustain any relationships. Depression is a major risk for the latter group because the Type A strategy defines the self through the eyes of others, and individuals using an A6 strategy, especially in the isolated form, have both defined the self as too negative for relationships and lost access to an outside 'mirror' with which to see the self. Sexual impropriety with children is also a risk both out of a desire for comfort and because age peers are too threatening.

A Dynamic-Maturational Model of Patterns of Attachment in Adolescence

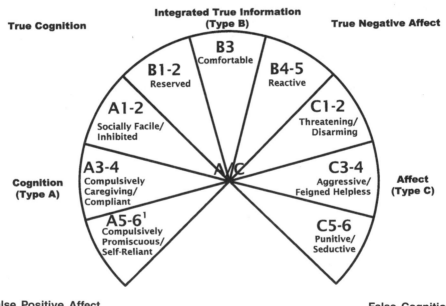

Copyright: Patricia M. Crittenden, 2001

Figure 3.2 The adolescent patterns of attachment

Opportunity

The central opportunity for adolescents is the chance to live in a world that is not defined by the characteristics of their childhood home. Their linguistic and cognitive skills, combined with an array of subtle affective signals used in regulated ways, enable adolescents to form many different relationships, develop their personal skills maximally, and prepare themselves to live independently of their parents and with a peer attachment figure. With self-awareness and abstract reasoning, adolescents can choose consciously to participate in the process of treatment.

Problems

Problems occur when parents retain too much authority, refusing to shift to the role of supportive adviser, or, conversely, prematurely abandon their adolescents as if they were fully mature.

The compulsive Type A strategies tend to function well in the school years. Because children are focused on pleasing adults by taking their perspectives and doing what they prefer, adults are pleased and reward children well. Although there are some long-term risks, they rarely announce themselves clearly before they strike.

> The Brightman family was exceptional. Seven children: six girls and then, after a gap, the youngest, a boy. Mr Brightman had risen to be the head of a small, but very successful, company; his wife cared for their children at home. Home was a well-kept, spacious house in the 'right' part of a small rural town. As the girls moved through the grades at school, one after another, they collected awards. All were exceptionally intelligent and each claimed her place on the academic honor roll. In addition, they were beautiful, graceful, and friendly. Each dressed in stylish clothing. No money was spared, but neither was it splashed – good taste was the standard in the Brightman family. By high school, each girl joined the right clubs (the debate club, future teachers club, a religious club, foreign relations club), and eventually each became head of a club. Each was voted by her classmates to represent them in the student government and, by their final year, each ran for, and several became, the head of the Student Council. Socially, the girls were selected by their peers as prom princesses and every one, in her final year, became prom queen. The girls were glamorous, poised, and successful.
>
> Mary, without question, was the most popular girl in her grade, always smiling, always speaking gently, but heard above the din of noisy adolescents, and always in a group of the brightest and best. Needless to say, Mary attracted the right sort of boys – although no one could recall whether she had a steady boyfriend or not. Mary was always proper, never skipping school or cutting class, never drinking, never cheating. The Brightman girls were 'good' girls, but still

fun-loving, humorous, and easy-going. As with her older sisters before her and her younger ones to come, Mary was marked at graduation by her bright future. She was headed to one of the best universities. Even later, when her classmates were queried, no one could recall being envious; she was much too nice and so obviously deserving.

In an amazing feat of achievement for her family, one couldn't find a cloud on her horizon, nor on that of her siblings. I often note to my audiences that when it's too good to be true, it isn't likely to be true. Is there risk in this story? If there is, what would it be? Is it too good to be true?

Of course, life doesn't end at the close of high school, but it is a natural break point. So we break the Brightman story here, to pick it up in the next chapter.

Risk

The riskiest time is early puberty when young adolescents do not yet know how to manage their new sexual feelings. Precocious sexual activity may both interrupt development and also result in dangerous sexual liaisons, sexually transmitted disease and permanent infertility, and premature parenthood. Lonely adolescents are especially at risk.

> When David was only 12 years old, he met a girl. Like him, she was quiet and lonely. Like him, she was uncomforted, but in addition, she was unsafe; her home was marked by violence to herself, her siblings, and her mother. At first, David and his new friend just talked and talked, excited to find someone interested in them. But the closeness they each needed and the new sexual feelings that came with puberty drew them to touching and kissing and caressing. After years of being untouched, they were breathlessly excited to find each other. They became a couple long before more accepted kids had left the groups of young adolescents to pair off. For David and his girl, there wasn't much playing the field; indeed, for them, there wasn't a field of possible choices. Just two lonely kids lucky enough to find each other.
>
> When they talked about the future, they created dream families that undid the fear and loneliness of their childhoods. David dreamed of taking care of his wife as his father had failed to do. He talked quietly about how wonderful his mother was and how much he hated his bullying, mocking, violent father. He would be different. Most of all, he said, his children would never go unattended and uncared for as he had. He would be a different sort of husband and father, a good, caring, and loving man. His girlfriend had similar dreams. She wanted a gentle and kind husband, one who wouldn't scare or hurt her, or their children. Because her father had been so distant and cold, she especially wanted a man who would be affectionate and involved with their children.

After the loneliness of childhood, sexuality created the possibility of warmth, affection, and intimacy for David and his girl. They felt incredibly lucky to have found each other. They married right out of school when they were each 17 years old.

David's developmental experience gives us the opportunity to think about variations in how sexuality is expressed *before* we become offended by David's future sexual contact with his children. Up to now, theorizing about sexual offenders has begun with the offense and worked backward to explain and predict it theoretically. Indeed, all the major theories of sexual deviance begin with the deviant acts or deviant men (e.g., Finkelhor 1984; Hall and Hirschman 1992; Marshall and Barbaree 1990; Ward and Beech 2006; Ward *et al.* 2006) This starting point can lead to a dehumanization of the men in which they become 'molestors', 'pedophiles', etc.; their behavior is labeled 'deviant'; and their characteristics are defined as 'entrenched' 'traits' (see Ward and Beech 2006 for this sort of usage). This sort of language, developed for adult sexual offenders, makes it almost impossible to see the whole man or even to think of aspects of the man that exist outside his offending behavior. Moreover, the language obscures the developmental process that generated the adult; this process, if it were revealed progressively as I have tried to do here, would be expected to yield compassionate feelings for the boy that would temper our feelings of offense and fear when the sexually inappropriate behavior is later exhibited by the man. Finally, a truly developmental approach, i.e., one that begins in infancy and moves forward (not backward from adulthood), can enable application of human developmental theory to all humans, as opposed to the need for a specialized theory for sexual offenders (or any vulnerable subgroup from individuals with personality disorders to those with psychotic breaks). One goal of presenting these vignettes is to clarify the humanity of parents who endanger their children and, in so doing, to approach a human theory of self-protection, reproduction, and adaptation.

Both the Brightman girls, with their compulsive performance strategy (A4–) and David and his girl, with their compulsive self-reliance (A6) and dreams of a different kind of childhood (possibly a bit of delusional idealization (A7) with compulsive caregiving (A3)), left adolescence with high hopes. Their strategies, however, carried risks for them during the transition to adulthood. To reduce their risk, they would need to gain awareness of the compulsive qualities of their strategies and access to the blocked-out information about their negative feelings.

The onset of puberty creates opportunities to meet, albeit belatedly, some childhood needs that have to do with attachment; in this case, a close and comforting relationship with someone who is not a threat. That sexuality can accomplish this is no surprise: the autonomic and sexual arousal systems are very similar, as are the behaviors that serve attachment and sexual functions. Moreover, both functions (attachment and reproduction) bring two people together, establish bonds of affection between them, and promote safety and comfort. Only sexual intercourse and reproduction differentiate the systems – and the opportunity for sex isn't usually rejected by adolescents!

The cortical development associated with adolescence permits adolescents to think about their experience and to make plans for their future. Both of these processes served David and his girlfriend well. The only worry that one might have – and David and his girlfriend didn't worry about this at all – is that reversal strategies often backfire. Unless the strategy is accompanied by a progressive series of changes in both behavior and information processing, there is a risk that the plan will function like the proverbial pendulum, going so far in the opposite direction that it becomes as undesirable as that which it reverses.

Even more complex forms of risk are those where the source of the problem is not clear and the risk created is risk to the self in the form of eating disorders and substance abuse (both are often associated with C3-6 strategies). Ironically these problems often occur when parents have tried to protect their adolescent from the parents' problem – by hiding the problem.

Nancy is a case in point. Two weeks before she was to begin high school in the middle-class district where her family lived, she received notice that she was being sent to the school in an adjacent low-income district. No appeal was possible. Life was rough in this metropolitan school; there were gangs, fights, high truancy, and drugs. Nancy lost access to her former friends and continued to struggle academically. Her after-school hours were lonely, and she sulked in her bedroom. Then she found a boy and – zip! – her life changed. No more afternoons shut up alone in her room. Nancy was in a crowd of kids and she was in love. Her grades dropped further. She wasn't attending school regularly any more, but her parents both worked and were unaware. She became moody and hostile – any questions were treated as intrusive accusations that pried into her personal business. Home became a tightrope of her parents trying to stay connected without 'butting in' and tripping her anger. Psychotherapy was tried again. But the therapist believed that talking to Nancy's parents violated her privacy and insisted on working entirely alone. He didn't even tell them when she cut appointments. What no one knew was that her moods and her defensiveness covered increasing alcohol use and then drug abuse. Nancy was facing dangers that exceeded her capacity for self-protection, but she had the skills and opportunity to hide the problems. Indeed, she even had the model for solving problems that way, an unintentional gift from her parents.

Nancy is a reminder that development is dynamic and not fully predictable. Her childhood began well enough, but took a downturn when she entered school. We can never be certain what caused what, but we can speculate.

Both her parents had had academic problems themselves. Did entry to school trigger fears that Nancy felt but no one could name? Both her parents had lost a sibling in childhood, but no one talked about this; indeed, the loss was actively kept out of sight by one parent and conveniently 'forgotten' by the other. Did her parents have inarticulate fears that made them want to keep Nancy nearby? Did her parents' strategy of silence around painful topics reduce the possibility that Nancy would be able to talk about her distress? Were they silent because no one had been available to comfort them or because they had never learned effective problem-solving and conflict-resolution strategies – or both?

Having a hypothesis generally is key to understanding such potentially complex questions and answers; this is what the DMM offers: a theory that addresses complex, interactive, and not fully transparent influences on development. In Nancy's case, the past lack of resolution was related to strategies of silence that then reduced her parents' ability, in their childhoods, to learn to resolve problems. That combination, plus their hope of doing better for Nancy, created the potential for problems that would be hard to define and harder to correct. What we know now is that Nancy thought she was supposed to be her parents' bright future – and she didn't feel up to the task.

Of course, Nancy's elementary schoolteachers contributed too. Any one of them might have become an auxiliary attachment figure, but instead they tried to rescue Nancy (in a bid for personal glory?). Then, when defeated, they isolated and taunted her, even calling her names in front of the class; they taught her to be a victim. We couldn't have predicted that from her childhood, nor from her parents', but her inability to articulate problems was surely learned at home.

The final blow was the change of high school that exposed her to dangers far beyond her ZPD. This occurred at a time when her parents were preoccupied with work and their own personal issues. They didn't know enough about Nancy's life, and, possibly, it was already too late for them to be helpful.

Another serious threat to future parenting capacity occurs when the adolescent's behavior is so unacceptable and dangerous to others that containment and punishment override nurturing responses.

> After puberty, Jackson combined romantic relationships with continued aggressive behavior. His fighting and vindictiveness resulted in his being dismissed from school, brought him to the attention of the police, and destroyed a series of placements until he was placed in a group home for troubled adolescents who had no other place to live. Jackson was becoming desperate and was still swinging between seeing himself as needing rescue and braggadocio claims of invulnerability. After he began cutting himself and attempted suicide, he was again placed briefly on a psychiatric ward.

Like many troubled boys (Tommy and Nick, for example), Jackson was a charmer. Indeed, he was almost charismatic. Consequently, when he met Janine, things took off quickly. As with David, it began as just talking and being friends, rather than dating. Jackson wasn't really looking for a girlfriend, and, when he found Janine, he wasn't playing the field. Instead, he was a loner who struck it lucky. Their comfortable friendship very quickly became an attachment. Sexuality was part of it, but it probably wasn't the basis of the relationship. To hear Jackson tell it, he became almost a member of Janine's family; indeed, once or twice in the retelling, he referred to Janine's parents as his parents. It seemed almost as if he wanted her family as much as he wanted her.

Nevertheless, there were serious problems between him and Janine in which Jackson seemed far more vulnerable to rejection or cheating than did Janine. This probably explains his verbal confusion, as he tells the story, about whether she was vulnerable and deserved protection from males or was the aggressor from whom he needed protection. That is, he seemed to confuse physical and psychological power.

After saying he had intentionally cheated on her to make her jealous enough to want him, Jackson said in rapid, run-on phrases: *Janine come down and started kicking off, and Janine used to beat me, quite severely, like black eyes, break my nose, bite me, pinch me, and kick me, you know, to the extent where I was in that much pain I could actually cry, you know, and I've been hit by full-grown blokes and I don't want to cry, but she actually put severe pain on me by carrying on hitting you, and, as I don't like hitting women, I just never used to do anything and we was down the park and she just kept hitting me and hitting me 'n' I didn't want to hit her, but I had to do something before she got past me to [incomprehensible], I know it seems nasty, but I had to stop, you know, it would have been a fight, and she just kept laying into me, and I basically pushed her away and grabbed her round the throat, not like you know crush, I got like – round the, like round the side there, and I – round the side there, flung her head under – round the back of me and put her in a headlock and it wasn't a headlock where you couldn't move. I knew what I was doing, and I did it so she could move, so it wouldn't hurt her or give her any marks...*

This excerpt, from Jackson's Transition to Adulthood Attachment Interview (TAAI) a year later, suggests the extent of his dangerousness, vulnerability, and psychological confusion in mid-adolescence. Professionals can find it difficult to engage with adolescents who present a mixture of dangerousness and vulnerability. Again, there is a tendency to reduce the complexity by omitting one part of the individual from representation, thus distorting the other by making it seem the totality. For some professionals, this yields compassion – and limited willingness to deal with the threat of the adolescent. For others, it results in a restrictive and punitive response that ignores the adolescent's history and current vulnerability. Neither approach is likely to work – because the situation is complex.

The similarities with David (a compulsive A) are substantial: a precocious love relationship, lack of any selection process, the overlap in romantic and attachment motivations, and the centrality of the relationship to the boy's self-image and future. All of these mark the relationship as a potentially ill-fated attempt to resolve in adolescence problems brought from childhood. But Jackson's relationship has differences from David's as well. The most obvious is the threat of violence; both the fight with Janine (when Jackson was 15) and the style of telling the event (the discourse when Jackson was 16) are very alarming. In addition, however, Jackson is more focused on the present, confuses it with the past, and is much less interested in planning for the future (all Type C characteristics). Moreover, he thinks only of himself, rather than expressing a desire to do better for his children. His speech is filled with evocative words, suggesting Jackson's intense and unpredictable arousal. Finally, there is uncertainty in Jackson's mind as to who is the perpetrator and who the victim (a C5-6 distortion). This may be tied to the triangulation and deception that he has repeated from his parents' experience (his mother's cheating). All of these suggest a different developmental pathway from David's; Jackson has the complexity of using both compulsive Type A strategies and obsessively coercive Type C strategies.

When young adolescents 'act out' against others in a misattribution of responsibility and revenge, they can cause a degree of damage that elicits moral approbation, custodial care, and punishment. Once that process begins, adolescents' opportunity to be the recipient of nurturant care and to shift developmental direction is greatly reduced.

The complexity of development in childhood

Once children go to school, life becomes much more complex. Surely this is true for children, but it is also true for professionals if they are called in to deal with problems. Three conditions are crucial for understanding this complexity: (a) the increase in the number and type of influences on children, (b) the 'sleeper' effects of pre-existing risks that do not become manifest until school activates them, and (c) hidden 'family secrets' or triangulating processes that affect parental behavior, but in ways that children and professionals cannot see and parents often don't even realize are occurring.

This chapter and its vignettes of children and parents suggest the nature of some of this complexity, but possibly the points made by the specific cases need to be summarized in a more generalized form, one that can expand the notion of developmental pathways. Let's 'pull it together' – let's integrate.

They say that readers can take away only three ideas. I offer 10! Choose your favorite three – and don't forget them! (I'll try to help by clustering them as child-related, parent-related, and professional-related. If you choose those three, you'll have them all!)

Ideas about children

1 *Timeliness*. Each developmental stage has different opportunities and threats (Sroufe *et al.* 1999). To the extent that parents function in children's ZPD, they can be helpful. But when parents are too involved or insufficiently involved (or alternate between these), children may find it hard to learn self-protective skills that can protect them from the stage-salient threats in their context. Type C children need to learn predictable causal effects in infancy before they can be expected to comprehend indirect causal effects; e.g., my mother is focused on her problems with my father so she yells at me. Type A children need to learn that negative affects that aren't displayed are still negative feelings that can motivate their behavior. Once a necessary step is missed, future development becomes more difficult.

2 *Unintended effects*. The non-B strategies have powerful effects on other people. Some reflect the function of the strategy, e.g., securing parental attention, whereas others are unintended. Among the unintended 'side effects' are recreating characteristics of the parent–child problems in the teacher–child relationship, as Nancy and Tommy did with their coercive strategy and all the Brightman children did with adults' high expectations. When the strategy is distorted (Type A or C), there is usually a discrepancy between how children feel and the effects they have on others. Children need clarification that both articulates effects, such that children recognize them in specific (concrete) instances, and identifies the precise feelings experienced by the child (such that inhibited feelings are made apparent and global feelings are differentiated.) For example, Nancy felt weak and powerless, but she had powerful effects on both her parents and teachers. This needs clarification to both Nancy (who needs to see her effects and discriminate her incompatible feelings) and professionals (who need to understand the complexity of Nancy's displayed powerlessness and inhibited, passive anger).

   Professionals might want to keep in mind that their strategies, too, can have unintended effects. For example, removing children from dangerous parents to safe foster parents may increase children's anxiety, teach them that they have no control over what happens to them, or, if repeated moves occur, cause them to treat professionals, cumulatively and generically, as attachment figures. Similarly, removing an undesirable symptom (e.g., outbursts of anger), without addressing the cause or function of the symptom, may generate a more hidden and self-damaging symptom (e.g., chronic intestinal distress).

3   *Comfort*. Comfort is as important to adaptation as is safety. When comfort is pervasively lacking, sexuality may replace it. That is, sex in the school years is usually not about sex. The 'comfort disorders' may have very severe effects on both the self and others, long into the future.

Ideas about parents

4   *Good intentions*. If we begin with the assumption that *all* parents are well-meaning, we may discover new explanations for their behavior. These explanations might guide us to more effective interventions. Of course, good intentions are not enough (this is true for professionals as well). Nevertheless, being seen as you believe that you are, and not as you are accused of being, can make it possible for a parent to want the help a professional can offer.

5   *Feeling good about oneself*. Children need to feel good about themselves; when they don't, they can become dangerous to themselves or others. Parents must feel good about themselves; hurt parents can be dangerous to themselves and their children. Professionals, too, must feel good; if they don't, they may become a danger to children and families. The principles of human adaptation are the same for everyone.

Ideas for professionals

6   *Appearances can be misleading*. Non-B self-protective strategies create appearances that can mislead. If we assume that aggressive children truly feel strong, we will be misled – and our treatments may fail. If we assume that weak children are only weak, we will be misled. If we assume that overachieving children are really perfect, we may miss serious problems entirely. To see below self-protective surfaces, professionals need both to be trained in observation and to have theory and empirical findings that suggest where to look for possible false appearances and how they function.

7   *Self-deception*. The distortions in the non-B strategies deceive both observers and the self. Ways of accessing more accurate information are needed and these are unlikely to be through direct questions.

Without guidance, children using distorted strategies will not understand why they act as they do. Asking them 'Why did you do that when you knew you weren't supposed to?' is unlikely to yield an answer that informs either the professional or the child. To get a useful answer, we must either be willing to accept true, but undesirable, answers or use theory to point the way, finding nonverbal ways to elicit the information. The latter is more likely to be effective. Without understanding their own motivations accurately, children will not be able to regulate their behavior adequately.

It is worth noting that no one ever asks children who do what adults want (as did the Brightman children) why they are doing that. This means, of course, that they are not urged to explain themselves and, if someday pleasing adults by being good doesn't motivate their behavior, they may be entirely unable to explain themselves.

8 *Causation versus effect.* Attention to the conditions that contribute to dysfunction may be necessary to resolve serious problems. Ridding a child or parent of symptoms may not be enough; in some cases, it can even make things worse. For example, behavioral feedback to reduce bed-wetting in a school-age child may, in fact, rid the child of the undesirable behavior. However, if the behavior is a symptom of a psychological issue (maybe excessive fear or unexpressed anger), removing the symptom will not correct the problem, which would be likely to appear in a different form later.

9 *Empirical feedback.* Unintended and untoward consequences can appear unexpectedly in spite of the best of intentions. This is true for children who organize distorted self-protective strategies, parents who try to protect children using ineffective or harmful strategies, and professionals who apply treatments. All hope for the best. Only professionals have the training to know that they need to collect feedback data to ensure that what they do is helpful and not harmful. They should do that.

10 *Complexity.* Dichotomization (into good versus bad, victim versus perpetrator, blame versus innocence, clients versus professionals, anger versus fear, etc.) distorts the actual complexity of most problems. A particular problem is overlooking the complicity of victims and of professionals.

The bottom line: false shortcuts usually fail

Developmental pathways are complex and must be understood and treated with enough complexity to represent reality with reasonable accuracy. They are not fully predictable from their starting point, nor are they trajectories. Serious disorder requires many contributions and some of them are unpredictable and out of anyone's control.

Too often, however, opportunities for beneficial change are missed by professionals through use of shortcuts that were intended to save time and money. Too often, shortcuts exacerbate problems, delaying their ultimate display until the complexity exceeds our capacity to understand and resolve them. When that happens, we professionals blame ... the disorder! It's incurable, it's genetic, it's ... not our responsibility to assess more thoroughly and design potentially expensive interventions that address the range of problems that a child, parent–child dyad or family might experience.

It is important to note that treatment need not address, far less correct, every causal condition. Service providers and their managers need to identify those conditions that require change (usually those that are dangerous) and those that can facilitate future change when undertaken by the individual. The notion of 'critical causes' (Crittenden and Ainsworth 1989) can help professionals to make choices regarding the focus of intervention. Critical causes are those conditions which, if changed, would initiate a cascade of naturally occurring changes. For example, addressing literacy in an illiterate adult can change everything: job, income, housing, etc. It is crucial, however, that professionals assess causation so as to decide which issues require intervention.

Professionals are responsible for implementing shortcuts, and this, therefore, is what we can change.

Notes

1 Deception appears to be an innately human behavior that has found an evolved place in our behavioral repertoire because it promotes survival (Dawkins 2008: 191–2).

Chapter 4

Becoming an adult: Leaving and loving

Historically, most people become parents at 16–25 years of age in the 'transition to adulthood' (although in technologically advanced nations this is delayed, creating a dyssynchrony between biology and culture). Young parents' major functions at that time become keeping the new baby alive until it reaches reproductive maturity and helping the developing infant to learn to protect him or herself. Of course, to do this, the parent too must stay safe. Attachment is how this generation-to-generation process is accomplished. What matters for a successful outcome is not how secure one's relationships with childhood attachment figures were, but rather:

1 whether the self-protective strategies learned in childhood function protectively in the current context;
2 whether they enable one to perceive and respond protectively to the needs of one's partner and children;
3 what information processing underlies them;
4 the extent to which that processing permits flexibility of strategy.

Adaptability and flexibility are the central issues in the transition to adulthood. One cannot know what the future will bring; to be ready, one must be ready to change. The point is not that the Type B behavioral strategy is best; it isn't. When one is dealing with dangerous deception or even erroneous sincerity, one must be protectively alert and responsive to the precarious situation. Open and direct revealing of one's intent and feeling might be very unwise. Put that way, it becomes clear that, in the transition to adulthood, a wise adult learns to differentiate balanced mental processing of information from behavioral enactment of the safest strategy. In other words, an adult who generally uses a Type B strategy will need to be able to use Type A and Type C strategies when faced with certain kinds of threat without losing access to the Type B strategy.

Transition to adulthood (16–25 years)

Strategies

The period from the mid-teens to the mid-twenties is when the potential of childhood is fulfilled. For those who have found safety, comfort, and psychological balance, fulfillment takes the form of economic independence and an adulthood family that will give birth to the next generation of humans. For those who are less fortunate, this decade offers possibly the best opportunity in life for change. For those who do not use this opportunity, this is a period of terrible risks that can destroy the rest of life or the lives of one's children. The stakes, in other words, are very high. All the serious disorders take shape in the transition to adulthood: the psychoses, the personality disorders, debilitating somatic disorders, and violent criminal behavior.

Two new strategies develop within the Type A group, delusional idealization (A7) and an externally assembled self (A8; see Figure 4.1). Delusional idealization is likely to occur when it has been impossible to escape the control of dangerous people, for whatever reason; that is, the individual might try and fail or fail to try because delusional idealization makes it possible to avoid awareness of the need for change. In any case, the person developing a strategy of delusional idealization takes the A5 distortion a step further by attributing protection and comfort to people who have severely endangered the self. These people can be childhood attachment figures or adult captors (e.g., the 'Stockholm syndrome' in which hostages take the perspective of the kidnapper and both justify his behavior and trust him to protect them) (Cassidy 2002; Goddard and Stanley 1994; Kuleshnyk 1984). Selecting endangering partners over safe people is a very distorted and dangerous choice. It can be observed among youth who are attracted to cults and similar groups, but may also occur in nongroup settings.

An externally assembled self (A8) is one possible outcome of having had too many caregivers and homes, none of which was permanent. One can't attach to a moving crowd, especially when the members of the crowd have no memory of one's past. Thus, adolescents who had numerous care placements across childhood are particularly susceptible candidates for this strategy. The strategy itself places all important information in others – in their minds, in their knowledge, and in their file drawers. Externally assembled individuals have gone beyond a false positive, parent-pleasing self to an absence of self except as others (especially professionals) define them to be. Because this strategy is the result of having no permanent attachment figures, it is often an iatrogenic strategy, one created by the professional service system when children have been moved from one placement to another too frequently.

Within Type C, there are three forms of very dangerous behavior that develop in the transition to adulthood (see Figure 4.1). The first is intimate

A Dynamic-Maturational Model of Patterns of Attachment in Adulthood

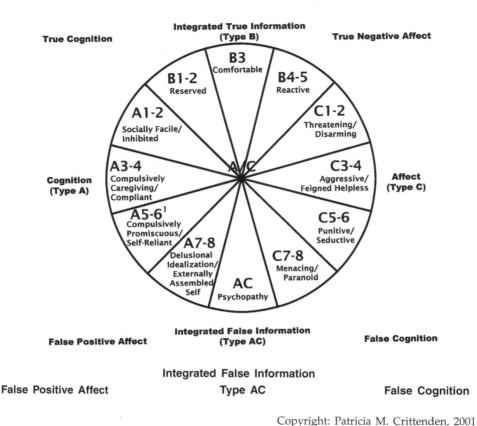

Copyright: Patricia M. Crittenden, 2001

Figure 4.1 The adult patterns of attachment

domestic violence, bully–victim relationships between partners that are maintained by both attachment and sexuality. In these relationships, sexual signaling and reproductive opportunity become confused with attachment needs for protection and comfort. Both partners try to attract and hold the other, both fear and expect deception, and women in particular use deception to get revenge against men's physical aggression. The deception that men fear most is sexual, that is, being cuckolded and deceived into raising another man's child; this fear is realized in an appreciable proportion of couples, but the exact number is difficult to establish (Bellis *et al.* 2005). The form of deception used most among women is to needle the man around his weakness – with a turn of phrase, a smirking look, and the like. The result is that the man is labeled the perpetrator and punished, and the woman is considered the victim and benefits from social sympathy. Even though both know that this dichotomization does not reflect their complex relationship accurately, neither can adequately articulate their interpersonal process – and the woman may be quite satisfied with the dichotomized view of her situation.

The second form of dangerous Type C organization involves a few very angry and fearful individuals whose Type C strategy will escalate to a menacing/paranoid (C7–8) strategy. At C7–8, the focused anger and fear that motivate C5–6 behavior become less focused such that more people are potential targets and more are feared. That is, the individual is angry, but also unclear about the source of the anger and, therefore, unclear about the target of aggression. In such cases, unexpected attacks that are justified irrationally will be plotted with subtly deceptive skill, using the sophisticated capacity of the mature adult brain. Very few people using a C7–8 strategy become parents, although when it happens, it can be very dangerous for the children.

In the third form, the vulnerabilities and psychological distortions of both the compulsive Type As and the obsessive Type Cs are combined in one individual. The result can be a combination of planned and controlled attacks (C7–8) with unplanned triggers (A4,7), i.e., intrusions of forbidden negative affect. The two probable forms of this are (a) a poorly organized set of A and C strategies, marked by intrusions of unresolved trauma, and (b) a highly integrated form of the strategy in which behavior is under very tight control, but marked by violent attempts to achieve closeness and revenge. The former can be thought of as similar to the diagnosis of borderline personality disorder and the latter to the diagnosis of psychopathy.

Service systems

Given these opportunities and risks, it is nothing short of astounding that our service systems provide less support during this decade than at any other point in life. Moreover, the greater the risk, the less the support. Adolescents whose homes have been too dangerous for them to remain with their parents and adolescents who themselves have been too dangerous to remain at home are both 'dropped' in the gap in services between childhood and adulthood. Neither child-and-adolescent services nor adult services attend properly to the needs of 16–25-year-olds.

Even when they qualify for services (usually through presenting with psychotic breaks, personality disorders, severe somatic dysfunction, or violent behavior), young adults are almost always treated as individuals and rarely treated in the context of relationships and families. This is linked to the issue in much forensic practice whereby 'dangerousness' is located within the individual rather than the individual in relation to others. The near exclusive focus on individuals, rather than individuals with a history of relationships embedded in more or less dangerous contexts, is a problem with much 'risk assessment' work. This, it is argued here, is not helpful, given that (a) their risk comes from their childhood relationships and (b) their emerging adult relationships will either maintain their state of risk or correct it, depending upon how partners are selected and relationships are managed. Only if they become parents, do they qualify for dyadic or family services and, if they are parents, much of the opportunity for change has already been lost.

Acknowledgment of the crucial importance to development and adaptation of the meso- and exosystems (Bronfenbrenner 1979a) is inescapable in the transition to adulthood. Were professional service systems (the mesosystem) and cultural values and priorities (the exosystem) managed differently, we should be able to reduce substantially the number of seriously mentally ill adults, children who will suffer from inadequate parental care, and adults who inflict sexual or violent harm on others (Crighton and Towl 2008).

Opportunity

To return to the pattern of the previous sections, the opportunity of the transition to adulthood is that, having a mature brain and being relatively able to care for themselves and not yet connected to a spouse and children, young adults have the possibility to orchestrate their own reorganization. They can choose to change themselves, with or without professional help, and do so without being constrained by either their family of origin or their future partner and children. The latter is especially important. However much one might hope to correct the mistakes of one's parents, few young adults who are at risk are able to attract balanced partners (Crittenden *et al.* 1991). Instead, they tend to select partners whose degree of risk is similar to their own (Kerr and Bowen 1988). Whether the risk is similar in Type or the opposite, the relationship is organized around distorted strategies, and this tends to maintain each partner's distortion. Engaging in a process of change with lighter psychological baggage from the past and without acquired baggage from the future maximizes the possibility that newly acquired intellectual competency can be applied productively to changing oneself and one's future.

Problems

Problems are maintained for individuals with mild or moderate risk when they do not seize the moment and, instead, move directly into establishing adulthood families. Both continuations of strategy and reversals of strategy, i.e., changes between Type A and Type C, occur.

In other cases, the problems can escalate to very serious conditions. If one stays at home too long or leaves too soon, the course of development may be changed in ways that endanger the self or others.

Some young adults are so invisibly entangled in their parents' functioning that both they and the parents know inexplicably that their departure will destroy the family, as would explicit expression of the problem and their negative feelings about the situation. For these young adults, expression of their distress is deflected such that it appears in nonfamilial interpersonal problems (i.e., a personality disorder), addictions that enable the perception of escape, somatic problems (e.g., eating disorders, chronic, stress-related somatic disorders), or psychotic-like disorders. In all of these cases, the problem is often 'externalized' in that a disease condition is 'blamed' for the individual's limitations. These strategies, in other words, can both be self-deceptive and mislead others. All have a component of intense negative affect, although this varies regarding whether it is an elaboration of coercion (C5–6) or an intrusion into a Type A strategy of forbidden negative affect. In most cases, the goals of treatment will be to change the misguided thoughts (the eating and personality disorders), end the chemical dependency, reduce the symptoms (the somatic disorders), or regulate arousal with chemicals (the psychoses). Nevertheless, treatment success with these disorders is very low, and the disorders tend to become chronic and sometimes crippling. In both cases, parenting casualties are high, with troubled children, divorce, and placement in care as possible outcomes.

Type C problems

There is a gradient of Type C disorders from which two examples will be offered. The first is the conclusion of Nancy's story.

> Nancy's transition to adulthood began with a stay in an alcohol treatment centre. Nevertheless, she graduated from high school. Six months later, however, she was living on her own; it was just too difficult for everyone for her to stay longer in her family. Living alone is lonely, and boys and alcohol ease loneliness. A pattern was begun that wasn't overcome for another decade. By then, she had two small sons who were affected as well.

At the turning points in development, things kept going wrong for Nancy. The early conditions, both hers and her parents, combined with unexpectable twists (misguided teachers, ineffective therapists, and a dangerous school) to expose Nancy to dangers that would take years to correct, with some outcomes (such as addiction and inability to establish enduring relationships) that would always hurt.

Is there a point where another direction could have been taken? We could hope that future parents wouldn't bring problems to their children, teachers wouldn't get frustrated, and school districts wouldn't be modified, but such hopes are unlikely to be realized. Is there a way out when development goes awry?

The best opportunity for change is in the hands of teachers and psychotherapists. How? By asking different questions, accepting unexpected answers, and connecting the dots of knowledge to see a different picture of risk and opportunity (because Nancy's well-meaning parents reflected opportunity as well as risk). Family-level assessment and a broad range of interventions need to be offered in ways that protect the parents' dreams while increasing the probability of their being realized. Because most parents have no idea what is wrong, we, the professionals, are troubled families' best chance to change the developmental pathway.

Eating disorders present a similar problem – with some twists.

Sophie arrived at the adolescent eating disorders unit emaciated and with her mother in tow; her father was busy elsewhere. Just when she should have been vibrant, sexy, and thinking about boys and going off to college, Sophie was scrawny, sexually unappealing, silent, and tied to her mother. Discussion among the staff quickly revealed dissension. Some thought Sophie should be treated as fragile and close to death; this group thought she should be cosseted and nurtured a bit. Others thought Sophie was powerful and manipulative; this group recommended a tough line. The ward was filled with discord. Behavioral plans were tried and discarded. Body image work followed; Sophie didn't gain weight and still didn't like her 'fat' body. As her weight dropped, her physician considered tube-feeding. With no disease condition, plentiful food, and parents who clearly loved her, Sophie was close to dying.

Prior to instigating the forced feeding, her doctor began a series of sessions with Sophie. How was she? What did she think about the unit, her disorder, her family, etc.? Sophie had almost nothing to say. In fact, her silences were so long that they felt extremely uncomfortable and even accusatory. For sure, they placed all the burden of finding a way forward on the doctor and let Sophie decide when to offer a monosyllable and when not. Sophie was rude, but in the most passive way. He asked about her childhood: 'I'm sorry. I have a really bad memory. I'm sorry.' She seemed so pitiful, but really! could she recall nothing? This sort of loss of information was startling; the doctor scheduled a Transition to Adult Attachment Interview (TAAI) to get a handle on how Sophie used information.

Sophie's TAAI was characterized by silence. The phrases that she used to describe her relationship with her mother came painfully slowly, but were all positive. Sophie treasured her mother. Or did she? When asked to supply evidence, Sophie had none. 'Wonderful, loving.' 'Always, she just was.' Nothing was concrete or memorable – except an illness she had had during the first months of life which, she was told, had cleared up completely. Still it came up several times, with a pattern of dysfluence around it – as if it were an unresolved trauma. The TAAI took only 25 minutes – a record for brevity. The doctor left with intense mixed feelings: frustration with Sophie, distress for being unable to understand or help her, and fear that things could go very, very bad if he didn't find the solution soon.

Meanwhile, the doctor found Sophie's mother as impenetrable as Sophie. She came. She smiled. She answered questions, always politely. But after each visit, he found he had learned almost nothing – and Sophie was taking his ward apart, invisibly creating wars among the staff. He began to dread the mother's visits without being able to say how she disrupted things. Well, if Sophie wouldn't talk, maybe mama would. He scheduled an AAI.

As he told me later, whenever he can't understand how a mother could be so unhelpful to her child, he suggests an AAI. After it, he has compassion for the woman and can begin to understand her experience as a mother. Only then can he engage her help. Sophie's mother was no exception.

The interview was long. Sophie's mother's words came slowly and carefully, as if each was considered before being spoken. Nevertheless, as the questions probed more deeply, both the story and her emotions appeared. She had been abused, repeatedly, then raped as an adolescent. Getting away from home in every way possible, she married a foreigner – who beat her and threatened her life. This was Sophie's father. She spoke in fragments, with unconnected images and tightly held emotions that erupted into tears several times. Here it was, the family secret, the thing no one knew and everyone reacted to.

When asked how childhood had influenced her adulthood, Sophie's mother could only repeat that she got past it – and would protect her daughter from anything like it at whatever cost. Suddenly her vulnerability filled the room. She seemed to think that if she had failed with Sophie, she had failed at everything that mattered.

This is where theory comes in – to connect the dots between the points of empirical certainty. How exactly did mother and daughter fit together? 'In silence' is the answer data offers (Ringer and Crittenden 2007). What the mother wouldn't say – for fear of passing the pain forward, the daughter felt – but couldn't understand. She felt her mother absent even when she was present. She felt the sadness and fear, but it had no cause. Being a child, she connected it all to herself: it's about me! She tried to shake the relationship with a nice threatening Type C strategy – and her mother almost disappeared. She tried to ask, to talk, but bad topics were swept aside behind professions of love. Even the ordinary problems of a child growing up found no words that could be shared. When all the other preschool-aged children were learning to tell episodes, Sophie and her mother were silent. Without shared words, Sophie had only images and routines with which to know and remember – and the most protective procedure was silence.

By the school years, Sophie had learned to get some attention and predictability by appearing helpless and ill (C4). She had also learned that words mislead, that good words didn't bring good feelings or clear contingencies. She became sullenly unhappy, withdrawing wordlessly, and that forced everyone to notice and try to placate her (it's about ME!). When other children were learning (integratively) to explain their motivations, Sophie was still without information, without an integrated guide (her mother), and with an exaggerated focus on herself. She was ready to escalate to C5-6.

This is where we met her, stuck in a family battle, symptomatic, unappealing, and unable to verbalize accurately what motivated her behavior. She truly idealized her mother (because she really, really, really cared about Sophie), but Sophie couldn't make that love work for her (because her mother was noncontingently unavailable in her preoccupation with her own traumas). Moreover, Sophie couldn't talk with her mother about it without risking hurting her feelings enough to destroy her. After all, if she said how unhappy she was, her mother would think she had failed. Without putting it in words, Sophie knew not to do that. Sophie couldn't go, she couldn't stay and she couldn't talk. No matter how much love her mother gave, it couldn't nourish her; silence fell where words might destroy. What was left was an incomplete coercive strategy combined with an incomplete idealizing strategy. Unable to discard her loving mother and unable to experience herself as real in her eyes, Sophie found herself, at the transition to adulthood, running out of options. Having unloving parents would free her to derogate and discard them, making a future without the parents possible.

Not all eating disorders are the same (Ringer and Crittenden 2007), nor do all children with a Type C strategy develop such severe disorder (indeed, the great majority do not). In another family, the girl would undercut both parents with false idealization (more common when marital problems are the family secret). In these cases, the young woman thinks she approves of one parent, but in fact that approval is merely used to point out the negative features of the other. There are even a few young women with an eating disorder who use a pure Type A strategy. What appears constant is the parent's attempt to protect the child by hiding the problem and the girl's implicit fear that if her unhappiness were expressed too clearly her parents might not be able to manage. If children do nothing else, they must protect their parents' ability to be parents. Now, in the transition to adulthood, that 'protection' risked destroying the daughter.

Comparable research has not been done, but it might be that aggressive delinquency in adolescent boys, who inarticulately cast their anger at people who have not harmed them, might be the gender equivalent symptom display for males.

Type C begins with uncertain outcomes that elicit mixed feelings. The display of feelings is later distorted, leading to a relationship defined by struggle and confusion of causation at every level: within the children, within their relationships, and among professionals.

Type A problems

Some young adults find meaningful and intimate relationships impossible to establish or sustain.

The full story of the Brightman children was never known; the family seemed to disappear after the death of Mr Brightman. But some stories came out at Mary's high school reunion, when she was 37 years old. Mary wasn't there, but she sent a long letter to her classmates, apologizing for her absence and explaining the reasons. She began with her achievements: a medical degree from the best university, work in the public sector, a husband and three children. Now she was earning her law degree, but that was on hold for the moment. She was struggling with chronic fatigue syndrome. It had gone on for several years, being diagnosed around the time of her divorce. Now her ex-husband cared for their children because she hadn't the energy to do it herself. Financially, it was difficult, so coming to the reunion wasn't possible.

I do discourse analysis. This letter stood out. Everyone had sent a short bio for a booklet. Mary wrote a five-page letter that, as I read it, felt like a personal explanation to, and connection with, each reader. The discourse markers? Long, run-on sentences without errors of person or time. An upbeat approach to distressing content. Compassion for her ex-husband and children and a total absence of blame or complaint. Assurances that she would work hard and recover and get her life back on track. Was Mary promising to fulfill everyone's expectations, even in the face of so much trouble?

The letter came with a newspaper clipping. The treasured son had died in adolescence in an alcohol-related automobile accident. The third daughter had dropped out of college and gotten messed up in drugs; no one knew where she was now. The oldest daughter, the most studious one and the one who had discovered the success strategy that her sisters would follow, had been found dead at age 25; this was what had made the news. Her nude body was discovered a week after her death, stuffed in the trunk of a car in a parking lot in a big city. The police treated it as a murder and determined that she had been working for an exclusive escort service. In the midst of this, Mary's father had died of a heart attack at only 58 years of age.

Is this merely bad luck, come in spades, or is there some developmental thread running through the Brightman family – and does it connect to the strategy of the Brightman parents? Surely, the compulsive performance strategy (A4–) seems to characterize all six of the daughters; did it constrain their development too much? Their small town and its high school would have reinforced the family's standards and could have made adolescent exploration of limits a publicly shameful experience for everyone, children and parents alike. Looking at the girls' failed relationships, their desire for distance and strangers, and their risk-taking after they left home for college, one wonders whether they had been exposed to too little danger. Surely, they were given all the best advice about safety, but did small-town life, combined with an overly protective and demanding family, limit the girls' opportunity to learn to recognize and cope with danger firsthand? Did the pressure to achieve hide a need to test limits and did the emphasis on appearance and happiness prevent recognition of negatives states? If a true self (including both positive and negative aspects of self) is not known, it cannot be shared with another person – and that prevents the development of genuine intimacy. It surely seemed that the oldest daughter was driven to a compulsively promiscuous strategy (A5) that used sexuality to claim the closeness that attachment did not yield. Was the precious last child, the treasured son, indulged in a way that his sisters were not, such that he accepted few limits and feared no danger (a probable coercive C strategy)?

How badly did the Brightman parents need to present themselves and their children as a perfect family? How much did they need a son to achieve this perfection? Did the girls try, one after another, to provide the success their father sought – from a son? Was the project doomed at their conception? After that, was everything a performance – and what price would they all pay for the show? And why? For that answer, we need to know about the parents, but, as is almost always the case, the details captured by the media are the gory ones, the sensational ones. The developmental processes that would explain it and make the characters human, like you and me, don't sell newspapers and aren't included. So we, the readers, don't learn very much that is useful to preventing the problem in future families. This is equally true – and maybe more so – when the news is about a criminal.

We never would have known about David except that his daughter's teacher reported that she suspected child sexual abuse. Needless to say, the investigation that followed was intense and included an AAI. Using discourse analysis to give meaning to the content produced the developmental history presented here. It is a history that is rarely known and certainly not told or thought about this way by most men who sexually abuse their children. Instead, we hear about what they did, about the child, and about the ineffectiveness of treatment to change pedophilia. Nevertheless, I have now read numerous AAIs of men convicted of incestuous sexual abuse, and the series of dangers along their developmental pathways is quite consistent: domestic violence, the mother choosing her husband rather than protecting her son, the father mocking the son for being 'soft', too much lonely time away from home, cruel punishment by the father for minor infractions (e.g., shooting the dog when the boy forgot to feed him), bullying and teasing by peers, precocious sexuality, early marriage, and a vow never to let his children suffer as he did. Telling David's story may help professionals to understand why some men sexually abuse their own children. Understanding that might change the way we manage treatment.

When the report of sexual abuse of his 6-year-old daughter reached child-protection authorities, they interviewed the children and confronted David. Did he admit to sexually abusing his daughter? David did not. He was silent and sad; he protested that he would never harm his child; he said she invited and liked their close affection. He absolutely denied that it was sexual abuse. He and his wife were told that he must leave, but no one wanted David to leave, neither he, nor his wife, nor any of their children. So the daughter was put in foster care until David was convicted and imprisoned. In prison, David was jeered at and bullied by other inmates. At home, his family suffered the loss of husband and father, an overwhelming sense of shame, and loss of income.

Discourse analysis of David's AAI revealed his self-protective and parenting strategy. He idealized his mother, transferring all responsibility for her failure to protect him to his father, whom he disparaged. He minimized or omitted entirely harm to himself and displayed almost no affect around his own suffering. Instead, he took his mother's perspective and showed compassion for her (A3, 7). His discourse also showed striking disconnections, especially of body parts from the person whose body it was. Hands hit, but the hands weren't attached to a body, nor did they hit a body. Where Sophie connected unconnected things and exaggerated feelings, David both kept connected things apart and mislabeled feelings.

A pattern of disconnections, plus one critical mislabeling, was crucial to making sexual behavior with his children possible without David perceiving his behavior as abusive: disconnection of his prescriptive semantic statements (what he said he should and would do) from his actions (what he did do), disconnection of his feelings from his actions, and even disconnection of his mother's love of him from her neglect of him. By keeping ideas apart, David was able to deal with absolutes. If his mother loved him, then she didn't neglect him (A7). If he loved his children (as he did), then he couldn't abuse them. Moreover, David had split parent and child perspectives, giving up his own perspective for that of his mother; this made it possible for him to be vigilantly attentive to his children's signals without understanding their meaning. In addition, David had mislabeled sexual feelings as feelings of affection and protection – because they had served that function for him. Finally, in an attempt to reverse their own childhood experience, both he and his wife had wanted him to be involved and affectionate with their children. Together, this set of contributing conditions opened the door to sexual enactment of attachment motivations with his children.

In prison, David acted as a good Type A would. He accepted what he was told by powerful other people about himself and his sexual attraction to children. He accepted his shame – as he had since early childhood when his father had jeered at him. He chanted back what he was told in treatment: he was entirely to blame, she did not invite it, he had groomed her. He completed the exercises about taking the victim's perspective; he acknowledged her suffering – and ignored his own. This common pattern of behavioral compliance illustrates the limitations of an excessive reliance on cognitive-behavioral techniques to elicit psychological change. Researchers involved in the evaluation of such interventions have perhaps weighted unduly such positive 'symptom-based' behavioral improvements. But David was a recidivist; once released, he offended again.

Sexualized attraction to children is thought to be nearly incurable. A story like David's (and David's story is not a unique story) raises questions that make professionals uncomfortable, but they are important for us to consider if we seek to help David and his children. Did David organize as a Type A compulsive caregiver to his mother and then, at puberty, find fulfillment of his attachment needs in sexual behavior? From the point of view of theory, did sex fulfill the function of attachment when attachment was blocked? Because his father and later his peers had shamed him throughout childhood, shame was nothing new for him. If so, possibly punishment and its inherent shaming quality had little probability of instigating change in David (cf. Thomas-Peter 2006). Was his feeling of being invited by his daughter an attribution of sexual meaning to coy signaling, i.e., a confusion between the attention-seeking and flirtatious functions of coy behavior? Did his 'grooming' reflect his desire to please his daughter, as his parents had not pleased him?

If we consider these transformations possible, then the common sorts of treatment that David was given in prison may have reinforced his Type A strategy, making it harder to get back to the true, but hidden, set of feelings and thoughts that actually motivated David's behavior. Wouldn't it be terrible if, with the best intentions but not knowing how incestuous child abusers come to engage sexually with their children, we offered treatments that *exacerbated* the problem?

The road to such criminality is not well understood. In the absence of knowledge, it can be easy to see monsters and innate evil where a developmental perspective could reveal humanity and suffering. Possibly following one boy as he grows up can raise questions about other boys and how they grow up to become dangerous.

Our first clear view of Jackson comes when he is 16. Like other children who have been bounced from home to home, Jackson treats professionals as attachment figures. He showed up unexpectedly at a former worker's office wanting to talk. Because he was happy to have a TAAI, we have a peek into his childhood and an assessment of his self-protective strategy and psychological processing. The transition to adulthood is, as said before, a crucial moment in time. It can give a boy like Jackson the chance to redirect his future. Four questions are of central interest as we consider whether this is likely to happen for Jackson:

1   What is his self-protective strategy in adolescence when almost the full range of strategies is available to him?

2   Does he show any potential for reflective functioning? This will be central to turning himself around.
3   Is he entangled in relationships that could catapult him into adult responsibilities or troubles, thus, stealing this precious developmental pause from him?
4   Is there anyone available to support and guide this process?

Careful analysis of Jackson's TAAI reveals pervasive danger and complexity. The danger has gone from very bad, in childhood, to much worse and much more complex, as he approaches adulthood. Does Jackson use a Type C strategy? There is a good argument for it; surely, we have aggression, blame and vindictiveness, supported by his descriptions of his own aggression and bullying. We also note that he perceives himself as a victim. In addition, however, there are vicious threats (e.g., to follow his ex-girlfriend if she goes out with someone else or to 'get' the boy who went out with her no matter how long it takes) that are both personal (to his ex-girlfriend and boys who date her) and impersonal (to all potential girlfriends). In other words, there is a suggestion of movement toward C7 (menacing). Nevertheless, his worker reminds us that Jackson is a charming, engaging, and likable guy. This combination of threat and likability is very ominous. Does Jackson use a Type A strategy? Compulsive caregiving and compliance (with the interviewer) are both clear. More startling is his oscillation between idealization, even delusional idealization (A7), of each parent and, at another moment, his derogation of each. Although he is aware of changing his mind, he seems unaware that such extreme dichotomies are likely to be distorted. Throughout he exonerates his parents and takes excessive responsibility for what has gone wrong. Finally, he refers quite often to what he has learned in his many bouts of counseling and therapy; we wonder whether he has aspects of an externally assembled self (A8). Putting it all together, our answer to the first question is A and C of all types, i.e., 'budding psychopath'. If we are going to make a change, we had better get started and be prepared to support Jackson for a long, hard process. If we begin and then let him down … no, let's not even think about the effect of that!

Reflective functioning is Jackson's strength. Throughout, he makes a number of insightful observations about the inexplicability of his own functioning. For example, about not being able to stay with his aging grandparents:

I cannot physically sit in that room, and see 'em because it just makes me want to cry and that's why I just walk out…;
About being separated from his parents:
Dunno, I was Mr Tough Guy, nothing used to affect me – I used to be, you know, anything, I'd just get back up and keep going, I never ever used to be able to be knocked down. How times change.

About feeling rejected:
No ... Well ... Well, they do, but they can't understand. I'm sitting here now laughing about my past, but it's like you always talk about the good things, you know, you never talk about the bad things that happen. I mean nothing really bad happened in my life until my mom started, you know, sleeping around 'n' things started going weird 'n', then when my nan died, then I just started, going crazy and then that's when everyone seemed to ... not care or not want to help me, or just used to push me aside (voice tones subdued).

Jackson has some insight, but is it more than talking therapy-talk to a therapist? Only taking the time to pursue a process of change with him could determine this.

Taking this time would require that Jackson be free of entangling relationships. It's not really clear whether he is or not. He says he has no girlfriend now, but he speaks about Janine as if she were his current girlfriend; this is so striking that the interviewer asks whether she is his *ex*-girlfriend. This, plus his attack on his father, suggests that he may not really be free of his past, nor able to pause for his future. What is clear is that the single most important thing to Jackson is finding a family with a home for him. He'd like it to be safe, but he'll accept it if it's permanent. Sex is fine, but what he wants is permanent relationships in a permanent home. Once this is articulated, it can be seen to underlie most, and maybe all, of his violence.

Finally, it is not at all clear that there are any long-term services for a young man like Jackson. All placements have failed, and he is living in a shelter for the homeless – at 16 years of age. He doesn't really fit child-and-adolescent services, he isn't an adult, nor is he a parent. It would seem that Jackson doesn't qualify for help, far less the long-term support that he needs. The next stop? A psychiatric hospital or, more likely, prison. Given his violence, drug use, self-harm, and occasional suicidality, someone is likely to pay a high price for our inability to seize these few years of opportunity.

For some young adults, the impasse between the need to stay home and leave home is absolute; they can't move forward, they can't stand still, and they can't deflect the problem onto others. In almost every case, these are compulsively compliant (A4) or delusionally idealizing (A7) individuals whose compulsive strategy has been expanded until it is applied everywhere and all the time in relationships with everyone, thus leaving the individual essentially no space for personal growth. Those adolescents who cannot move forward at a time when development insists that one start a family, and our society insists that one leave the childhood home to do this, face a crisis.

The risk is that the inhibitory strategy will break down and, in that moment, two decades of inhibited anger, fear, or desire for comfort will suddenly be unleashed. In many cases, the moment is highly destructive;

in all cases, it is so uncharacteristic of individuals that they seem out of their mind, not themselves, crazy. Further, because these extremely compulsive Type A individuals have no experience in regulating the display of negative affect, they are at the mercy of the displayed feelings, usually until they exhaust themselves or can be downregulated by pharmacological interventions. Depending upon whether the outbursts threaten the safety of themselves or others, these young adults will be treated by the mental health or criminal systems. In either case, regaining their inhibitory capacity is usually the goal.

Albert entered the room with 15 doctors, psychologists, and other staff seated in a circle watching him. He was strikingly calm, almost as if we were not there. At 22 years old, Albert had been hospitalized for the third time and, in this meeting, a foreign specialist was going to evaluate him – in front of all the floor staff. His symptoms included both brief periods of mania and motor arousal that sometimes were associated with mental speed and sometimes with limited sensory awareness and periods of extreme tiredness, stupor, and muscular weakness that interfered with concentration to the point that Albert couldn't discern individual words or understand sentences. He had been diagnosed with schizophrenia. Neither medication nor supportive therapy had helped, and sometimes the medications worsened his condition.

Albert was a slim, shy, quiet young man who lived alone with his single mother, his father being a married sailor who had been 'in port' briefly. He had done well in school, but had had no friends or extracurricular activities. He had no interest in girls (or boys) and was not sexually active. He was now a medical student functioning at the top of his class, but seeking a year's leave of absence. His mother, according to the staff, was a caring, but unremarkable woman.

Prior to this meeting, Albert had been given the AAI and the consultant had classified it. Now Albert sat in the only empty seat, next to the head psychiatrist who leaned in closely toward Albert and proceeded to interview him. Albert sat motionlessly with lowered eyes, answering in a soft, clear voice; the only sign of stress, even when the psychiatrist suddenly shook his finger near Albert's eyes, was an almost imperceptible tremble in his thumbs. Three things were striking: his obedience to the psychiatrist, his gentle attitude, and his acceptance of such public exposure without either distress or playing to the audience. He behaved like a specimen.

The AAI gave a developmental and psychological context to this amazing performance. Asked about his childhood family, Albert opened with a startling statement: *'Well, I am kind of such … illegitimate child … so such so Mom gave me birth out of marriage … was not … married to this person.'* The entire first response is about his illegitimacy and his unknown father. His mother is present only as his source of information.

His first memory was from age 3 or 4 years: '*I ps ps pulled over myself a bucket with hot water. It was very hot, I had a skin burn ... well and ... I was taken to the hospital ... well and ... such ... memory ... stayed ... only the first one ... well really of the hospital, moreover of erm ... (several unclear sounds, slight stammering) ...ff ...nnnot of bed there, but surgery table ... that dressing table well and there ... I naturally lay on the back and saw, you know, surgery rooms have that kind of such ... such big round lamp and there are several ... well erm ... just a moment, lamps, yes.*' Like his initial response, this one is filled with meaningless sounds. If we remove them, the meaning and the gaps in meaning become clearer: '*I pulled over myself a bucket with hot water. It was very hot. I had a skin burn. I was taken to the hospital. Such memory stayed, only the first one, really, of the hospital, moreover not of [my] bed there, but surgery [the] table ... that dressing table. I naturally lay on the [my] back and saw ... [Usually] surgery rooms have such [a] big round lamp and there are several ... just a moment, lamps, yes.*'

We note the lack of affect except in the dysfluence, the disconnectedness of the images (the only connected phrase is his taking responsibility for pulling the bucket on himself), the emphasis on how hot the water was, the shift of his attention to the lamps that are usually in surgery rooms, and the use of the present tense ('are'). His mother is completely absent from his episode. When asked why he recalls this event, he says: '*Well hard kind of [to] explain logically, I can't even give any interpretation, no nothing, frankly speaking...well, [I] could have come up but erm ... [I] really can't say anything ... unfortunately ... why it stayed in memory, that such small, that nothing except for this lamp, such strange thing a bit.*' We note that Albert gives logic a prominent place in his response when, in fact, it is less relevant than affect, which he neither displays, nor thinks about. That is, in this recalled experience, affect (e.g., pain) is crucial, but it is not treated as relevant to communicate in the event, nor to recall when looking back to understand oneself. His final five words are an inconclusive metacognition. That is, he finds the crucial bit, recognizes that it is discrepant, and then doesn't pursue its meaning further. We would call this an unresolved and dismissed trauma, but Albert did not think about it that way.

Discussing the relationship with his mother, Albert worked hard to find five phrases with which to describe it. When he got them, they were highly positive synonyms (which he noted) for which he could not recall any episodes. Nevertheless, we learn generically that he (a) had trouble beginning school and was taken back home, (b) worried when his mother was late picking him up from school, and (c) sometimes wandered away from school. It is hard to follow even the basic ideas, however. For example, this is what he said about the first day of school: '*She let me know that she is also upset ... well being upset united in this case ... from outside it became ... kind of ... well ... simply it became outside ... understanding and desire kind of came up, that is, complete understanding, that is, of these reasons ... that is, it promotes ... easing up ... of so to say ... negative well if for other reasons to try to explain to mom something ... does not always turn out, not always able to find right words ... and not always ... for adults, in general, it is clear why such ... worry ... not good one.'* A possible translation, based on taking out distracting phrases, might be: *She let me know that she is also upset, that being upset united us from outside [people]. Understanding and desire, that is, complete understanding, promote easing up of negative [feelings]. To try to explain something to mom does not always work out. For adults, in general, it is clear why one should try [to take their perspective].'*

For the word 'self-sacrifice', he talks in general about how much money he has cost her and how he limited her opportunities. 'Care' is learning to eat porridge. In the section on childhood troubles, however, we learn that in the school years, his mother slept in his bed because he couldn't sleep and that he was in a sanatorium where he was diagnosed with atypical epilepsy. His discourse is convoluted, abstract, reflective of his mother's state and perspective, and extremely cautious regarding what should be said.

In a convoluted and repetitious statement that is reduced here, Albert said that he forgets the negative and doesn't know why: *'No, any memories did not stay, some pictures, but they are not related well ... there are very negative emotions, they were present in what I was telling. There is only remembered something positive, the negative gets erased from memory. Exit to all these negative emotions. They generally were forgotten ... though not always, of course. This position existed for a long time, it doesn't work all the time, of course. For some reason, I don't have anything negative left. When ... mom came to take ... but the rest are calm memories.'* We note both awareness and disconnection, particularly of his mother coming to take ... [him].

Asked whether his mother rejected him, Albert responded (with most of the communication-obstructing dysfluence removed): *'Only that [she] had to place child [himself!] in the corner to think. Suddenly there appeared distance between mom and me. Anyway, there was [I made!] some offense. This presence of distance elicited such serious feelings, such uncomfort [in me, that I] redressed right away, [I] asked for forgiveness, when everything ... normalized.'* In this, the threat of losing his mother (his entire family!) is palpable, while his acceptance of offending – without knowing how – and the need to beg forgiveness flatten the feeling.

About being angry with her, he said: *'Well, I think that [exhalation] ... you know, when ... had to go shopping with mom, naturally often child starts asking for something, to buy something, well, you know, it is a natural thing absolutely, well and start showing, he starts all that there [laugh], naturally [he] will feel himself unhappy, well little child [...] ... well, then it all calmed down.'* This discourse is notable for the two bits of displayed affect (exhale and laugh). We presume that anger is a hot point that is in conflict with the essential state of being calm. In a follow-up response, we learn that his mother's response to the tantrumming child brought the neighbors out. We wonder what she did.

Albert clarified that his punishment was psychological. Again, the pauses and intruding words almost hide the meaning, but removing them, Albert says: *'Psychological punishment ... negative feelings of distancing. I had very difficult feelings of offense and something else, anger so ... frightening.'* His anger at his mother frightened him.

His response about being sexually abused was disturbingly ambiguous: *'No, this did not happen, not happen because then, as far as I know ... by the way [I] read in magazines that it is rather seriously influencing psyche ... later very severely influential when you are adult.'* The 'because' and 'as far as I know' make consideration of sexual abuse possible, and we recall that his single mother sleeps in his bed – up to the present.

When asked about deaths, his style of speech changed completely, and he spoke at length and cogently about the neighbor woman's death, mentioning that he now wishes to be a pathologist.

Asked how his childhood influenced his personality, he responded: *'Well, in childhood ... erm ... erm let's say such ... well ... features formed, that now have to ... well struggle with them really ... that is, overcome ... there refuse, well, so that is ... because they are absolutely ... for instance, I stay being infantile person ... that is, don't dare to make any decision independently ... in general have to struggle against them unfortunately ... they will not leave by themselves.'* He assigns these features to *'genetic or constitutional specifics'*.

Reading these excerpts in their original form is exhausting. One is inclined to skip over them as gibberish. But if one takes out the filler words, adds his mother and himself where they are the implied subject or object, and connects the remaining phrases, the meaning is clear enough. Albert knows what he must forget. He knows what feelings he must not show, and when he can't contain his anger or fear any longer, he is diagnosed and sent to an institution. All of this, it appears, is to protect a vulnerable, possibly depressed mother, who on the surface looks OK. Although we could consider him depressed with unresolved trauma and using a compulsive caregiving and compliant strategy, the hints of sexuality suggest the role reversal may more accurately be a spouse-like relationship. Now, on the cusp of adulthood, Albert professes his love of his mother and disregard of girls, and when he goes mad because of all that he is giving up, he takes a vacation on the psychiatric ward.

Understanding how his compulsive strategy had functioned to protect his mother, and thus him, in the past could help explain why it had become dysfunctional in the present when it is time to leave home and find a new love.

Can this alternate set of attributions open the door to change? Moving from *intra*personal to *inter*personal systems can show how Albert handled the irresolvable conflict between his mother's need to have him stay with her and his own need to establish an independent life. He wavered between agitation that prevents focus and depression that prevents focus and, from time to time, escaped to the hospital for respite. Because outside forces (such as genes) were treated as causal, attention was directed away from the problem between mother and son, and the balance, the psychotic balance, was maintained. Diagnostic shortcuts that fail to explore the function of behavior, and attribute meaning without understanding family members' experience, can render resolution of problems impossible (Procter 1981; Stratton 2003).

There are several important features of this case. First, neither mother nor son could tell this story by themselves. Second, the son's story was told in distorted ways that had protected him in the past. Only thorough discourse analysis of the transcribed AAI revealed the discrepancies and inconsistencies in Albert's narrative that allowed this interpersonal narrative to be constructed. Third, the near complete absence of affect suggested that Albert had almost lost access to important information that could have motivated him to confront his mother and seek an appropriate sexual partner. Fourth, a developmental perspective suggested that Albert's problems had not come to light earlier because at younger ages Albert needed his mother more than he needed independence and the conflict was not yet irresolvable. The AAI and Albert's behavior in the psychiatric interview revealed an unexpected family process – one that was quite different from the stories of biological anomaly that professionals and families tell each other about schizophrenia. The new story, however, fits the understanding of psychoanalytic and early family therapists quite well (Bateson 1972; Bettelheim 1967; Haley 1976a; Laing and Esterson 1964); it differs in being derived from new methods of data gathering and analysis and the identification of different developmental processes.

The DMM emphasizes the functional nature of all attachment strategies, especially highly distorted strategies, while recognizing that what may have been functional in one context may be dysfunctional or even dangerous in others.

Risk

The riskiest time is when the young adult comes to professional attention. If the developmental and interpersonal/familial components of the individual's problem are overlooked or if behavior change (e.g., symptom reduction, abstinence, or avoidance of reoffending) alone is sought, long-term resolution of the problem is unlikely. For sure, the severe problems in this period are not easily corrected. The question becomes how the professional system will respond.

The riskiest condition is when social intolerance is combined with risk of severe harm to self or others. Harm catapults the case to a crisis status where physical or pharmacological containment is applied immediately and intensively. Social intolerance has the undesirable characteristic of defining blame and responsibility, and, almost always, these are simplified and dichotomized. Social disapproval limits the resources available to help the distressed young adult. Such disapproval can routinely be reflected in the responses of some professionals.

The transition to adulthood can create a pause in the onward rush of development, one that can reduce the complexity that has been accruing through the school years and onset of sexuality. If young adults can support themselves or be supported without family entanglements, and especially if they can find a helpful mentor during this period, there is a possibility of substantial reorganization that can change the young adult's developmental pathway and that of his or her future children.

Yesterday's children

Yesterday's children, healthy or hurt, become today's parents. These three chapters described an array of self-protective strategies that are learned during childhood. One or more of these is used by parents to care for their children. Of course, the strategies should not be considered absolutes, boxes into which individuals must be stuffed – whether they fit or not. To the contrary, the strategies reflect a dimensional continuum that is expressed uniquely by each individual.

Under the best of conditions, grown children were protected and comforted when they were vulnerable, but guided to do for themselves what they were ready to learn to do, and relied upon to care for themselves independently when they had the needed skills. Among those skills are (a) recognizing and using the full array of self-protective strategies and (b) using reflective and integrative mental processes to decide when to use each strategy. If the parent was safe and comfortable growing up, the primary strategy is likely to be near the top of the model (see Figure 4.1). If the parent was unprotected and uncomfortable or, worse, harmed and uncomforted, the primary strategy is not only likely to be further down on the model, but there is also less flexibility among strategies.

A few important ideas can be drawn from the theory and cases presented here. First, developmental pathways are not fully predictable from the starting point, nor are they trajectories. At each step, however, previous development influences what follows. Second, serious disorders require a series of developmentally salient, untoward events. That is, each life stage has different threats. Some are tied to development at a previous stage, but some are random occurrences. Serious disorder requires both a series of these threats and also progressive self-generated strategies that protect the self while distorting understanding. Development, therefore, is explicable in hindsight, but not fully predictable from its roots. Third, families seem to be involved in every case, both vertically (parents and children) and laterally (siblings). Fourth, sexual behavior is much more complex than it appears; at a minimum it can serve both reproductive and attachment functions and need not do so similarly for individuals sharing an instance of sexual contact. Almost all serious disorders have both attachment and sexual problems. Fifth, changes in attachment figures (especially when figures are lost permanently, as opposed to separated as in divorce), too frequent change of domicile, and too early departure from a childhood home are all indication of risk of psychological distress and maladaptation. Sixth, chemical addition (including dependence on prescribed medications) both disrupts learning at important periods and changes brain functioning in some permanent ways. When alcohol and drug usage begin in early- to mid-adolescence, there may be serious implications for both immediate understanding of causal principles (in a generalized and abstract form as opposed to concretely, instance by past instance) and also affect (in terms of discriminating states, predicting how they will motivate behavior, and regulating expression of that motivation). Finally, cortical integration is central to being able to reorganize in ways that increase the probability of safety and comfort for both oneself and one's children. Each of these points has implications for parenting, both in terms of its probable success and in terms of the interventions needed if problems arise.

Experience with danger is proposed to be central to parents' caregiving because it influences (a) which mental representations are deemed most predictive of future conditions and (b) the process by which conflicting representations are resolved into behavior. This leads to the unexpected conclusions that (a) preconscious memory systems regulate important aspects of parental behavior because they promote safety, and (b) reflective, integrative, and verbal processes may be infrequent, especially among risk parents, because integrative processing itself can expose parents and their children to danger. This is the topic of the next chapter.

Chapter 5

Remembering the future: The process of mental representation

The only information we have is information about the past, whereas the only information we need is information about the future. This chapter is about how humans take information learned in the past and process it to generate representations of the probable future. On the basis of those representations, we act.

Of course, no one knows the future for certain, and each time we act, we hope we understand the situation accurately and have responded appropriately. Our understanding, however, is tied to what we have experienced in the past. That is, we take in sensory information about the present, but we give it meaning on the basis of what we know from the past. That meaning organizes our behavior. Because the past will never recur, we must adapt past information to current conditions. These 'transformations' make the information less accurate about the past, but function to make it more applicable to the future. Because everyone has different past experience and history of mentally using information to extract meaning from the past, different people experiencing the same conditions may arrive at different understandings of how to act. Without understanding how each individual transforms information and derives self-relevant meanings, we cannot understand why parents do what they do.

This chapter addresses two aspects of organizing behavior: (a) transforming incoming sensory stimulation to give it meaning and (b) using the transformed information to organize a possible response.

Five transformations of information

The two basic transformations of sensory stimulation to meaningful information are 'cognition' and 'affect'. When these result in action, the outcome provides feedback about the meaning of the information. On the basis of this, the meanings are transformed further. Five transformations are proposed: truly predictive, erroneously predictive, omitted from prediction, distorted prediction, and falsely predictive. Each, used in the right time and place, can guide the individual to behave in ways with a higher probability of being protective than if the information were untransformed.

Truly predictive information

Information that is 'truly predictive' is transparently accurate. That is, it means what it appears to mean. For some children, a parent's upraised hand means that they are going to be hit – and they are hit. The cognitive (temporally based) sequence truly meant what it appeared to mean. Similarly, the intensity of the mother's screaming (affect) signals that the mother will do something extreme and the child should prepare to protect him- or herself. When the mother starts throwing things, the affective information is seen to be truly predictive.

These two examples show self-evident cognitive and affective information that is truly predictive regarding danger.

Erroneously predictive information

Information that is treated as being meaningful but has no predictive value whatever is 'erroneously predictive'. To use the example of the parent with the upraised hand, if the child notices that the parent is wearing purple and if that is unusual, the child might think that purple clothing predicts being smacked. That would be erroneous because the parent's clothing had absolutely nothing to do with the punitive behavior. Nevertheless, if the child became fearful every time the parent wore purple, we would conclude the child had made an erroneous transformation. Then, if seeing purple, the child responded with protective behavior (for example, being very good, giving the parent a little gift, etc.) *and* wasn't hit, the child would be negatively reinforced for the erroneous attribution and would be unlikely to correct it. Simply feeling very aroused, if treated as truly indicative of threat, can produce erroneous affective information. In the song phrase from Radiohead, 'Just because you feel it, doesn't mean it's there'.

Omitted information

The opposite of erroneous information is information that has meaning but is treated as being meaningless or irrelevant. Such information is omitted from further processing. For example, in the raised hand example, the child might feel very angry, but discover that expressing the anger led to more violent punishment. In the future, the child might reduce the probability of this dangerous outcome by omitting awareness of being angry from further processing. The child would omit the affective information, thereby losing potentially valuable information in the long term, but protecting the self in the short term. Similarly, the child might have done something to elicit the parent's upraised hand. If he or she omits that cognitive information from further processing, it will both protect the child from self-blame (an unpleasant thing!) and increase the probability that the sequence will be repeated with the outcome of more hitting.

Distorted information

When information is omitted from awareness, the remaining information exists in the absence of contradiction. That is, if negative affect associated with the parent is omitted, then all one's feelings about the parent are positive. This distorts the representation of the parent – who is positive, but not entirely positive. Similarly, if we omit from awareness our own contributions to negative events, we have a distorted basis for blaming other persons entirely and feeling extreme wrath toward them.

False information

Some information means the opposite of what it appears to mean. For example, Jackson said he would never hurt a woman and he put his girlfriend in a headlock. Some smiles cover fear, anger, and an intent to attack. These two examples reflect false cognition and false affect, respectively.

These transformations are self-protective and necessary. All people use them and must try to recognize them in others. They are the means by which what one has experienced in the past is made relevant to the future. That is, having once treated all information as truly predictive, one learns to predict in more sophisticated ways. When dealing with children, however, one must keep in mind that they do not have all these transformations (yet). If parents who were endangered as children carry forward into their caregiving of their own children all that they have learned about predicting hidden danger, they are likely to endanger their own children.

Dispositional representations (DRs)

Understanding why parents behave in ways that endanger their children requires understanding how people generate and select 'dispositional representations' (DRs). DRs are the outcome of mental processing of information. They dispose us to behave in particular ways. This term is used as a replacement for the older and less precise construct of 'internal working models', both because it clarifies the 'disposing to action' function of representation and because it emphasizes the transient, in-process quality of represent*ing* (as opposed to the retained and static quality of models).

This chapter addresses several ways that people can represent the relation of self to context. A memory-systems perspective (Schacter and Tulving 1994) is used. These different ways of knowing are described in a developmental framework in which neurological maturation interacts with experience to generate developmental pathways (Bowlby 1969/1983). The outcome, at any given moment, is an emergent, ever-changing set of DRs that (a) shape individuals' perception of the world and their relation to it and (b) guide the transformation of mental representations to enacted behavior. The complex ways in which multiple DRs interact to generate parental behavior are the focus of this book

From a mental-health perspective, understanding the minds of parents whose behavior is maladaptive is crucial to enabling them to change. Change requires that we build a bridge from their reality to ours and then help them to cross it back to the safety of normal functioning. To do this, we must carefully differentiate behavior from its meanings because the former is objective, i.e., we can all agree on what happened, and the latter is unique to each viewer.

That is, for any exchange between parent and child, the parent's intent provides meaning from their perspective, whereas the effect on the child provides meaning from our perspective. It is easy to see that these meanings might be quite different such that, if we try to communicate at the level of attributions, we will often miscommunicate. This is especially likely because professionals' terms often imply moral censure of maltreating parents' behavior (e.g., 'abuse', 'abandon') and a lack of meaning for mentally ill parents' behavior (e.g., 'chaotic', 'personality disorder', 'bipolar', 'psychotic'). If parents do not share these meanings, our terms will build walls of misunderstanding, rather than bridges to cooperation. This can be a real problem when particular diagnoses are viewed as defining a moral state, such as 'psychopath', or an unchangable and intolerable limitation, such as various 'personality disorders'. The emphasis in this chapter will be on describing parental behavior and discerning its meaning to parents.

Much of our approach to intervention and treatment is based on symptoms and focuses on behavior change. To use the examples in the previous chapters, Luke's father was thought to have abused Luke by breaking his arm, and, because he wouldn't admit to it, Luke was put in foster care. His foster mother reported that he wet the bed, had nightmares, and cried a lot before and after visits to his parents. On the basis of these reported symptoms, he was diagnosed with PTSD and treated for that by having fewer parent visits with increased supervision. Meanwhile his father tried to demonstrate how much he cared for him by accepting counseling. In that process, he slowly came to recognize that his own experience of being very severely abused as a boy was affecting how he raised his children, especially his attempts to protect them. In fact, he discovered that misplaced protection had resulted in Luke's broken arm. How did his childhood reach so far into his parenthood that he harmed his own child? We will discover that the foster mother's childhood self-protective strategy with her blind mother affected her choosing to foster, her relationship to Luke, and the meanings she attributed to Luke's behavior. How did professionals overlook this bias?

By school age, Nick's behavior was really out of control. He couldn't play with other children and sometimes attacked them – for no apparent reason. Neither his teachers nor his parents understood. Long parent–teacher conferences made clear that his mother cared tenderly for him and tried her best to make him happy. Moreover, his father had appropriate standards for behavior, used contingencies well, and wasn't excessively harsh. Still, Nick's behavior was getting more and more aggressive. Only much later would it become clear that each parent was 'right', but, together, they were 'wrong', and they were together because each found in the other a way out of the limitations of their own childhood. Their solutions worked for them, but not for Nick. How did their childhoods reach through their marriage to harm their son?

Nancy's problems kept her from learning in school, reduced her access to normal peers, and created intense distress for her parents. They learned to back off, feeling helpless to do anything but make things worse. By high school, Nancy was on the fringe; her friends were in trouble, too, and together they found alcohol and drugs. These made daily life with all its failures easier to bear. In another family, one where the parents didn't back off, Nancy might have developed an eating disorder. In either case, Nancy – or Sophie – would know not to complain directly. Instead, her behavior would have to tell their story – and behavior, for all its apparent clarity, can mislead. If we want to change these disorders, we need to understand why each girl does what she does and, for this, we need to know why her parents, most often her mother, kept certain things out of sight. Most often these are threats the mother experienced from which she wishes to protect her child. How can an attempt to stop the spread of distress create new forms of distress that can't be understood by the protective parent?

Jackson needed more than one strategy, and, in the end, no strategy protected him from physical harm, psychological cruelty, and abandonment. Deception and implicit triangulating involvement in his parents' marriage and divorce left him feeling unable to trust himself or others. How do we understand the motivations that regulate his highly variable and unpredictable behavior? How do we help him to understand and regulate these motivations? Why did his home and caregivers change so many times that, in the end, he had none? Whose DRs were operating then? Under what conditions will Jackson know when and whom he can trust? What actions on our part can foster that process – and which actions are likely to hinder it?

All of these cases demonstrate that focusing too exclusively on the presenting problem and prematurely attributing meaning to it, especially in cases of very severe disorders, can misdirect the response, making potentially resolvable problems seem unresolvable. Parents' problems carried forward from their childhoods had unexpected, unwanted, and usually unrecognized effects on their children. These parents, like most parents, had wanted the best for their children. When they can't deliver that, we, as professionals, need to look at what is happening psychologically between intention and action.

If the basis for behavior lies in the information processing that precedes action, our interventions might better be targeted on the point where the process goes awry, rather than solely on outcome behavior. The mental processing that leads to behavior is referred to as 'representation'. The neurological and psychological aspects of representation are discussed first, and then they are applied to inadequate or dangerous child-rearing.

Mental representations

Mental representations, however much we think of them metaphorically (e.g., as 'internal models'), are actually networks of firing neurons. The neural response to externally generated information represents the state of the *context* at that moment. The neural response to internally generated stimulation (from the muscles, skin, inner organs, etc.) represents the state of the *self* at that moment. Together, these generate the neurological representation of *'the self in this context now'*. This representation motivates and organizes individuals' behavior; in Damasio's terms, it *disposes* the self to a particular response (Damasio 1994). Although the process is not yet fully understood, consideration of how past representations affect the array of DRs can inform our understanding of how parental behavior is organized.

To see the impact of these representations, compare the probable representation of self of Nick and Albert. Nick acts, and, depending upon which parent responds and how they feel at that moment, Nick is cajoled, placated, yelled at, or punished. Until he is old enough to sort out those contingencies, there isn't much information to guide his behavior. On the other hand, as he escalates from complaining to tantrumming, the sensory information generated by his body becomes more and more intense. The information sent to the brain screams 'Emergency!' and Nick organizes his behavior accordingly. Albert, on the other hand, has learned that any action risks a negative response, particularly any display of negative affect. He knows exactly what to do (usually 'nothing' until told what to do) and he displays no evidence of feeling. This reduces the amount of bodily arousal and similarly reduces the information about his own state that is sent to his brain. Without information with which to represent himself, Albert disappears from his own view.

What is retained from past experience?

The brain does not keep or store memories (or internal models). Instead, the array and strength of synapses and patterns of firing among neurons reflect past experience (Baddeley and Hitch 1974; Mongillo *et al*. 2008; Schacter 1996). Both frequent reactivation and intense stimulation strengthen synapses (Schacter 1996). Strong, numerous, interconnected synaptic networks are more easily triggered than those with fewer and weaker connections (i.e., long-term potentiation). Thus, what is retained over time is not an 'internal model', but rather a potential neural network, with each connection having a probability of firing in response to certain stimuli. In any given moment, these probabilities generate chains of activated neurons that represent 'the self in this moment in this context', that is, the *who, when*, and *where* of existence. Because danger is an intense experience, it increases the attentional focus of the right orbitofrontal cortex. Focused attention is required for neuroplasticity and parcelation of pruning in the nervous system (Doidge 2007; Schore 2003). Consequently, danger has a disproportionate impact, compared to its frequency, on the strength of chains of synapses and, thus, on information processing and DRs.

These ideas hold the potential to provide a means of evaluating interventions for changing attachment as well as for evaluating treatment in general. In both cases, the evidence of change would be changed neural processes, particularly processes when individuals feel threatened or feel their children to be in danger.

In addition, there is a difference between rich and impoverished neural networks. Lest the previous example suggest that Type C is equivalent to 'more' and Type A to 'less', let's reverse them for this example. Let's compare Sophie (who had anorexia) with Mary Brightman (who had chronic fatigue syndrome) and Luke (whose father broke his arm). Sophie's mother found it difficult to stay attentive to Sophie whenever Sophie tried to express negative feelings or whenever her mother was already preoccupied with her inner thoughts. For Sophie (who used a C5–6 strategy), this resulted in learning to inhibit negative affect, not transforming it into words, and not constructing contingency-based cognitive explanations. Sophie's neural network for coping with distress was impoverished; it contained little variability and few effective responses. For Mary, it was the opposite. Her breadth of performance (social, academic, and interpersonal) brought approval and praise – both at home and at school. She had a rich network that supported further compulsive behavior in many settings and with many people. Luke's father presents a somewhat different picture. His behavior seemed entirely normal, both with Luke and siblings, until Luke did something dangerous *and* ignored his command to stop. In that moment, Luke's behavior triggered a rich, but narrowly focused, neural network established in his father's youth when he was abused by his father. Once triggered, this representation disposed his action quickly and out of his awareness. As a child, this was protective; as a father, it resulted in his jerking his son and breaking his arm.

What kinds of DRs are there?

Six types of representation are described below. They vary in (a) whether they are 'cognitive'[1] (temporally based) or 'affective' (intensity based); (b) whether they are preconscious and nonverbal, or conscious and potentially verbal; and (c) whether they are available in the early years of life or only later. Figure 5.1 displays these six ways of representing the relation of self to context graphically.

Implicit, preverbal representation

The temporal order in which sensory information is perceived is crucial. In Piagetian terms, this is sensorimotor representation. In information-processing terms, it is *procedural memory* (Tulving 1979). Behaviorally, it is

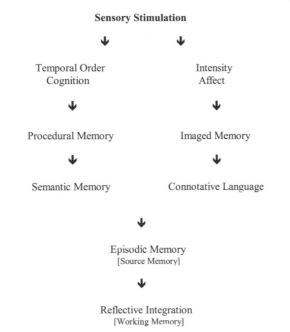

Sensory Stimulation

↓   ↓

Temporal Order   Intensity
Cognition   Affect

↓   ↓

Procedural Memory   Imaged Memory

↓   ↓

Semantic Memory   Connotative Language

↓

Episodic Memory
[Source Memory]

↓

Reflective Integration
[Working Memory]

Figure 5.1 Six memory systems as a function of cognitive and affective information organized in both developmental order and order of psychological complexity

learning theory (Skinner 1938). Temporal order is also the basis of implicit causal attributions (Crittenden 1997; Schmahmann 1997). For example, a young child may learn that, after he makes noise, his mother hits him. Such a child may learn to inhibit vocalization both without awareness of the reason and without limitation regarding the context or circumstances.

> Luke's father had learned that to disobey led to very severe punishment. That sequence, begun when Luke didn't respond to his command to 'stop', together with his fear for his son's immediate safety, increased his arousal dramatically and led to a 'preventive' re-enactment of his own father's angry behavior. That is, to protect Luke from the street and from his own flashback-like memories of his father's abuse, Luke's father acted. The intent was protective; the outcome was harm.

Alternatively, the child may discover that being helpful reduces the probability of being hit – even if one has been noisy. This child may become compulsively helpful, again without being able to put the idea in words. Procedural representation is rapid, preverbal, and preconscious – and it may be inaccurate. It is information about *when* in the sequence of events a particular event might occur.

Changes in the intensity of stimulation activate the limbic structures (LeDoux 1994).[2] This affects somatic arousal, i.e., heart rate, breathing rate, etc., in ways that heighten sensory awareness and prepare the body to fight, flee, or freeze (Cannon 1914; LeDoux 1994; Selye 1976). Changes in the autonomic state produce sensory stimulation that is itself processed through the limbic system. This can produce an escalating feedback loop of self-arousal; for example, rapid breathing feeds new somatic stimulation back to the brain, thus leading to even more arousal. Associative learning connects sensory aspects of contexts with experienced outcomes, thereby increasing the set of sensory stimuli that elicit arousal (Pavlov 1928). For example, a child who was punished in the headmaster's office might later feel uncomfortable in any office.

> In Nancy's case, anything associated with school became threatening to her, such that her future ability to care for herself and raise her children was jeopardized.

Arousal changes how individuals feel, literally; psychologically, it gives rise to 'feelings' (Bowlby 1980; Damasio 1999). In Schacter and Tulving's terms, this is 'perceptual memory' (Schacter and Tulving 1994); in the terms used here, it is *imaged memory*.[3] Imaged memory represents sensory aspects of the context, and, like procedural representation, it creates a disposition to act that is preverbal and preconscious – and possibly erroneous. Imaged representations are information about *where* an event might occur. For example, the smell of a dentist's office elicits fear and motivates one to run away. Both procedural and imaged representations are probabilistic and reflect past experience with predictability.

> Both Jackson and Albert had strong images of danger. Jackson's were visual ('*He had a big red bag. My father's one big man, huge! Really a bear-like man*'), auditory ('*She had the cheek to say, "Why d'you call me a bitch?"*'), and animated ('*because my arm actually come up and like up there over [showing]*', snapping his fingers during emotionally intense sections of the AAI). In addition, the animated image of snapping had connotative qualities that kept his arousal high, kept his listener aroused through the startling quality of the snapped fingers, and evoked the suddenness with which danger struck in his home and for which he used the word 'snap'.
>
> For Albert, the images were few and visual ('*a big, round lamp; well, there with green liniment, well, brilliant green, also kills Gram-positive bacteria; with scratched knees, well, no joints, that really badly scratched … I think of asphalt scratched badly*'), or medical ('*stomach inflammation, uterine inflammation, stenocardia, cardiac fibrillation*'). In order not to have these imaged DRs activate behavior, the images were kept unconnected to people, either the self or the dangerous other person, and in the case of the medical symptoms of bodily distress, highly abstracted and in medical lingo that distances one from actual feeling.

Images can vary on a gradient from absent or disconnected (Type A processes) to exaggerated and animated, i.e., acted out by the speaker (Type C processes). Their function is to protect. For example, a week ago, a screeching fire alarm went off in my hotel room. I froze, unable to continue my activity. Then I leapt up and dashed to the door, and then realized that my running shower had produced so much steam that it had set off the fire alarm. I raced into the bathroom, drenching my head in my haste to turn the water off, and then stood shaking for 5 more minutes until the alarm turned itself off. Half an hour later, my heart still beat noticeably faster than usual – in spite of my complete safety.

The fire alarm signaled an actual change in safety and functioned to alert others to the need to help. In other cases, actual and undistorted images can be given 'erroneous' (magical or superstitious) powers – for example, the nighttime protection of the low, soothing voice from far away in the warmly glowing plastic radio that seemed to keep a child's bed safe from intruders all night.

Somatic images are among the most crucial because they address the state of the self directly, both the physical self, e.g., pain from a wound or disease condition, and the psychological self, e.g., the wrenching intestinal cramps of a distressed child waking to face another day. Images can also distort stimuli until the image, rather than the person generating the image, is animated. Such images are delusional, i.e., sensory hallucinations. A sickening taste (that accompanies everything) or a foul smell (that no one else can perceive but which goes everywhere with the child, even sticking to his skin) might reflect the disgust of others or the fear that the child experiences, especially when the child imagines himself to be the rejected thing, or when no safe place or protective action can be imagined.

Delusional images can also be thought of as representing a disposition to act, with the source of the forbidden disposition being placed outside the self; for example, in the words of an imagined speaker in an auditory hallucination. Visual images can take on delusionally animated qualities. For example, one deeply depressed adolescent perceived trees, telephone poles, and oncoming cars as 'pulling' her with enormous magnetic force such that she almost couldn't resist the urge to lock eyes on the deadly object and slam her foot down on the accelerator. Her escape was to give up driving. In a mixed auditory and visual hallucination of suicidal intent, open windows several stories above a courtyard appeared to be 'calling' one man, such that to be safe he had to stand well back from the windows, in the middle of the room.

Sleepwalking could be considered an animated and delusional image; e.g., a 'sleeping' child standing in the open front door at night or swaying at the top of the stairs leading away from the bedrooms, and then returning to bed having not acted on the desire to escape the craziness of home or the sexual abuse of the uncle in the next bedroom. Although sleepwalking is thought to be genetic or at least familial, it is associated with perinatal risk, child behavior problems, and parent psychopathology (Gau and Soong 1999; Shang *et al.* 2006).

The extensive functional variation among the images given as examples makes clear the variety of ways that the mind can retain, connect, and use experienced or observed danger. Further, the language with which these paragraphs are written exemplifies the difference between abstract denotative language (which captures ideas, but is not emotionally 'moving') and affect-eliciting, connotative language (see below).

Explicit, verbal representation

Procedural and imaged representation are functional in humans at birth. With maturation, both can be processed further in ways that make them verbal. Beginning in the third year of life (i.e., 2 years of age), cortical processing can render procedural information verbally explicit in the form of generalized, context-free information (Tulving 1987). The classic form of semantic representation is a *when/then* or *if/then* statement. For example, Luke's father said, '*If you done something wrong, [then] she'd say, wait till your father gets home, and she'd make dad punish me*'. *Descriptive semantic memory* consists of generalized descriptions of how things are.

On the basis of statements of contingency, individuals construct notions regarding how one *should, ought to,* or *must* behave. Thus, *prescriptive semantic memory* generates verbal DRs regarding how things are – or ought to be. For example, Albert, speaking about his mother, said, '*She always must know what happens to me … well, that so … erm … it is always, that is, ..to protect me.*' Such representations are often used by parents to instruct children and to explain parental behavior.

On the other hand, Type C individuals use prescriptive semantic memory either to blame someone else (they should …!) or in confusing, illogical or misleading ways. For example, Sophie said this about eating: '*If I couldn't control anything, I could control my eating and it's like a real tool, like a self-destruction thing as well, like that I don't deserve to eat so why should I?*'

Whereas procedural and imaged information is always self-generated and self-relevant, verbal information can be generated by other people and remembered without corresponding sensorimotor experience. Therefore, semantic DRs can be 'borrowed' from others and implemented without self-relevance. To take Jackson again, he makes many statements such as: '*I know it's selfish. Everyone calls me selfish.*' These are borrowed semantic statements. Often, however, the source is not given, and it's not so easy to determine that this is not a self-generated semantic idea. For example, if Jackson had said, 'I know it's selfish; I'm a very selfish person,' we wouldn't know whether he believed that or he believed someone else who believed that.

The verbal form of imaged information is *connotative language* (Crittenden 2002). Connotative languages increases or decreases the impact of affect on both speakers and listeners. Connotative language begins to be experienced, in the form of stories, rhymes, and songs, in the preschool years and to be generated by children during the school years. For example, school-aged children's taunting chants have the power to elicit strong emotional reactions in other children. Some connotative language is very arousing and *evocative* (that is, it evokes feelings in the listener). Jackson's description of fighting with Janine in Chapter 3 has evocative language. At the other extreme, connotative language can be *dry and artificial*; this use of language lowers arousal. For example, Jenny's mother said, as her son leaped toward her and Jenny, '*umm*'. Like semantic information, connotative language can be self-relevant or borrowed; both can generate emotional states in the self or others. That is, the way we tell our stories affects the way we and others feel and thus what we are disposed to do.

Cortical integration

By about 3 years of age, all four sorts of DRs (procedural, imaged, semantic, and connotative) can be integrated to yield episodic recall of specific events. Episodes contain the temporal order of events and the sensory context in a verbal form. Young children cannot construct episodes without guidance in the form of questions and elaborations by parents (Fivush and Hamond 1990). In teaching children to construct and tell episodes, parents both influence the representation of the episode (with omissions, additions, and distortions) and teach children what should be omitted, added, and distorted when constructing an episode. This affects how children attribute meaning to experience.

A good episode should have a sequence of events (a beginning, middle, and end). It should have characters, some descriptions, and the central feelings regarding the action.

> I can remember, I can remember leaving home one day. I don't know what it was about. I remember saying I was going to run away and I packed this big suitcase which was under my bed and I took this fabulous dress which my cousin had just handed onto me because I thought she was the bees' knees [laugh] and my new shoes. And that was all I took in a suitcase, and I remember walking off down the road and thinking, I hope someone comes and gets me, because I will actually have to give in and turn around and go back because I didn't have the faintest idea where I was going. I was obviously wanting to make a statement. And actually Dad came and got me, Mom didn't; Dad came in a truck. And picked me up and said, 'Well, you need more than your new dress and your new shoes, so you better come back home so that we can pack your bags properly'. [laugh] And we went home, and I didn't run away again, until the next fight, I suppose. I can't even remember what it was about.

This episode is complete in every way – in spite of being about a dangerous event. It is told in the first person. It has a beginning, sequence of events, and an end. It has imaged details and expressed feelings. It contains both the speaker's perspective and that of her parents. There are dysfluencies, but they don't transform the meaning. Finally, the speaker actively reflects on her experience and draws conclusions about her psychological state at the time that she couldn't have fully drawn in childhood.

A subtype of episodic memory is source memory. Source memory is the ability to recall precisely when and where an event occurred or the precise source of semantic information (Schacter 1996). It tags all types of memories with a code for the occasion when this information came to be one's own. The source may be an occasion, what another person said, or the conclusions that one drew oneself. Knowing the source of information is crucial to being able later to evaluate its likely accuracy or veracity, given current circumstances. Two conditions of source memory are particularly relevant to parenting problems.

Confusion of information from different sources (e.g., the self now, the self in the past, one's mother, one's religious guide, etc.) is considered 'disorientation' in the DMM. It is associated with maladaptive and nonstrategic behavior because the person acts in concordance with the motivations of different people or of the self at different times, and these motivations can be incompatible with one's interests in the present. Disorientation is often observed in the parents of child psychiatric patients. Because source memory develops after about 6 years of age and isn't fully mature until mid-adolescence, disorientation is a relatively late-developing mental disorder. Rather than affecting the process of representing, disorientation affects the integrative process by eliminating one of the bases for evaluating the probable validity of the various dispositional representations. People who are disoriented appear less obviously abnormal than people with transformations generated earlier in life.

Misattribution of self-generated information to an external source is considered delusional. Because delusions reflect errors of source memory, delusions, as used here, cannot properly occur before school age. Delusional information is proposed to be generated by the mind when the gap between what is known about dangerous and safe conditions and what needs to appertain is so discrepant as to make self-threatening danger an imperative concern. Delusions function to permit the self to feel safe when in danger or to behave in otherwise forbidden ways that are self-protective.

Working memory is the fitting of a representation from another memory system (procedural to episodic) to immediate physical circumstances; for example, thumb sucking as a self-comforting behavior is a procedure, but to be implemented, working memory must fit the movements to the positions of the body in real time.

Integrative functioning, on the other hand, combines DRs in ways that change the meaning of information. Procedural, imaged, semantic, connotative, and episodic DRs can be compared, contrasted, and integrated cortically to yield a best-fitting representation of the relation of self to context at this moment.

Integration, however, is a slow, all-encompassing process that depends upon multiple, concurrent inputs from all over the brain. The advantage of integration is that it permits the best fit of self to current circumstances. The disadvantage is that it consumes the breadth of the brain (thus leaving little capacity for scanning the environment) and progresses slowly (thus leaving the individual relatively unresponsive to external stimuli for a long time). Under these conditions, danger could come close without the individual's being aware of it. Thus, the closer in time and space the danger is perceived to be, the less the individual will dare to dally in reflection and the more likely he or she will be to act on a less fully processed and possibly erroneous DR from procedural or imaged memory. Integrative capacity improves as a function of maturation into the mid-thirties (Doidge 2007; Gazzaniga 2005; Sowell *et al*. 2003). Thus, self-protective integration will require maturation, sufficient safety to promote reflection, and sufficient exposure to threat to provide relevant information about danger.

Selection of a DR upon which to act

If all the DRs provide a similar picture of the relation of self to context, behavior proceeds unimpeded. All the excitement occurs when the various dispositions are in conflict. For example, the procedural representation predicts dangerous outcomes (so the individual is disposed to act defensively), whereas in imaged representation the individual feels comfortable (and, therefore, is disposed to attend to other things). But, semantically, one has rules that require (or forbid) certain actions, and episodically one recalls a similar situation and how one acted, and that it turned out badly (or well). As one considers these possibilities, one tells oneself a story, using minimizing (or arousing) language. Each of these representations generates a disposition to behave. Given sufficient time, the mind can sort through these, evaluating, combining, and contrasting them so as to generate an integrated and comprehensive solution to the problem.

Time is crucial. More complete processing takes longer. Under conditions of perceived danger, time cannot be wasted and processing may need to be aborted in favor of protective action (Damasio 2003). This is desirable because it reduces the probability of injury or death. It is undesirable because it occurs before full analysis of the ambiguities and uncertainties has been completed. As a consequence, the protective action may be based on inaccurate information and may not be necessary. There is, in other words, a trade-off between accuracy and speed.

Talisha (from Chapter 1), who hit her daughter to punish her just as her mother had spanked her, and Luke's father provide an interesting comparison. Both had procedural, imaged, and episodic DRs of punishment from their childhood. But they differed in their semantic DRs. Talisha thought spanking was appropriate whereas Luke's father wanted not to be similar to his own father. Both were too rough with their children, but, for Talisha, the smack was intentional and noninjurious. Luke's father, on the other hand, grabbed Luke on the basis of affect-laden 'trauma' DRs that he had no time to consider in the situation of fearing his son would be harmed. For Luke's father, there was a semantic discrepancy that he was unable to use to initiate integrative processing. It may be worth noting that it was in the case of unexamined discrepancy that a child was injured.

The outcome of these constraints on integrative processing is that older and less endangered people will engage in more reflective thought than others. Parents who were exposed to danger in their childhood would be expected to overestimate the probability of danger and more often to abort integrative processing in favor of self- or progeny-protective action. Thus, they would have fewer alternative and less elaborate DRs. When low intelligence is added, the risk of inappropriate behavior rises.

Pain

Pain is treated here as a special topic for the following reasons:

1 it is crucial to danger to the self;
2 it has both cognitive and affective components;
3 it can be represented in all of the memory systems, with each contributing something to how pain is tied to behavior;
4 it is more complexly processed than other sensory experiences.

The evolved function of pain is to protect the self (Damasio 2003; Diatchenko *et al.* 2007). Pain elicits reflexive, self-protective action and can be considered the body's last-ditch effort to protect the self in that it occurs only after the attack has begun. That is, one can think of smell as the best distal signal of danger, with sight and sound functioning similarly but not quite so directly, and taste and touch as signals of proximal danger. Pain, however, signals that harm to the self is underway.

In memory-system terms, innate withdrawal reflexes and learned sensorimotor responses are *procedural* responses to pain. Usually, these occur very, very quickly, roughly 30 milliseconds before the pain is even felt as a 'feeling' (Hermans 2002). For example, soldiers in war who suffer horrendous injuries sometimes report no immediate experience of pain. Moreover, exposure to overwhelming trauma in combat results in sustained periods of analgesia. Solders wounded in battle require much lower doses of morphine than in other types of incidental injury (Beecher 1946). Like other procedures, pain reactions can be inhibited as both an innate 'freeze' response (LeDoux 1994; Scaer 2001) and as a learned response. When the latter occurs, the process of inhibition has been highly and broadly developed.

As would be expected, pain leads to a sharp increase in arousal (Doidge 2007). As an *imaged* response, pain is the feeling of the body (searing, burning, throbbing, piercing, etc.) that both produces autonomic changes in the body and, as afferent feedback, escalates the process of somatic self-protective change, i.e., the fight or flight response. When afferent feedback is absent, there is impairment of the emotional response (Critchley *et al*. 2001). Emotional responses, however, can be modulated by expectation and attributed meaning and, at very high levels of arousal, by reversals of the valence of arousal; that is, painful stimuli can be perceived as pleasurable (Rhudy and Meagher 2001). In common experience, this is the confusion between laughing and crying, but in more extreme conditions, it may open the door to masochistic behavior.

Both placebos (that affect expectation) and hypnosis (a combination of certain types of connotative language and arousal lowering, monotonous procedures) can be used by the self or by a therapist to lower arousal, thus, increasing tolerance of pain (placebos: Wagner *et al*. 2004; hypnosis: Molton *et al*. 2007; Wickramasekera 2008). In addition, negative emotions can lead to inhibition of awareness of pain, but only when they are highly arousing, whereas moderate negative emotions with low-to-moderate arousal facilitate perception of pain (Rhudy and Meagher 2001).

Pain itself can be experienced physically or emotionally, or observed empathically. All three conditions produce activity in some of the same brain structures, i.e., the anterior cingulate cortex (Botvinick *et al*. 2005; Eisenberger *et al*. 2003), but pain experienced empathically does not elicit a neural response in the sensorimotor cortex (Singer *et al*. 2004). Further, pain is associated with several other affects, particularly fear, but also sadness, and these are processed separately. Finally, the stimuli that elicit emotion-based pain appear to be unique to each individual (Vogt 2005) with prior extreme experiences, such as abuse, modifying response to pain, both by raising the threshold (i.e., increasing inhibition) and lowering it (i.e., augmenting the response) (Ringel *et al*. 2008). Finally, it is worth noting that necessary as pain is, our responses are evolved to enable us to avoid it or its precipitating stimuli. That complexity is reflected in all levels of our response to pain from neurological to behavioral.

Levels of awareness

The detailed information of the previous sections can be summarized developmentally and functionally in terms of three levels of awareness. These, in turn, can guide the selection of interventions when change is needed even before a full evaluation has been completed.

Preconscious functioning

The brain is organized structurally and ontogenetically first to carry out simple and rapid transformations and, then, as development, time, and previous experience make it possible, to elaborate the transformations, in an increasingly complex and slow process. The process moves from preconscious to highly self-reflective.

Babies and young children actively process information, but are unaware of it; their knowledge is preconscious (referring to extent of processing) and implicit (referring to how it is known).

Awareness

Consciousness, depending upon how one defines it, begins sometime in the preschool years (roughly 2–5 years of age). With awareness, it is possible to have both greater control over one's mental processes and also a more extensive array of transformations of information. Conscious awareness makes some information, but not all, explicitly known. The clearest evidence of explicit information is that which is verbalized in language. Even then, however, discourse contains implicitly known information; the discrepancy between the implicit and explicit aspects of verbal information makes discourse analysis possible.

Beginning around 7 years of age, simple concrete forms of integration of information take place. The logical aspects of this process have been studied very extensively whereas the integration of feelings with logical thoughts is less fully explicated. Nevertheless, integration of cognition and affect is central to the DMM understanding of psychological balance and personal adaptation.

Conscious integration

Reflective functioning, i.e., the integration of both concrete and abstract information from the various memory systems, does not begin until adolescence and is not complete until the mid-thirties when brain maturation is complete. Reflective functioning permits integration around specific problems to be distilled and generalized so as to be applicable to many situations, including some that have not yet been experienced.

The most sophisticated form of conscious thought is metacognition, which is the ability to think about how one thinks. Recognition of thought processes, together with a process of giving meaning to discrepancies in how one is thinking, gives individuals the greatest range of self-control.

Each of these levels of awareness is useful in adult life, less aware functioning producing behavior more rapidly and reflective integration producing more precise behavior. As always, there is a trade-off, and the proximity of danger (in time and space) together with its consequences (in probability and severity) suggests which compromise is likely to be most beneficial.

Conclusions

The crucial points to take from this discussion of information processing are that:

1 Many sorts of DRs are generated by the brain.
2 The most rapidly protective DRs are preconscious and, therefore, vulnerable to error retained from the past.
3 The more one has been exposed to danger in the past, especially in the first years of life,
   a. the more facilitated preconscious protective neural networks will be;
   b. the less experience one will have with integrative processing;
   c. the fewer alternative DRs one will have available to apply to current circumstances.
4 Pain is extremely self-protective and can be transformed in many ways, some of which may inhibit protective action or elicit pain-seeking behavior.
5 Degree of consciousness varies, often as a function of the immediacy and severity of danger.

Notes

1 The term 'cognitive' is used here in the restricted meaning of 'based on temporal order'. It does not, as used here, refer to a wider range of cortical processes.
2 Innate, genetically based differences in the perception of change in intensity contribute to temperamental differences in emotional lability.
3 The term 'imaged' was selected because it reflects both subjective experience and usage in the trauma literature.

Chapter 6

How do parents affect children's representations?

The terms 'pattern of attachment' and 'quality of attachment' have been used to refer to the ABC patterns described by Ainsworth (1979). They are also considered strategies for eliciting care from attachment figures and internal representational models of how to elicit care. That is, as Ainsworth's work developed, it moved from being strictly descriptive (patterns of attachment) to awareness of the interpersonal function of the patterns (strategies) to awareness of the mental processing that underlies behavior (inner working models and, now, dispositional representations). Although academic discussion of these reflects a historical progression, the three are inseparable and co-occurring aspects of the same phenomenon, a trinity, we might say. This chapter considers both what constitutes a self-protective strategy and what the array of possible self-protective strategies looks like in behavioral and information- processing terms. The chapter closes with a transgenerational look at the cases introduced in Chapters 1–5.

From representation to strategy

An expanded model

The first four chapters presented the DMM of attachment strategies in the form of case examples. In the section below, the strategies are presented in a concise and abstract manner that (a) ties behavior to the underlying information processing and (b) presents some general clinical problems tied to the distortions of information inherent in the strategies.

Type A strategies

Individuals using the Type A subpatterns organize their behavior around cognitive procedural and semantic contingencies and discard as unreliable or misleading imaged and connotative information (i.e., affect). In infancy, this is displayed as inhibition of desire for comfort, anger or fear, and is accomplished by keeping the attachment figure out of perception (by 'avoiding' looking at the attachment figure). By the end of the second year of life, maturation gives children the ability to inhibit even when perceiving the attachment figure, and the Type A strategy becomes more subtle. Children using it look at the parent, but with an object raised between them. This keeps the adult from feeling rejected while still avoiding intimacy. Also in the preschool years, children learn to substitute displayed false positive affect for inhibited negative affect, e.g., smiling when angry or frightened, and to use coy behavior to disarm parental anger. Finally, the onset of sexual arousal in adolescence can give adolescents an arousing affect that is acceptable – particularly in males.

This can mean that males using a Type A strategy can express other forbidden affects in sexual ways. Sexual desire in both males and females is closely related to affection and achievement of comfort. In addition, sexual arousal in males may be related to angry and fearful arousal with all three states (desire for comfort/affection, anger, and fear), resulting in penile arousal (Laws *et al.* 2000; Marshall and Hucker 2006; Schwartz and Masters 1994). Functionally, this will mean that some males using a Type A strategy will display affect, anger, and fear with sexual behavior; that is, the function of the sexual behavior will not be sexual/reproductive, but rather attachment/safety. This can result in harm to others. For females, the problem is more complex. Display of sexual desire is less acceptable in females; instead, in some cultures, it is often distorted and can appear as compliance with or submission to men's sexual desire (Impett and Peplau 2003). This, too, can lead to risks, but more often it will involve the self being harmed than the self harming others (Donnelly and Fraser 1998; Peplau 2003).

The distortions of cognition begin in infancy as highly predictable behavioral responses. By 3–4 years of age, these cognitive distortions begin to take verbal form as exaggerations of probability. Such distortions can often be identified by such 'absolute' words as 'always', 'never,' 'very, very', etc. A particular problem for Type A individuals is how they name feelings. Because individuals using a Type A strategy omit forbidden feelings from awareness and function verbally, access to feelings is semantically regulated. As a consequence, the label given to an act or feeling may be more defining than the function. For example, if sexual behaviors have been used for their function of 'comfort' or 'affection', they may be applied where sexuality would be forbidden without creating a semantic discrepancy between the semantic prescription and the labeled act, as was described for David in the previous chapter.

Moreover, as the numeral of the pattern increases (from A1–2 to A7–8), the extent of distortion in cognition increases, as does the compulsiveness with which the strategy is applied to daily problems. That is, an individual classified as A1 (idealizing of attachment figures) or A2 (negating of self) uses a strategy that is mildly biased toward temporal contingencies but, in the face of clear, disconfirming information, can change strategy. On the other hand, an individual using an A7 or A8 strategy (delusional idealization or externally assembled self) relies almost exclusively on temporally organized and distorted information and applies the strategy without variation to both appropriate and inappropriate conditions in spite of clear, strong, and highly self-relevant disconfirming information. That is, strategies are considered 'compulsive' to the extent that they require the individual to act in a rapid, reflexive, and unchanging manner. The intermediary substrategies are A3 (compulsive caregiving/attention), A4 (compulsive compliance/performance), A5 (compulsively promiscuous), and A6 (compulsively self-reliant). The cognitive distortion is in the direction of taking responsibility not only for one's own contribution, but also for other people's contribution. That is, individuals using a Type A strategy hold themselves responsible for things they didn't cause and can't change. That gives them perception of control (which is healthy), but they must often experience failure because the control is false. This leaves them vulnerable to depression and, in extreme cases, delusion.

Four points are important. First, cognition takes two forms, procedural action and prescriptive semantic guides. Second, as the numeral increases from A1–2 to A7–8, the source of semantic prescriptions becomes increasingly outside the self (i.e., parental directives to the moral/religious standards of people claiming to represent or be the source of guidance). Concurrently, language moves from dry (A1–2) to borrowed parental speech (A3–4) to artificial and abstract (A5–6) to borrowed professional jargon (A7–8). Third, semantic words and ideas define acts more than the feelings associated with the act. Semantic memory, in other words, is the entry to recall and thought. Fourth, as the numeral increases, there is an increase in both the extent of distortion of information and also the uniformity with which the strategy is applied to all perceived threats, appropriately and inappropriately (see Figure 6.1).

Type C strategies

Individuals using the Type C substrategies are biased toward acting on the basis of their feelings (i.e., affect, as represented by imaged and connotative information) and find temporal contingencies to be unpredictable or misleading. Type C is a more complex organization than Type A. In infancy, it is experienced as simple arousal leading to mixed feelings of desire for comfort, anger, and fear. These motivate approach with requests for comfort, approach with aggression, and escape, respectively. Any one of these responses might be the most adaptive response to a given situation, but, used together, they are incompatible and ineffective. Moreover, they confuse the parent.

By the end of the second year of life, maturation gives children the ability to regulate these feeling states both internally (such that behavior becomes focused) and interpersonally (such that displayed affect is used to regulate others' responses). Thus, a preschool-aged child might usually approach problems with angry aggression, but, when faced with adults'

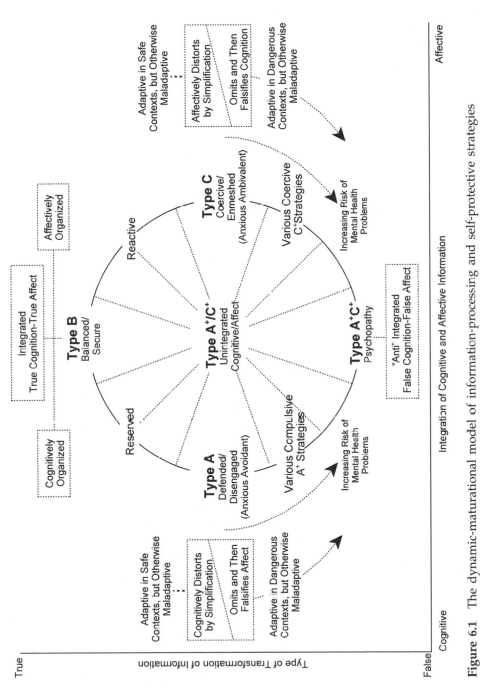

Figure 6.1 The dynamic-maturational model of information-processing and self-protective strategies

anger, shift to disarmingly coy bids for comfort (while hiding evidence of anger). Similarly, a coyly coercive child will shift threateningly to anger when faced with the parent's frustration over the helpless display. The Type C strategies include C1 (threatening), C2 (disarming), C3 (aggressive), C4 (feigned helpless), C5 (punitively obsessed with revenge), C6 (seductively obsessed with rescue), C7 (menacing), and C8 (paranoid).

Because coercive children do not display the full range of states that they actually feel, observers do not see evidence of the inhibited feelings. When they describe the child's feeling in words, they do not name the hidden feelings. This leaves the meanings of words murky to the child who, looking angry and feeling fear and desire for comfort as well, is given the word 'angry'. 'You are "angry".' But when feeling fear and inhibiting anger and desire for comfort, the child is told, 'You are "afraid".' But the child felt similarly in both cases! Only the display was different – for strategic reasons. An adult could understand this. But a child cannot and the child is only learning the language. If this occurs, as it does for many children using the Type C strategy, the child will find language ineffective to express feeling with precision. Nonverbal expressions may be maintained longer than for other children. When sexual desire is added in puberty, the indistinct mixture of arousing feelings can become more complex, with nonsexual desires being negotiated interpersonally with sexual signals and behavior. This, of course, adds to the complexity and ambiguity of relationships, thus, increasing the probability of discord and disappointment that cannot be resolved verbally.

Individuals using the Type C strategy omit awareness of their own contribution to events. In the short term that feels good; the other person is responsible and the self is an innocent victim. Long term, however, such false innocence prevents one from seeing what one could do to fix the problem onself. Without that knowledge, the problem will remain and may recur. One can get angry and angrier. But it doesn't solve the problem, and one feels more and more vulnerable. Splitting responsibility in this way puts too much control in the hands of other people – and this is then resented by the coercive individual. As with the Type A distorted distribution of responsibility, failure to acknowledge one's own contribution to events can lead to failure and possibly depression or, in very extreme cases, delusion. If people do not recognize their own contribution, they cannot correct it.

Three points are important. First, desire for comfort, anger, fear and pain constitute a gradient of increasingly arousing affective states that transform arousal into coherent action. The more arousing states become more prominent as the numeral increases from C1–2 to C7–8. Second, as the numeral increases, these states are increasingly generated and maintained by the self. Third, as the numeral increases, there is an increase in both the extent of distortion of information and the uniformity with which the strategy is applied to all perceived threats, appropriately and inappropriately (see Figure 2.2).

A/C patterns consist of any combination of A and C strategies, e.g., A1–2/C1–2, A3/C4, A1/C5. Individuals who organized an A/C strategy could think that they had all the information, took both perspectives, and both kept and gave responsibility. They might not notice that they had failed to integrate these so as to find a balance. Without that, they would swing from one extreme to its opposite, never finding the most predictive information, nor organizing the most adaptive response. Such people could become very bitter, very vulnerable, and very dangerous to themselves and others. When the 'others' are their children, the harm done can be substantial.

Reorganization, trauma, depression, disorientation, and intrusions of forbidden negative affect

When individuals are exposed to danger, they have the opportunity to garner new information on its antecedents and context, their own behavior and feelings, and the consequences of their actions. That information can be used in many different ways. If individuals discriminate accurately that information which is unique to the specific situation (i.e., dismissing the irrelevant information from the current representation) and that which is general and, therefore, relevant to the future (i.e., carrying forward the relevant information), they are considered resolved with regard to that dangerous experience. If in addition, they can integrate the dangerous experience without distortion into their understanding of their life's experience, they may be or become balanced. Alternatively, the whole strategy may undergo a change.

Specifically, there are five ways in which a strategy can be modified by exposure to danger.

Reorganization

Sometimes resolution of exposure to danger changes individuals' understanding of the relation between themselves and their context such that both their internal processing of information and their strategic organization of behavior are modified in ways that increase the fit of person to context. That is, exposure to danger can be the impetus to correction of omitted, distorted, erroneous, and falsified information, such that individuals *reorganize* in a more adaptive manner. In terms of strategies, a reorganizing A7-8 might move toward an A3-4 or even a B by correcting the erroneous, falsified, omitted, and distorted information. Similarly, an obsessive C (C3-8) could correct information-processing errors to move in the direction of Type B.

Unresolved trauma

On the other hand, if individuals make errors in discriminating self-relevant information from information that is true but not self-relevant in the present, either dismissing that which is relevant or carrying forward that which is not relevant (or both), they are considered *unresolved* (U). In the DMM, 'danger' refers to events and 'trauma' to certain kinds of psychological responses to dangerous events.

Overall, there are ten ways that unresolved trauma can be described in the DMM. Most, however, are observed infrequently and all can be clustered as dismissing of the self or preoccupied with the self. The dismissing of, or distancing from, self forms of lack of resolution include *dismissing* lack of resolution, which causes signals of danger to be omitted from representation. Other forms of distancing from the self responses to unresolvable trauma are *displaced* (on to another person, often a sibling) and *blocked* when there is no conscious awareness of the event, but the markers of psychological trauma are present. The preoccupying forms of lack of resolution tend to increase the range of stimuli that elicit a self-protective response. *Preoccupying* lack of resolution causes people to respond as if there were danger when there is not. Other forms of trauma that make danger excessively real are *vicarious* (when the self shows psychological trauma for an event occurring only for one's attachment figure), *anticipated* (when there is evidence of psychological trauma around an event that is irrationally thought to be imminent), and *hinted* (when the individual dare not articulate an accusation, but offers evidence that will cause the listener to state the accusation). Both distancing and involving errors make prediction less accurate, the former by underestimating the probability of danger and the latter by overestimating its probability. Three more general forms of trauma are *delusional* (when the traumatizing event simply could not be as stated), *depressed* (when the self believes nothing can be done to restore the self to a functional condition with regard to the traumatizing event), and *disorganized* (when several events are confused temporally, in terms of involved persons, and psychologically in terms of responses).

Depression
Depression (Dp) occurs when the individual has concluded that no action will effect any change in any aspect of their life; arousal drops, sometimes in life-threatening ways. Depression is assessed in all six memory systems and consists of procedural lack of protective sequences, flat expressed affect, and lack of engagement with others (without actively rejecting them or struggling with them). Depressed images are not self-relevant. Semantic statements indicative of depression express futility or the fatefulness of events, i.e., lack of self-efficacy. Depressed connotative language is heavy, sad and flat. The episodes of depressed individuals tell the whole story of what went wrong without complaint or any opening for changing events in the future. In terms of reflective functioning, all the information seems present, but the problems seem intrinsic to the situation. That is, knowing clearly does not open doors to rethinking the situation or arriving at new understandings.

Disorientation

Disorientation (DO) occurs when sources of information are confused such that individuals' behavior is sometimes in their own best interest and sometimes not – without their being able to identify this. Instead, without knowing it, they may act on DRs from earlier ages or from other people, especially attachment figures. When adults are not oriented toward specific interests (their own or others), behavior becomes incoherent.

Intrusions of negative affect

Intrusions of unregulated anger, fear, desire for comfort, sexual desire, or pain occur when inhibited negative affect intrudes explosively and without a coercively alternating display of negative affects that function interpersonally. Intrusions increase arousal rapidly and intensely. Such intrusions (a) are only possible in a compulsive Type A (inhibitory) strategy, (b) can function to reverse depression, and (c) are sometimes associated with psychotic breaks.

To summarize, as individuals deviate away from Type B, they become increasingly locked into a strategy without sufficient regard to current circumstances. Cognitively, they distort probabilities and responsibilities. Affectively, when feeling, function, and linguistic label do not coincide, there will almost certainly be misdirected, misunderstood, and maladaptive behavior. Sexual feelings are particularly prone to this sort of confusion. Transformations of information used in strategies that were self-protective when they were developed can prevent safe and comfortable relationships in the long term. When the long term in question is raising one's children, correcting the distortions and reorganizing one's information processing become crucial.

Using integrative processes, on the other hand, reflects mental balance with regard to the type of information used to generate behavior and this, in turn, creates the greatest probability that (a) discrepancies will draw attention, (b) distortions in representation will be discovered and corrected, and (c) occasion-specific and effective self-protective solutions will be found to life's threats. That is, psychologically balanced individuals have the greatest probability of being safe and feeling secure. Put another way, the Types A and C strategies use past representations to organize behavior (with working memory fitting the old solution to the current context, rather than considering *whether* the solution fits the context). The Type B strategy, on the other hand, is a strategy for using information to generate new solutions to problems.

Sometimes, Type B is treated as a state that, once entered, is protective across the life span. It can seem as if, having once achieved the safe land of security, one is forever out of the water. However, once one considers how information is processed and the effects of the context on one's physical and psychological safety (including the unpredictable effects of changes in the context), then safety looks less like a permanent spot on a sunny beach and more like knowing how to swim very well. Predictable currents flow though life and unpredictable storms can appear out of nowhere. One is always swimming for dear life and is never 'home free'. For sure, Type B shows the greatest empirical continuity across life and even across generations. I think that this is because people using the balanced strategy work their strategy daily to achieve balance in the context of an ever-changing set of life challenges. When one is habitually and actively adapting all the time, one is rarely so far out of synchrony with the context as to be in danger or to endanger one's children. Type B is not assurance that one is safe, or that one will always be comfortable. It is simply the strategy of stacking the probabilities in one's favor.

Maturation of the brain functions to repeatedly create opportunity for reorganization, with the most propitious opportunity coming in the transition to adulthood when the cortex of the brain is finally mature and able to achieve the full integrative potential of humans. At that point, a person can care for themselves, has two decades of experience (more or less), and can think. This moment of opportunity is very special and what happens in it is of great import for each person's children.

How does perception of danger affect behavior?

The attachment literature treats parental representations as being different from attachment representations (George and Solomon 1999). The perspective offered here is more general. Representations are simply networks of firing neurons that represent the relation of self to context at a particular moment in time and dispose the self to some response. DRs elicited when safety or reproduction are threatened are more intense and temporal relations are learned in fewer trials than when DRs are not related to attachment. That is, stimuli signaling danger to the self, progeny, or opportunity for sexual reproduction receive preferential attention.

Threatened individuals often take extreme risks to protect themselves and their children or to gain access to reproductive partners. That is, many of the things that one does to protect oneself – or one's children – are themselves dangerous. What except extreme danger would make a person jump from an upper floor window – as some people did from the World Trade Center on September 11? Why would parents send their children away to be raised by strangers – as did some Jewish parents in Nazi Germany? Why would anyone permit their body to be cut open – as is done in surgery? Why would a man beat his wife – as many husbands do? What would cause people to hit their own children – as far too many parents do? The answer to all of these questions is most often the same: fear of greater danger if this very dangerous action is not taken.

Applying this notion to the first three examples is straightforward. The second example, however, is important in showing that parents treat children as an extension of self such that their survival can be more important than protecting the self. That is, children are parents' genetic future and thus are protected as a part of self (Dawkins 1976). The final two examples, spousal and child abuse, are more perplexing because they seem counterintuitive and morally reprehensible. Nevertheless, the most common reason for spousal abuse is fear of sexual unfaithfulness (Dobash *et al.* 1992; Wilson and Daly 1992). That is, the attacking man is protecting his reproductive opportunity and refusing to be cuckolded into using his resources to raise another man's children. The most frequent reason for striking children is to teach them not to do something that the parent believes is dangerous (Holden and Zambarano 1992). Framed this way, these relatively frequent forms of danger can be included in the same motivational model as more extreme and unusual forms of risk-taking.

Thus, one principle can account for a great deal of dangerous human behavior, including most forms of inadequate child-rearing:

The more dangerous the threat is deemed to be, the more risk will be incurred to prevent or overcome the threat.

Further, the greater the perceived danger, the more rapid and incomplete the processing of information and, therefore, the more vulnerable the representation is to error. Finally, the specific error is likely to be one that treats current conditions as being similar to past conditions.

How do parents' strategies affect children's strategies?

The heavy contribution of the past to current psychological and behavioral functioning might suggest that parents who were mistreated in childhood would necessarily repeat that process with their children. That is, one might assume both that what was done to the child, the child as a parent would do to its child and that the parent's strategy would be used by the child. This notion of 'transgenerational transmission' of constancy/sameness is prevalent in both the maltreatment literature and the attachment literature. In maltreatment, it has been widely assumed that if you were maltreated, you will maltreat your children. The data do not confirm that notion ((Kaufman and Zigler 1987; Monaghan-Blout 1999). Instead the findings are more complex. If you maltreat your child, you almost certainly were maltreated. But if you were maltreated, it is more likely that you do not maltreat your own children. So only a small proportion of maltreated children (30 per cent) become maltreating parents (Kaufman and Zigler 1987), but almost all maltreating parents were maltreated (Blumberg 1974; Friedrich and Wheeler 1982). The effect, in other words, is important, crucially important, for preventing harm to children, but spontaneous 'recovery' is more common than not. Things get better on their own – in most cases.

The same transgenerational hypothesis is widely articulated in attachment work (Main and Goldwyn 1984). Further, there is empirical support (Benoit and Parker 1994; Kanemasa 2007; Kazui *et al.* 2000) for the notion of continuity of pattern of attachment from mother to child. Nevertheless, in a meta-analysis of studies reporting the correspondence between mothers' and infants' patterns of attachment, the data leave the majority of the variance (78 per cent) unaccounted for (van IJzendoorn 1995). Moreover, if one looks closely at the 22 per cent representing continuity, one discovers that it is accounted for almost entirely by cross-generational continuity within Type B – only Type B. That is, more often parents' DRs do *not* match their children's, and the parents most likely not to match their children in pattern of attachment use the Type A and Type C strategies. In these cases, both corrections (toward Type B) and reversals (to the opposite A or C pattern) of the parental error are common. To understand this, one must consider the process of 'transmission' of DRs.

What is transmitted?

Beginning with communication between two adults, each adult has all six kinds of DRs. One DR regulates behavior in a particular moment, and the first person acts. That is, what gets out of the mind is not the representation itself but, rather, behavior. The other person perceives this behavior as sensory stimulation: temporally ordered stimulation and intensity-based stimulation. Perception, itself, however, is colored by previous experience, such that one perceives what one expects to perceive; according to Gregory (1998), 90 per cent of perception is memory. The second person's brain processes this already distorted information as networks of activated neurons and generates a set of DRs. On the basis of one or a combination of these, the second person acts – producing behavior that the first person perceives as sensory stimulation, etc.

The DRs (i.e., the networks of firing neurons) never get out of the person's brain. They exist only in the moment of synaptic firing and cannot be directly shared with another person. What 'gets out' is behavior, but even behavior isn't transmitted directly, but rather is perceived in the form of temporal order and intensity of stimulation. At this point, the recipient's brain begins transforming the incoming information to generate its own DRs of the relation of self to the other person. These representations may – or may not – be similar to the first person's representations, but they are never identical.

Parent–child transmission

The situation between parents and children is the same – with one exception. Parents, being adults, have six functioning memory systems. Infants have only three and older children are developing the other forms of representation. Anything the parent does, no matter how complex, will be represented in a simpler form by infants and children. That is, infants' and children's DRs *cannot* be the same as their parents'. Parents cannot give or transmit their *representations* to their children. Instead, parents act, creating an environment in which infants and children perceive certain stimulation and then generate their own representations of the relation of self to context. Like parents' representations, children's representations vary in the emphasis on temporal or affective information used to organize behavior, and this may reflect – or reverse – the parents' emphasis.

A few familiar examples

Some of the case examples used in the previous chapters have both parent and child attachment data. These few cases can suggest some of the parent-to-child patterns that might be found, but they cannot, of course, indicate the probability of the patterns, relative to other possibilities, nor is there any reason to believe that these are all the relations that occur. The examples do, however, suggest the complexity of the parent–child relationship.

The data on Luke and his parents are extensive. His father's AAI was classified as reorganizing from an unresolved and dismissed trauma in a compulsively self-reliant strategy (A6) toward a recognition of the trauma and its effects and a simple A1 strategy, i.e., much nearer B, but not yet balanced. With him, Luke almost used a secure B strategy – and definitely did not use an A or C strategy. Luke's mother's AAI was classified as a simple A1–2, without traumas. If both parents settle at A1–2, there should be no risk for Luke or his siblings, because A1–2 is a normal strategy with only a slight transformation, one that is corrected under dangerous circumstances. With his foster mother, Luke used a coercive aggressive strategy (C3), whereas his foster mother's AAI was classified as unresolved trauma and loss in a preoccupied and anticipated form with a compulsive caregiving strategy (Utr&l A3). So Luke used a Type C strategy in response to a Type A strategy from the foster mother. The foster father used a coercive feigned helpless strategy (C4). These two families demonstrate both matching patterns between the spouses (the biological parents) and opposite, but complementary, patterns (the foster parents). They also demonstrate that children can use different strategies with different attachment figures and that these strategies can resemble the parents' strategy (with the father) or strongly and negatively react in the opposite manner to it (the foster mother). It is expected that strategies nearer the balanced part of the model would more often match and those nearer the middle of the model, where information is omitted, would be complementary opposites.

Jenny's mother's AAI was classified as partially depressed but using only an A1 strategy, with a bit of caregiving. Jenny displayed a coercive aggressive and feigned helpless strategy in an effort to activate her mother's protection. Because her strategy was not working, we can expect it to escalate in the direction of greater risk-taking (as the brother showed) or, possibly, a reversal to compulsive caregiving – especially if the mother recedes into a more pervasively depressed state. This last statement is a reminder that development is dynamic and can be responsive to change.

We also know about Sophie and her mother. Sophie used an entrenched coercive punitive strategy (C5) with an imagined trauma (she erroneously blamed an early illness for her eating disorder). Her mother had unresolved trauma about which she was both dismissing and preoccupying in a compulsively caregiving strategy (Utr(ds&p) A3). In this case of anorexia, we have a reversal of strategy from parent to child. It should be remembered, however, that in other cases, the parent and child strategies can be the same, e.g., both parent and child using a coercively punitive and seductive strategy (Ringer and Crittenden 2007).

Finally, in the case of David, we have a coercively punitive father (C5) and a coercively seductive and helpless mother (C6). By adulthood, David had organized as delusionally idealizing of his apparently helpless mother (A7), failing to acknowledge that she, too, harmed him, in her case by abandoning him to his father's fury. In addition, however, David had a series of unresolved traumas both in and out of his home. David, in other words, was both on the opposite side of the model and more extreme than his parents, probably because his strategy did not function to make them more protective or comforting.

Conclusions

The chapters in Part 1 set out the dynamic-maturational meta-theory of attachment and adaptation. They did so developmentally, showing how the strategies develop as maturation changes the brain and culture changes the contexts in which children live. New contexts offer greater variety and call for new self-protective strategies. Case examples were used both to give an imaged representation of the strategies and to demonstrate their relevance to clinical conditions.

In addition, Part 1 outlined the information processing that underlies strategic behavior, describing how information processing can explain the complex relation between parents' and children's strategies. Even when the strategies match, however, we should keep in mind that the parent's strategy is not 'transmitted' to the child. Only behavior is expressed by the parent and only sensory information reaches the child; children must use that to construct their own strategy.

Part 2 will focus on parents' strategies for protecting children, especially in cases where children are not protected or comforted adequately. In order to understand parents' intent, we will need to get 'inside' these strategies. That is, having read how they develop over childhood and what sorts of transformations of information occur to generate them, we will need to try to think and feel like someone using that strategy if we are to understand parents who harm their children. Once we can do that, we may be able to join parents meaningfully and guide them safely to a less dangerous reality. Without understanding them as they understand themselves, we may not be able to help.

Part 2

Raising Children

Chapter 7

Representation and child-rearing that endangers children

Part 2 has two purposes. The first is to provide a perspective on why parents raise their children as they do, especially in cases where parental behavior has harmed the children or put them at risk. This will help professionals to have a focused and compassionate perspective on parents. This, in turn, is essential to successful treatment. The second is to rank the explanations in terms of the extent of distortion of information processing, representation, and self-protective/child-protective strategy. This will help professionals to individualize and shape the treatment plan, and that also is essential to treatment success.

Why parents behave as they do

In Part 2, we will try to take the *parent's perspective* to understand parental intentions. Intentions precede behavior. Intentions are DRs and, as shown in Part 1, each of us has many intentions. The intention that is of interest is the one that motivated the actual behavior. If we want to change behavior, we must change that intention. Most often, however, professionals ask about intentions *after* the behavior has occurred and only in cases where the outcome was undesirable. When that happens, there are three sorts of intention to think about. We are interested in the intention that preceded action; that will be the most difficult to uncover. Especially in cases that challenge all rational notions of 'protection', the disposing DR will actually be the confluence of several DRs, almost always including procedural, imaged, or peripheral/somatic DRs that are not consciously known to the individual. In practice, professionals often assume intention based on the outcome of the behavior. Because that was not necessarily the parent's functional intention, it is not what we are seeking. On the other hand, professionals do ask parents what they intended, and that answer, too, is not what we are seeking.

Why not? Because that answer is likely to be a prescriptive semantic DR (about what one *should* do) that is generated after the event in the context of knowing (a) how things turned out and (b) that a professional is evaluating the response the parent gives. Once the action has produced an outcome, the representational context is changed – for everyone. It can be difficult to see what you intended when it didn't turn out and you are to blame for something bad. Only the most balanced people can recreate their predisaster state of mind and deal openly with the discrepancy between what they intended and what happened. This is especially true if they harmed their child. Instead, they (we! because everyone does this) seek an acceptable answer, one that portrays us in a good light and makes the outcome seem a random, unexpectable, or inexplicable event. This, of course, is exactly what children do when they answer their parents' questions about why they did what they shouldn't have done. When there are negative consequences hanging in the balance, both children and adults (including professionals) seek an answer that will please a powerful or threatening listener.

Instead, we want to know the parent's intention *before* the consequences of the action were known. If the points made in Part 1 about transforming information, memory systems, and representations are correct, then many parents and almost all troubled parents will be unable to tell accurately why they did what they did when they did it. This will be especially true when they know they should not have done it or when it turned out poorly. Therefore, it will usually be futile – and often be misleading – to ask the parent directly why they did what they did. Only well-integrated people can answer the question, and, even then, it can take considerable thought. In addition, if the questioner is a threat to the parent, as child-protective services and the courts are, the immediate context of the question changes the context of representation substantially. Under such circumstances, the parent shifts from trying to solve a problem with the child to trying to solve a problem with the professional. Nevertheless, changing parental behavior will be accomplished best if the actual basis for the behavior with the child is discovered, i.e., uncovered, and changed.

If we can't assume on the basis of consequences and we can't simply ask, then it will be necessary to seek alternative ways of accessing the parents' DRs. From the array of representations, we can explore both what is represented and also which representations are acted upon in the crucial instances when things go awry. Having person-specific hypotheses regarding the content and selection priorities among representations should be helpful in choosing treatment strategies with the potential to change the representations or the process leading to acting upon them.

Current practice

At present, evaluations of parental competence are made largely on the basis of particular behaviors that are deemed maltreating or not. That is, the terms 'abuse', 'neglect', and 'sexual abuse' are used to define cases of inadequate child-rearing. Once maltreatment is substantiated, the response of the service system is to offer services to correct the deficiency or, if change is deemed not possible, to place the child in another care context in the hope that this will protect the child from the effects of the parent's inappropriate behavior. Four aspects of current practice are important.

First, as said earlier, if we use these pejorative terms, parents will almost always deny the abuse or neglect. In large part, I think, it is because the harmful outcome does not match their intention. Fear of censure and shame at the outcomes or revealing of their behavior are of course other components of parents' denial of abuse. These latter reflect the parent's interest *after* the fact.

Second, the type of maltreatment strongly affects the initial response of professionals. Sexual abuse tends to elicit the strongest and most rapid response overall (Higgins 2005). Very often it results in family separation even prior to other services being initiated (Brodsky-Jones 2003). Given that, prior to adjudication, fathers cannot be forced to leave their homes, one or more of the children are often placed in foster care (Havez 1992). On the other hand, in all except the most serious cases, instances of physical abuse usually begin with home-based services, but sometimes result in later removal if the services are ineffective. The course is different, however, if the abuse is identified in a hospital setting. In that case, removal of the child from parental custody and discharge from hospital to a foster home are common. Child neglect less often results in removal (as a percentage of identified neglect cases; US DHHS 2006a), and when removal occurs, it is usually delayed longer than for abuse. Psychological maltreatment exists as a type of maltreatment, but is rarely invoked even for the provision of supportive services, far less out-of-home placement (Fluke *et al.* 2005; Higgins 2005; US DHHS 2006a). This suggests that professionals believe that the immediate threat to children is greatest for sexual abuse and least for psychological maltreatment (Crittenden and Claussen 1993; Fluke *et al.* 2005; Higgins 2005; US DHHS 2006a). Because data to support that conclusion are limited and sometimes contradict that conclusion, it might be that other factors, such as moral censure, are operating to dispose professionals' behavior. That is, even in the case of professionals' behavior, intention can be difficult to establish – especially if the outcome is harmful to a child, as foster care often is.

Third, the services most frequently offered are parent education and cognitive-behavioral training (CBT). This suggests that professionals believe that maltreatment (or inadequate parenting) results from lack of information or lack of skills, or both. Again, the evidence indicates that maltreating parents who abuse their children are as knowledgeable about children's development and parenting practices as adequate parents of similar socioeconomic background (Friedrich and Wheeler 1982; Larrance and Twentyman 1983; Wolfe 1985); this is less true for neglectful parents. Alternatively, it might be that these sorts of interventions are offered because they are specifiable in a programmatic way that permits direct service personnel to measure outcomes in a reportable manner and enables decision-making agencies to account for their actions and justify their recommendations. Indeed, we could even argue that, like parents, when there is a crisis, a feeling of impending danger, professionals (from front-line workers to policymakers) act quickly, intuitively, and sometimes without deep reflection on the complexity of the problem. What might instigate the professionals' crisis? Media reports of harmed or killed children combined with the reaction of politicians. The points are that (a) professionals' behavior reflects the same psychological principles as parents', (b) the threat to professionals comes from outside the service system, and (c) there is no reward and there may be punishment for grasping and dealing with the actual complexity of failures to protect children. Again, this suggests the need for professionals to be very explicit with themselves regarding their intentions and the influences on their intentions.

Fourth, certain types of important child-rearing dysfunction are overlooked when evidence of maltreatment is the basis for professional involvement. Three sorts of conditions are relevant. The first is that of children of parents with mental illness. Such children are often not identified at all when instances of maltreating behavior are the primary basis for evaluating parental competency. Second, problems tied to compulsiveness are not only often overlooked but also are highly approved of by school authorities and parents alike. Consequently, compulsively organized parents and children (e.g., the Brightman family) may pass unnoticed when their behavior is actually a signal of serious problems that threaten both adult and child safety (Honoré 2008; Marano 2008). The third group consists of children diagnosed with a disorder that is misunderstood as being an individual characteristic when in fact it reflects the outcome of a distorted parent–child developmental process. These cases do come to professional attention, but the parental and dyadic aspects of the cases often escape notice, in spite of professional guidelines that require both a history and observation of the parents (Josephson 2007). The interpersonal quality of the disorders may be missed both because the processes are subtle and because our diagnostic methods focus on individuals' symptoms, thus not directing professionals' attention to parental or dyadic qualities. The third of these conditions is the most provocative, controversial, and 'politically incorrect'.

Interpersonal disorders in children

The conditions in children that might be tied to aspects of parent–child interaction include a wide variety of puzzling disorders, ranging from Munchausen's syndrome by proxy (now known as factious illness by proxy) to ADHD, PTSD, autism (and its spectrum), chronic fatigue syndrome/ myalgic encephalitis, the personality disorders, the psychoses, and violent and sexual criminality. Increasingly, genetic, neurological and biochemical explanations are sought for these relatively intractable disorders. There have been, however, familial and contextual/developmental explanations offered in the past by such great observer-theorists as Bateson, Bettelheim, Freud and Watzlawick. Some of their ideas proved to be flawed when put to the test, whereas others were dismissed because empirical data were lacking and because the ideas were deemed 'mother blaming'.

Genetic influences

On the other hand, our current notions of individual pathology are not yielding to either empiricism or treatment, and exculpating mothers may shift the burden of responsibility for the consequences of the condition from the family to their children. Empirically, findings of heritability are often based on familial co-occurrence of the disorder; this could be explained as well by developmental and interpersonal processes as by genetic factors. Moreover, in some cases, hereditable is confused with familial, and we now know that the twin designs used to investigate this difference seldom paid attention to the age of adoption or to genetic differences, including those in the 'promoter' regions of genes, in monozygotic twins.

Even when significant genetic effects are found, they are usually disappointing because they explain very little of the variance between disordered and non-disordered children. Moreover, to date, most findings are only of group differences with causation remaining an untested hypothesis. For example, a study of genetic contributions to autism (Weiss et al. 2008) reported finding a gene associated with autism; this gene was found in 1 per cent of cases of autism versus 0.1 per cent of the general population. One reviewer concluded, 'Autism may represent the summation of a series of rare events, whose detection will require screening tens of thousands of patient samples' (Jasny 2008: 1311). Another way to look at such findings is to say they are accurate statistically, but unlikely to be relevant to the causation or amelioration of autism (cf. Rutter et al. 1999). Another hypothesis might be needed.

In another example, ADHD is currently assumed primarily to be a neuropsychiatric disorder present from birth, but not immediately identified by clinicians. Nevertheless, as with autism, the evidence is not there to substantiate that hypothesis. Instead, the disorder may be based on psychosocial factors, including prolonged parent–child separation (Joseph 2000; Schachar and Wachsmuth 1991). This notion is evident in the follow-up studies of the Romanian children's home adoptees. Pervasive ADHD was initially observed in these children and attributed to their early care. However, the ADHD persisted only when the children were adopted too late for the initial severe deprivation to be remediable through later interpersonal experience and specific intervention efforts (Kreppner et al. 2001).

Pharmacological treatment has been the primary focus for treatment of ADHD, but, again, the studies are methodologically limited. There are in fact no double-blind studies in which neither researcher nor patient is able to say, after taking the drug, whether the patient took an active substance or not. Classically, placebos have been chosen as 'neutral' substances, rather than as substances that are indistinguishable from the substance under investigation; for a stimulant, this means that they need to experience an effect from the placebo, albeit one which is seen as irrelevant to the condition being investigated. In the existing studies, patients (who are not told) quickly perceive that there is no effect of the neutral 'pill' placebo. Only when drug therapy is compared with an active ingredient that does not affect ADHD symptoms can we know the actual effects of the drugs that were tested (Andrews 2001).

On the other hand, emerging work that has considered both the long-term and potentially negative effects of medication on ADHD is finding that medication (a) has no effect compared with no intervention after 2–3 years (Jensen *et al.* 2007; Molina *et al.* 2007; Swanson, Elliott *et al.* 2007) and (b) produces reduction in growth rates (Swanson, Hinshaw *et al.* 2007).

Epigenetic influences

A more promising route is through gene–environment interactions. Current studies of epigenetic processes suggest how context can change the *expression* of genes (Hanson and Gottesman 2007). A crucial aspect of context is variation in the danger, i.e., threat to survival or reproduction. This is a reminder that Bowlby (1969/1983) tied attachment behavior to an 'environment of evolutionary adaptedness'. Logically, as the environment in which an individual or group of individuals (e.g., a culture) lives and reproduces varies, so might the display of attachment behavior. That is, the functions of protection of self, reproduction, and protection of progeny would remain constant, but the strategies (and information processing underlying the strategies) that promoted these functions might vary in environments marked by different dangers.

Current technology makes possible sophisticated studies of genetic and biological contributions to disorder. Recent work is focusing on how inherited and acquired modifications of DNA modify genomic expression (without changing the DNA sequence itself), e.g., for major depressive disorder (Mill and Petronis 2007), psychosis (Kan *et al.* 2004), and schizophrenia (Petronis 2004). A crucial element is the influence of context, particularly the context of danger, on phenotype and heritability of phenotype. Further, this inherited moderator of gene expression appears to be reversible when the contextual threat is modified (Weaver *et al.* 2006). These perspectives return to the idea of behavioral adaptation to the context of experienced dangers.

Similarly, however, current video technology makes possible new exploration of interpersonal processes. Both psychoanalytic theory and family systems theory were prepared to address such hypotheses, but have backed off in recent years. In family-systems work, the reason is to retain a metaperspective to the family. Consequently, conclusions about the quality of parental care are rarely made so as to avoid pointing at anyone or evaluating anyone. Possibly, however, our inability to tolerate the results that close observation might offer denies families the very thing that they seek from psychological and psychiatric treatment. Possibly, we cannot help families if we see only what we think we *should* see or imagine that they *want* us to see. Maybe humans need to be seen accurately and assisted to change what they wish to change to fulfill their own intentions. Possibly, we could comfort troubled families better by offering truthful statements about behavior that they, too, can observe and evaluate.

Treatment approaches tied to interpersonal behavior

It might be more productive to enable family members to see what they actually do procedurally as compared with what they intended to do, or think they did, or explain to themselves about how things went badly. Video feedback, such as is described for some of the cases in this volume, can enable family members to see accurately what they do. This can enable them to take greater control of their behavior and change it, thus changing their interactions and relationships. Combined with the family systems idea of 'restorying', this can permit them to tell a new story to themselves about what has happened in their family. Often this will be a painful story of misunderstood intentions and missed opportunities to connect. Nevertheless, this accurate narrative can have a happy ending when accurate perception leads to behavioral change. 'Restorying', in this framework, leads to two new stories: correction of the misperceptions of family members, followed by behavioral change that leads to more empathic and synchronous experience – the new story. The crucial bit, however, is adding correct procedural information. Simply retelling painful narratives in more positive ways is unlikely to prove helpful because it adds fantasy on top of error. People, be they patients, researchers, clinicians, see what they (we) expect to see, and that is often driven by both memory (for implicit DRs) and desires and expectations (for semantic and connotative DRs).

To borrow from Piaget, theory should change in keeping with knowledge; it should both assimilate and accommodate. The issue becomes why we discarded the older unsupported interpersonal hypotheses and embrace equally unsupported biological hypotheses about anomalous genes or processes. To consider this question, we might need to ask who is advocating the research, i.e., putting pressure on funding institutions, and who is writing the research proposals that are funded. Anecdotally, at least some of these people (advocates and researchers) are parents of children with poorly understood disorders. Such people both have special insight and lack objectivity. It is very difficult to retain the necessary objectivity in such a situation, regardless of how well trained one is in the scientific method. Might not their status as parents or patients influence the types of solutions they would seek? Might they have DRs that would distort responsibility, externalize blame, and seek 'victim' status? If that is even possible, the ethics of disclosing conflicting personal interest in the work being done should extend beyond formal and financial relationships with institutions and companies to personal factors that might generate bias in the choice of hypotheses, analysis of the data, and framing of the findings.

The ideas proposed here and elsewhere in this book are based on clinical experience and are derived from data from many countries. They do not constitute experimental or controlled empirical evidence, but in the absence of good evidence for any hypothesis, these clinical findings constitute powerful 'practice-based', case study evidence. Case studies can complement evidence drawn from experimental research findings well when the cases use rigorous observation that is methodologically defined (as opposed to uncontrolled observer perceptions). Further, 'action research', which clinical practice offers, is the opportunity to test theory by observing the impact of different interventions (Dallos and Smith 2008). This, too, is a powerful form of evidence that has informed DMM theory and the specific hypotheses offered here.

If any of these very serious disorders (ADHD, the psychoses, autism, etc.), most of which are increasing in prevalence, have a familial component, then identifying and treating that component will reduce suffering. This is not mother-blaming. To the contrary, throughout this volume, I am asserting that, when understood correctly, even parents who harm their children intended to protect and comfort them. Freeing those who have not achieved that goal to act differently can reduce both their suffering and their children's. That is the single most important goal of this volume.

To conclude, current practice reflects society's representation (as interpreted by professionals) of the child's interests, and these are defined by outcomes of children. Whether these are actually children's interests has been a matter of dispute for some time (cf. Goldstein *et al.* 1973, Goldstein *et al.* 1996). Parents are viewed as the vehicle for meeting children's needs, and they face disapprobation, with legal consequences, to the extent that they fail to do so. In this volume, I seek a greater balance of parents' developmental experience and current context with children's needs.

Assessing transformations of information and DRs

There are very few assessments developed specifically for the purpose of assessing representations, and those that exist are not usually part of a child protection and forensic assessment protocol. Such assessments, however, offer several advantages over a traditional 'battery' of psychological assessments.

The most widely known of the assessments of representation are (1) the Strange Situation (Ainsworth *et al.* 1978) for 1-year-old infants and (2) the Adult Attachment Interview (AAI) (George *et al.* 1985/1996; Main and Goldwyn 1984) for adults. Working with Ainsworth, I created the CARE-Index for infants less than 1 year old (Crittenden 1981, 1988c, 2005a) and expanded the Strange Situation classificatory criteria to fit maltreated infants (Crittenden 1983) and, later, preschool-aged children (Crittenden

1992c; Crittenden *et al.* 2007). I have also expanded the AAI to fit better the range of variation in clinical populations (Crittenden 1999a) and adapted it to younger adults in the transition to adulthood (TAAI) (Crittenden 2005d). Finally, an assessment for school-aged children is now in the series (Crittenden 1997–2005). With this addition, we have an almost complete developmental series of assessments of (a) attachment, (b) self-protective strategy, (c) transformations of information, and (d) crucial bits of history tied to danger and lack of comfort.

These assessments have several characteristics in common. First, all are interpersonal. That is, none assesses individual characteristics and all assess how the individual functions within a specified relationship. The only exception – and it is only a partial exception – are the discourse assessments (SAA, TAAI, AAI). These yield information regarding both how the relationship is with each individual and the speaker's current strategy and transformations of information processing. The speaker's current strategy is enacted in three ways: in the use of discourse, the display of affect, and the relationship with the interviewer. Second, an important feature of these assessments is that they represent the subject's perspective, albeit, often in a manner that is not explicitly known to the subject. Third, another common characteristic is a lack of transparency. That is, the individual who codes, classifies, and interprets the meaning of the assessment is looking for evidence of DRs rather than seeking the explicit answers to the questions. Finally, another commonality is use of the DMM classificatory model, defined, of course, by the development of the person being assessed. That is, the outcomes of the assessments are framed by the DMM. The DMM expands Ainsworth's model from A1–2 and C1–2 in infancy, to A3–4 and C3–4 in the preschool years, A5–6 and C5–6 by adolescence, and A7–8 and C7–8 by adulthood. This expansion is applied to each assessment at its appropriate developmental level.

In the chapters that follow, we will be looking for the *parents'* DRs, particularly those that motivate their behavior in moments of threat to their children. In most cases, the information will be drawn from AAIs, TAAIs, and Parents' Interviews, but some information will come from parents' behavior in one of the videotaped procedures for young children.

Ranking transformations of information

In Part 2, the ideas about information processing are combined with observed problems in parenting to (a) create a gradient of increasing transformation of information (from truly predictive, through distorted predictions, to falsely predictive), and (b) hypothesize what sorts of parenting problems are most frequently associated with these distortions (see Box 7.1). It is important to keep in mind that these are normal human processes that are used excessively by parents whose caregiving endangers their children. This gradient is organized by *psychological functions*, and not by parental

Box 7.1   Parenting clusters: a clustering of parental representations organized around a patterned gradient of covarying psychological processes

---

Distortions of normal child-protective behavior
(1) Parents whose competing representations too often reflect self-needs, thus *minimizing* recognition of child needs (and thus underprotecting and sometimes neglecting their children)

(2) Parents who exaggerate the probability of danger to their children by relying on past contingencies (thus overprotecting and sometimes physically abusing their children)

Distortions that emphasize self-protective behavior
(3) Parents who transform desire for comfort into sexual desire and respond to children's needs with sexualized behavior (thus sometimes sexually mistreating their children)

(4) Parents who fail to perceive children's signals or to attribute a need to protect the children to the signals (thus sometimes physically and psychologically neglecting their children)

Distortions that substitute delusional information for accurate information
(5) Parents who misconstrue powerful forces as threatening both themselves and their children (thus sometimes severely injuring or killing their children)

(6) Parents who implicitly believe that the children threaten their own survival (thus sometimes deliberately killing their children)

---

behavior, outcome to the child, maltreatment of the child, or psychiatric diagnosis (see Box 7.1). Nevertheless, associations with maltreatment and psychopathology are offered to help the reader to visualize six different clusters. The purpose, however, is to tie distortions of information processing to endangering parental behavior.

Self- and child representations

All representations contain two represented components, the self and the nonself. This discussion is structured around how parents integrate *self-*representations with representations of their *child* to organize parental behavior. The interplay among DRs determines what and whose needs are given priority, what meanings are attributed to them, and what action is taken. The clusters reflect three co-occurring and interrelated gradients:

1 extent of awareness (from reflective to explicit to implicit);
2 extent of transformation of information (from truly predictive to distorted and omitted to falsely predictive);

3 frequency of nonstrategic behavior (unresolved trauma and loss and modifiers of depression, disorientation, and intrusions of forbidden negative affect).

It is not expected that Type B parents would be unaware with grave transformations and substantial nonstrategic behavior (except in rare cases when actual threatening conditions elicit rapid protective measures without 'wasting' the time needed for integration).

A set of hypotheses

The basic hypothesis is that *as past threats become more prominent and children less accurately a part of parents' DRs, parenting will become less adequate.* At the extreme, a delusional representation of the child may motivate behavior that protects the parent at the expense of the child. Although the gradient is structured around psychological functions, there is a rough concordance with symptom-based diagnoses such that parents fitting clusters 1 and 2 rarely carry a diagnosis or, if they do, it is a mild Axis I, stress-based diagnosis, whereas parents in clusters 3 and 4 often have additional diagnoses (comorbidity) and personality disorders (Axis II, enduring and maladaptive personality characteristics) and many parents fitting clusters 5 and 6 have had delusional or psychotic episodes.

It is noteworthy that these hypotheses are often consistent with what maltreating and mentally ill parents say about themselves and inconsistent with what the professional literature says about them. As presented here, they reflect an attempt to reconcile parents' words with the evidence of their harmful actions in ways that might (a) change professionals' understanding of the parents, (b) permit parents to recognize themselves in the descriptions (thus reducing denial), and (c) change the sorts of interventions that are offered. Throughout, the goal is to explain existing evidence with a set of new and potentially informative hypotheses.

There are four bases for the hypothetical clusters offered:

1 empirical studies, especially of physical and sexual abuse and neglect;
2 observations of parent–child interactions, Strange Situations, SAAs, TAAIs, and AAIs of disturbed children and adults;
3 clinical experience with troubled families, especially in child protection;
4 theory regarding self-protective attachment strategies (Crittenden 1997, 2000a, 2000b, 2002).

The clusters are intended to connect what is known empirically with the richness of clinical practice and the meaning-generating function of theory.

Chapter 8

Distortions of normal child-protective behavior: Marginal maltreatment of children

Information processing follows a series of steps that are both linear (each happens in order) and nonlinear (early steps may re-enter the sequence or later steps may be omitted when action is precipitated quickly; Crittenden 1992c). The way those steps are managed is, however, tied to past experience of what deserves attention and how far to carry the processing before ending it and acting (or not acting). In order for child-protective behavior to be initiated, the following series of psychological steps must occur:

1 Specifically, the information (cognitive or affective or both) about the state of the child must be *perceived*.

2 Then it must be identified as *relevant* to both the self and the child – otherwise no action on the part of the self regarding the child will be needed.

3 Next, the parents must *generate meaning* for the information (e.g., I should tell him to stop, he needs my help, or he can do it alone so I'll let him do it).

4 Next, the parent might consider all that they know about this moment, comparing alternative responses, and *select a response*. Parents who distort information (by omitting cognitive or affective information) are unlikely to engage in this integrative step because they have no alternative representation to create a discrepancy and thus a comparison.

5 Having chosen a response (either implicitly, explicitly, or after consideration), the parents might or might not *implement* it, depending upon what other DRs they have at that moment.

Our interest is knowing where and how in this sequence something went amiss in the parent's processing such that the action taken or not taken by the parent endangered the child. We want to know this because it suggests where we should focus the intervention at the beginning of treatment. Knowing *what* information (cognition and affect in greater or lesser distortion) was used will help to define what the intervention should address. Neither, however, is sufficient to tell us how the intervention should be organized, i.e., the type of intervention to use, although both can contribute to that decision.

Cluster 1: Parents whose competing representations too often reflect self-needs, thus minimizing recognition of child needs (thus underprotecting and sometimes neglecting their children)

Parents who neglect their children err in the direction of underestimating the danger to the child or its implications for their own behavior. Neglect occurs in many forms (Crittenden 1993); this section addresses the most common form, which I have called 'marginal maltreatment'. (More serious forms of neglect are described in Chapters 9 and 10.) Marginally maltreating parents raise children in crisis-ridden, multiproblem, conflictual homes.

Marginally maltreating parents know what to do; that is, they could answer questions about parenting correctly on a test, but still they do not do it, do it in a timely manner, or do it consistently. Chronic failure to do what the parent knows ought to be done is one form of neglect. If queried regarding their failure to act, some parents respond apologetically, saying, 'I meant to do it but ...' This suggests a problem at the transition from step 3 or 4 in information processing (selecting a response) to step 5 (implementing it). Because interference with appropriate responding occurs relatively late in the stages of information processing, it would be presumed to occur in less pervasively neglectful families. A pattern of competing parent versus child priorities typifies marginally maltreating families (Crittenden 1988a, 1998b).

Failure to implement a selected response might happen if the parent were distracted by other priorities. For example, just as the mother was reaching to pick up her crying baby, she heard a pot boil over on the stove. Instead of attending to her infant, she rushed to the kitchen, forgetting entirely about her infant. Of course, such interference occurs occasionally in every home. Some parents, however, behave in ways that maintain the chaos rather than looking ahead to prevent it.

The central problem generating repeated crises is the parents' failure to act so as to prevent problems.[1] Instead, parents respond only when the intensity of the signal is very high, i.e., when it elicits affective arousal in the parent. Consequently, when moderate signals elicit no response, conditions can escalate, become urgent crises, and force the parent to choose, under pressure, what to attend to (for example, the crying baby, the overflowing toilet, the eviction notice, the gossipy neighbor, or the fighting preschoolers). The parent's behavior appears erratic unless one notices that intense sensory input and impending danger capture parental attention preferentially. So, in the example, the baby and preschoolers vie for the mother's attention while her interest is in gossip, and the eviction notice gets no response – until the family's belongings are on the curb.

Sharon and Sean had five children: Jasper was 8, Carley was 6, Lee was 3, Missy was 1½, and Brian was the newborn. A call had come in indicating that the children were dirty and seemed hungry, and that no one was watching them when they were outside. When the worker went out, she saw a household in chaos. Piles of laundry, dirty dishes in the sink, old food sitting out, roaches running rampant, unmade beds, and the sound of the TV with the intense emotions of a soap opera. Sharon was talking on the phone while heating the baby's bottle and keeping an ear cocked to the story on the television. The baby was in his rocker and fussing intermittently. From time to time, one of the older siblings offered him a toy or patted him gently and he calmed a bit, but without really engaging with his sibling. Meanwhile Lee and Missy played and fought – with equal vigor for each activity. Sean was outside, tinkering with the car.

The worker waited a bit and, in a break in the action, got Sharon's attention enough to explain why she had come. At first, Sharon was all puffed up and defensive, talking rapidly about how it hadn't been like that and, at the same time, about how the neighbors were always butting into everyone else's business. *'You can't do anything in this place* [a public housing community] *without someone calling the police or calling the child protection ...'* She was off and running, talking up a storm. She was outraged and made no secret of it. She was happy enough, however, to talk to the worker and, in fact, seemed to rather enjoy the company and to assume the worker's agreement with her position.

Then the screaming from the street grew louder and Jasper burst in, crying about the boy next door bullying him. Sharon forgot the worker entirely as she yelled threats at her son for disturbing her, then suddenly stormed out the door to defend her son.

When Sharon returned, she was all stirred up. Each time the worker tried to focus her on the problems regarding the children, Sharon started to respond, then she took the topic far afield, tumbling rapidly from one idea to another until there was no connection to the original topic at all, but lots of aroused feelings with a diffusely inclusive focus. Nothing was finished, completed and resolved, and a feeling of futile exhaustion lay close by under the surface of agitated arousal. At one point, Sean yelled, *'Will you shut those kids up?'* The children paid no heed, but Sharon looked concerned and called them all inside, bribing them with sweets if they would be good until dinner. It was only a few minutes, however, before they were scrapping again and then leaking back outside without Sharon noticing.

The worker tried to plan. When could they meet? In the office where it was quieter? Sharon was willing enough, but she didn't know what she'd be doing on Tuesday, it all depended ... and anyway, she'd need to bring Brian. Could the worker find someone to take care of Lee and Missy so she wouldn't have to bring them? And did the worker know who could sort out the electric bill; they were threatening to cut the power off … and Sharon began rummaging though piles of papers to find the bill.

The worker eventually left, not sure what she had accomplished, quite tired herself and not feeling ready for her next appointment, but also feeling that Sharon was open and willing to work with her. Still, everything had been so fragmented that she was unsure how much Sharon had understood.

Back in the office, a look at the record revealed that Sharon had had service intermittently since Carley had been born. A parent education course, homemaker help, help with budgeting, and a few sessions of couples work when Sean had given her a black eye. In fact, on closer view, Sharon's mother had been known to the services when Sharon was a child. The complaints were never about serious abuse or neglect, and the children were never put in care, but, on the other hand, even when intervention had seemed to help, the problems always reappeared, often within weeks of the close of service.

There are many, many families like Sharon and Sean's. They have numerous minor complaints, absorb services like sponges, seem to know what they should do, but are unable to organize their household in a way that prevents minor problems from ballooning into urgent crises. When this happens repeatedly, one must ask whether the parents' behavior is strategic and how it functions for them.

Together, Sharon and Sean had a Parent's Interview in which they had the chance to talk about their childhoods, their marriage, and how they raised their children.

Sean took control by letting Sharon answer first, then watching to see how the interviewer responded to her answers. After Sharon answered, he sometimes corrected her. She didn't protest, although she sometimes looked up as if to say, 'Oh, God, there he goes again!' There was a bit of swagger in Sean's attitude. He had lots of ideas about raising children, mostly conventional rules suitable to a strictly run household. His role as head of household was absolutely clear, and, in fact, Sharon rarely followed through on anything he disapproved of. Sean's was a world of semantic 'should' pronouncements that conflicted with his behavior. 'A man's role is to take care of his wife and children.' But Sean was often out of work and left Sharon to manage the children and sometimes hit her when he got too frustrated to express himself any other way.

In the content of his childhood history, his own father hadn't been there much. He'd been a bit brutal, and Sean sounded a bit scared even now, talking about it. He couldn't recall much love and no one had been especially gentle with him. Sean was clear: *He* was a good father and his children would have better!

Sean was moderately coercive, showing the strong stereotypical male role, but feeling quite small and not so powerful. In the episodes from his childhood that he told, the other person always took advantage of him and harmed him unjustly.

Sean never found his own contribution to the outcome. Reason might tell us that surely sometimes he did something that elicited the unpleasant responses that he got. But Sean *felt* like an aggrieved victim, and, in that feeling state, he could not easily find his own contribution (Blaney 1986). Not knowing what he contributed, Sean couldn't act so as to change the sequence that ended with his being blamed or punished. Then he felt doubly the victim, unjustly punished and also unable to change future conditions. He couldn't figure out what caused what, and it made him angry. Feeling innocent but being put down left him with the proverbial chip on his shoulder. That is, he came to expect putdowns and found them where they were real – and where they were not as well. In the end, sometimes the only way he could feel on top of things was to see who was lower – or to put them lower.

Sean's putdowns could be sarcastic and demeaning. Mixed with his openly expressed pride in and love for his children and wife, they left his family engaged, but wary. With Sean, there was always a hidden price to pay for the good stuff. It should be noted, however, that Sean did not carry grudges; he was simply quick to identify a slight and attack back. Nor was he deceptive about his anger. Put another way, Sean's aggressiveness was visible and open, albeit overready; he did not meet the criteria for a punitive, obsessed-with-revenge strategy (i.e., he used a C3 strategy, not C5).

When he described his role as a parent, Sean talked about rules and rewards. He'd given his kids all sorts of stuff and he listed toys and video games and lots of non-essential stuff. He didn't want to talk about the things that held him back: his confusion about how to manage so many children, the issues of money and getting a good job – and keeping a job. Now that he was a husband and father, Sean was both proud and scared. His home was his castle; he might be a nobody at work, but, at home, he was the king. Respect was what he hungered for, recognition of his intentions. Fear and feeling small and inadequate were what he didn't want to show.

Rather than acting weak (as he felt), Sean split his feelings of desire for comfort, anger, and fear and displayed exaggerated (distorted) anger. In his marriage, he needed Sharon to accept his leadership and, when she didn't, he fought back explosively, as if wounded. This coercive oscillation between too strong and too weak is something that *we* recognize strategically in Sean, but was exactly what Sean was trying *not* to notice in order to avoid feeling vulnerable.

A few quotes from Sharon convey her perspective as well as the atmosphere of this family. This is how the Parent's Interview began:

You know that we're interested in how people raise their children. We've asked you about who is in your family and who can help you if you need help, and we've watched some of things you do with Missy. Today we'd like to learn a little more about what you think about being a parent, what are the rewards and what are some of the problems … OK?

It ain't easy [slight laugh and smile]. Being a parent is not easy. I mean you have days when you want to leave and everything, I mean, I've felt like that quite a few times … like Friday night … my old man [Sean] came home. I mean he was tired. Well, I couldn't see his point, and I said, 'Well, I'm tired too, I've been here with the kids all day', and, well, we both come together on punishment 'cause, used to be, we'd let 'em get by with it, let 'em have their way, fine, they wasn't bothering us, and now when I punish them, he doesn't let them have their way. When he punishes them, I don't say anything, and, with Missy, that's kind of hard to punish her cause she'll look at you all sad-eyed like, 'Momma, I didn't do nothing', when you know she done it. But she'll sit down and go to sleep quicker than she will if you sit her in a corner. Now Lee, you got to put him to bed or stand him in a corner 'cause he doesn't like to be punished.

What kinds of things do they do that they shouldn't?

Throwin' rocks, biting one another, pulling one another's hair. That's what she's famous for [nodding to Missy], pulling hair and biting.

If one listened to the content only, one could become alarmed. The discourse analysis tells a somewhat different story. Sharon tells everything; she doesn't distort very much and she doesn't hold information back. What you see is what you get with Sharon. This is much less concerning than parents who omit information, thus saying more of what we want to hear. On the positive side, Sharon can take her husband's point of view and she knows the effect of the children's nonverbal communication. She also differentiates her behavior for one child as compared with another. We note that she thinks in the form of recalled episodes made more lively by quoting speech, but in fact she does *think* about being a parent.

Do you think you look or sound like your mother?

Oh, yes. I scream at them, you know, better. Carley will look at me and she'll start crying 'cause it scares them when I scream at 'em. It used to scare me when my momma screamed at me. But then – that's how I get the anger out of myself, plus I don't hurt them. By just screaming at her I get the anger out. And then I'll sit down and explain to Carley, 'Well, Momma didn't mean to scream at you, it's just that you aggravated me.' I says, 'Would you rather me scream at you or whip you?' And she says, 'I'd rather you scream at me.' And screamin' hurts, she says, but it don't hurt half as bad as whippin' does. And I've learned to control myself. 'Cause I know one time I hit her with my fist ... that's how mad I was and Sean and I were having trouble, we didn't have but one child and I hit her with my fist ... and then I said, 'Wait a minute you got to get yourself together', and then, now I feel like I got myself together better than I did have then.

[Loud knocking on one-way mirror; the mother looked, gasped, big issue over child poking objects at power points (that were safety covered). This was one of about 10 high-intensity interruptions from children during the 1-hour interview.]

Again, Sharon's openness is startling – and should put us at ease. No, we professionals don't like what we heard, but we can be fairly certain there isn't more that is worse. Sharon doesn't keep her icebergs out of sight. Instead, she thinks about her behavior – after the fact and in very concrete ways. She doesn't notice, however, that her rapidly changing feelings motivate her behavior more than her ideas about what she should do or changes in what her children are doing. We also notice that her children use danger to get her attention and it doesn't always work.

Is there anything that you really wouldn't want your children to grow up to be?

Mm hmm, to be alcoholics. That's one of the things I don't think I'll have to worry about with Carley. 'Cause she says, 'Momma, I see what it does to Gramma, I see what it does to Daddy.' And you know, she's had to deal with this, he drinks. And she – through her seein' him and Momma, that stuff will make you sick. And I told her that when a person drinks, a lot of times it causes them to do some things they normally wouldn't do. Like her daddy used to beat me [incomprehensible], and she would see him and she would naturally wonder why, and now that she's old enough to understand, I sit her down and explain it to her. I have to tell her the truth. 'Cause why lie to her about it? Later on, when she gets old enough to really understand, she's gonna tell me that she remembers it, so, you know, I want to tell her the truth ... [goes on talking about Carley going to school].

The positives here are (again) Sharon's openness and her desire to help her daughter to grow up with useful understandings. Sharon doesn't seem to understand, however, that Carley needs different explanations at different ages (not all the 'truth' when she is very young). Nor is Sharon fully aware of how pervasive and detrimental to the family her troubles with Sean are. In fact, they come up again and again in her responses. Finally, we notice Sharon's run-on quality of speech and how she drifts through topics, and her inability to talk clearly about Sean's beating her. What she can't say coherently suggests what she doesn't understand.

A question that is asked toward the end of the Parent's Interview reinforces points I've tried to make earlier.

What would you say your goals are for raising your children?

To teach them right from wrong. And let them know it's not right to go over there and steal or hit somebody in the head, like one of the kids has gotten by with it – I don't uphold my kids in nothing they do. And I think if you teach them right from wrong, they'll turn out halfway decent. But if you let them get away with it, they'll turn around and let you have it in the face full blast. And they're not going to respect you.

Sharon's goals are normative – and respect is an important way of knowing that your children will do what they should. But as always in this family, the real power was in a somatic image (in the face full blast).

To summarize what we learn from the discourse analysis, we learn that Sharon has access to all the information and can put it in words. She also can think in concrete ways about what she and her family members do. On the other hand, she isn't consistent, is strongly motivated by her changing feeling states, and doesn't fully understand multiperson effects, e.g., the effect of the state of marriage on children. Finally, she can't think about Sean's violence to her. Put another way, she doesn't understand the cumulative meaning of daily experience and its complexity well enough.

Sharon's strategy was a bit different from her husband's. She didn't confront Sean often, but her face told two stories: pride and disparagement. She had fallen in love with Sean's strong, braggadocio appearance and his romantic softness. After nine years of marriage, she saw through him and was still a bit disappointed that the strong protector had turned out to be both weak and intimidating. She couldn't have put that in these words, but her nonverbal communication was clear enough. We could read it and so could Sean. Sometimes he lashed out when 'that look' made him feel he wasn't man enough for her or father enough to protect their children. The effect of Sean's aggression was to reduce her challenges to his authority.

Instead, Sharon's attention was all over the place, sometimes to deal with issues and sometimes to avoid more difficult issues. She was close but hard to hold, directive but unclear, and affectively involving throughout. The effect of Sharon's behavior was to focus everyone on herself. Where Sean took the offensive to avoid being threatened (based on a hidden feeling of being weak), Sharon meddled and invited and filled her world with demands and demanding people. This created endless conflict that she couldn't resolve, but also kept her constantly in touch and touched, in the literal sense, at least by her children.

What was Sharon seeking that hadn't happened and that, even now, she could neither make happen nor articulate directly? If we rephrase the question as 'what did her tales lack?', we discover that Sharon was loved and protected (enough, but not more), but not comforted. Did Sharon, more than anything, desire comfort? Did her need to be the center, the recipient of comfort, interfere with her being able to stand back a bit and make 'executive' decisions about what would benefit her family most in the long term?[2] Did this desire make even Sean's sarcasm and occasional slaps seem like a price she could tolerate for the benefit of his romantic warmth and the tenderness of his apologies and promises?

As with Sean, it is worth noting what distortions Sharon did not use. She did not fake incompetence or illness, nor did she undercut people who tried to help her. She was unusually sensitive to desiring comfort or assistance, but she was also grateful and pleased when she received it. This rules out the seductive, obsessed-with-rescue strategy (C6) and makes even the C4 only partial.

Parental behavior and DRs

The problem for parents such as Sharon is that there are competing triggers to parental action. Of course, that is true for everyone, but when powerful motivations from childhood remain active in adulthood, then there is the risk that children's needs will become confused with parents' desires. This could interfere with acting protectively and comfortingly toward one's children. In this cluster, the most compelling DRs are those tied to parents' own feelings. Parents run from crisis to crisis, solving problems and soothing children in a just-too-late pattern that maximizes everyone's arousal. In addition, the children's intense focus on the parent satisfies the parent's own need to feel important and loved.

Nevertheless, these parents care for their children and try to protect and comfort them. That is, when children are prominent in the parents' DR, they are cared for more or less adequately, but achieving and holding that state is difficult and, often, not fully under the children's control. Instead, competing sensory signals interfere with parents' attention, and causal semantic information is not used to predict children's needs. Consequently, the parents respond only after the children have imposed themselves, in intensely imaged ways, on the parents. The response itself, however, can be both unpredictable and ambiguous. For example, the mother might shout angrily at the shouting children, grab and cuddle a crying child, or both admonish and smile lovingly at a child whose hug around her neck was choking her. In this context, children tend to focus on getting a response and ignore its unpredictable nature.

When the parents do respond, they do so with a sense of urgency that precludes access to semantic ways of framing the situation or reflective thought that could integrate competing DRs. Then, because their behavior was organized preconsciously, the semantic explanations offered later to professionals often fit poorly and raise doubt in professionals about the truth of what they have heard. The professionals may then express nonverbally that they don't believe the parent, and the parents will not understand that response either. At this point, the parent–professional relationship begins to flounder and possibly even fail.

Sean's strategy is slightly different. He, too, is motivated by vulnerability, but he covers this and acts tough. This pushes people away, with the result that few people put him down, but as well few comfort him. For men like Sean, sexuality creates a way to attract others (usually women, but this applies equally in cases of homosexuality). Sharon is attracted to the strong, romantic, 'I'll take care of you' approach of Sean. She fusses and flirts and flatters him. He loves it. But when she's disappointed, he strikes out. Professionals know this too – and they prefer to deal with Sharon.

Outcomes for children

The problem for children in marginally maltreating homes is that they find it difficult to predict when, how, and to whom their parents will respond. That is, the children experience their parents as inconsistent and unpredictable, but also loving and protective.

Under such circumstances, some children learn to soothe and care for the parent. They become little parents to the parent (A3) and enjoy their grateful parent's approval, warmth, and, of course, dependence. This was Jasper's strategy with Sharon. If the family has other children, as Sharon's did, they may choose other strategies. Some might learn to be vigilant regarding parents' attention, to heighten their signaling (to exaggerate evidence of their presence), and to compete with siblings (C3-4). They exaggerate and alternate displays of negative affect and engage in either provocative/risk-taking behavior or feigned helplessness. In Sharon's family, both Sean and Sharon liked tough little Lee (C3), but when Missy tried to compete directly with her mother around being helpless (C4), she was often overlooked. Possibly Sharon didn't buy into helplessness because she knew (intuitively) how it could be manipulated?

By the school years, competition for parental attention may become competition for teachers' and peers' attention. Once others habituate to the intense signals, children must take even more extreme attention-getting, protection-eliciting action. They must exaggerate their behavior further to elicit a response. This becomes part of a dynamic process between parent and child. This 'coercive strategy' (Crittenden 1992c) can lead to disorders of attention, arousal, and conduct, and these, in turn, can prevent academic learning and satisfactory peer relationships.

Parents' DRs

These multiproblem homes can be described as those in which affect is dominant and cognition is minimized. Feelings motivate behavior; that is, family members organize their behavior in terms of how they feel. More intense feelings attract others' attention more effectively than less intense feelings. Although failure to act can occur at any point from sensory perception to cortical reflection (Crittenden 1993), in cases of marginally neglectful maltreatment, parents' self-DRs interfere with their perception of their children's needs. This means that parents respond to children only after they have forcefully imposed themselves, in imaged ways, into the parents' priorities. That is, such children must work very hard to become part of the parent's DR. When the parents do respond, they do so with a sense of urgency that precludes access to semantic ways of framing the situation or reflective thought that could integrate imaged and semantic DRs. To change their behavior, the pressing priorities of the parents need to be reduced, so that the children's needs are proportionally more compelling.

One might think that the opposite approach should be taken: teach the parents more about children. Emphasize the importance of parental behavior. Slow the information-processing sequence down (count to ten before acting). These things will produce desirable changes, but only in the short term. As soon as services are withdrawn, problems will reappear that pull professionals back in. If service providers don't function as transitional attachment figures, helping parents in their ZPD, these comfort-seeking mothers and respect-desiring but frightened fathers will revert almost immediately to behavior that keeps the services involved.

Notes

1 It is worth noting that the autonoetic consciousness that enables 'mental time travel', i.e., to look into what might happen in the future, is thought to depend on frontal lobe functioning (Siegel 1999, 2001), which, in turn, depends upon the caregiving and comfort given in first two years of life.
2 Frontal lobe functioning, autonoetic consciousness, and 'mental time travel' depend upon the individual's having been adequately comforted during frontal lobe development (Schore 2002). That is, we should expect exactly the constellation of behavior described for Sharon (including especially lack of anticipation of the future and unmet need for comfort) if Sharon herself had not been comforted as a child.

Chapter 9

Distortions of normal child-protective behavior: Physical abuse of children

Cluster 2: Parents who exaggerate the probability of danger to their children by relying on past contingencies (thus overprotecting and sometimes physically abusing their children)

Most child abuse occurs in the context of punishment (Holden and Zambarano 1992). Most punishment occurs when parents want to teach children who are behaving dangerously or disrespectfully to behave safely and respectfully[1] (for a review of this literature, see Crittenden 2005c). This is true regardless of whether they scold, spank, or hit children hard enough to hurt them. Strangely, these explanations are accepted when there is no injury and yet rarely believed when the child is hurt. Nevertheless, outcomes do not define motivations, and the same psychological process can account for both ordinary physical punishment and injurious punishment (but see sections below for parents who attack or kill their children without apparent cause).

Assessing risk implies assessing dispositional representations

Ordinarily, an evaluation of whether a parent's action was appropriate or not depends upon both the outcome of the child and also our evaluation of the precipitating danger. For example, if a parent broke a child's arm by jerking him off train tracks in front of an oncoming locomotive, most people would consider it a justifiable act that saved the child's life. The same event might be considered abusive if the child had been pedalling a tricycle toward an empty street. This example highlights that it is not simply severity of injury that defines child abuse, but rather a comparison between the parent's DR of the situation *prior* to action and an authority's representation *after* action is taken (Crittenden and Claussen 1993).

Injurious physical punishment can lead to charges of child abuse in ways that do not closely reflect parents' threat to children or, more generally, the threat of further violence. A review of the literature on severity of injury by parents indicates that the strongest correlate of severity of injury is the age of the child (Crittenden and Claussen 1993). That is, younger children, being smaller, sustain greater injury when hit or jerked than older children. There is no evidence, however, that their parents are more disordered, have greater psychological disturbance, etc. Nevertheless, severity of injury weighs heavily in judgments regarding child abuse.

On the other hand, for older children, who rarely receive as much concern, the threat might be greater than the lack of severe injury indicates. This is because use of physical punishment is normative with younger children, especially when they have done something dangerous, whereas physical punishment of school-aged children, especially adolescents, is considered inappropriate by almost all cultures. With older children, the threat becomes that of the child (a) attacking the parent or other children (Heide 1992) or (b) leaving home. These risks are not central to the evaluation of parental behavior, but are relevant nevertheless. Put another way, the behavior of parents who strike older children is more deviant culturally than that of parents who strike young children; this suggests a psychological process that is more distorted than that with younger children - in spite of the lesser injury. It is the former, the psychological processes that precede action, that need to be understood better if we are to prevent further suffering to children.

Parental behavior and DRs

Parents who abuse their children are not usually mentally ill (Kolko 1996). Instead, it is proposed that they make errors in estimating danger and its implications for their own behavior. That is, they imagine trucks when others see an empty street; it is the imminence of danger that differs, more than the fact of danger. Such errors are hypothesized to be drawn from their experience of having been exposed to danger in their own childhoods (Zigler and Aber 1981). Abusive parents are likely to *over*estimate the probability of danger and respond protectively too frequently and too forcefully (Crittenden 1998). For such parents, mildly threatening situations may elicit recall of very dangerous consequences (i.e., procedural DRs that initiate compulsive behavior) or strong sensory images (i.e., imaged DRs that elicit intense arousal), or both.

What happens next depends upon the extent to which parents integrate representations from the past with those of the present. When parents both mistakenly accept their childhood DR without question and place themselves in the adult role (as they should), they may be disposed to act in an authoritarian manner, possibly repeating the sorts of behavior used by their parents. Alternatively, parents may have reflected sufficiently upon their experience to have decided to raise their children differently. In these cases, parents may take the child's perspective and behave too permissively, thus, reversing the pattern. Although this protects the child from physical abuse, it carries risk of its own, specifically mild child neglect. Finding a safe balance between past and present conditions and between adult and child perspectives is difficult and requires extensive and ongoing integration (Crittenden *et al.* 2000).

Parental behavior

Abusive parents tend to be attentive to their children; indeed, they are often vigilantly focused on identifying misconduct. In these cases, the 'trigger' to parental processing of information and enacting of a DR is the state of the child: the child is perceived to be doing something endangering or failing to show respect for parental authority (Crittenden 2004). This elicits a protective response. When the response is authoritarian (cf. Baumrind 1971) and involves frequent or harsh physical punishment, the outcome will sometimes be injury (Krug *et al.* 2002). It is important to understand that the punishment was intended by the parent to be protective and is deemed abusive by others. The error that the parents have made is an implicit assumption that current circumstances are as dangerous as the past is remembered or felt to be. Luke and his father are an example of this.

Most abusive parents have clear and meaningful representations of children as needing protection to the point of being vigilantly focused on identifying (dangerous) misconduct or disrespect. The problems in organizing a response on the basis of these representations are (a) simple procedural distortion of overestimation of danger based on past experience, (b) intense imaged fear of negative consequences that impel a quick response, and (c) a limited array of response alternatives. That is, there are too few alternative neural networks activated and too much perceived urgency to take the time to evaluate them or generate new responses. Without time to access verbal representations (i.e., semantic, connotative, and episodic DRs), the array of possible responses is diminished and reflective integration is precluded. This impoverished set of procedures may trigger a protective, albeit authoritarian, response that can lead to injury. It is important to understand that the punishment was often intended by the parent to be protective and is deemed abusive by others.

Although verbal DRs are not accessed in moments of perceived urgency, abusive parents as a group use semantic memory in highly conventional ways (Crittenden *et al.* 2000). Moreover, they often set very high standards of performance for both themselves and their children.

> Vanessa had 2-month-old, healthy twins. She was a single mother living alone. A neighbor made a child-protection complaint, saying that the children cried a lot, their mother screamed a lot, and that Vanessa had tried to choke the infants by placing them side by side on the bed and pressing a broomstick against their throats. Medical examination confirmed the pressure, but no physical damage was identified. Evaluation of Vanessa's parental competence was ordered.
>
> The initial visit was without an appointment, not even a phone call. The purpose, of course, was to see how conditions were ordinarily.

The twins were awake and quiet. The home was a bit messy, with baby paraphernalia scattered about, but it was clean. Vanessa accepted the worker in a friendly, but anxious way, beginning immediately in urgent and fast speech to explain her behavior, her parenting strategies, the things you should do with babies, etc. She seemed both eager to talk and eager to display her competence.

Her discourse was characterized by not being an interpersonal dialogue; instead, it was more like a fast-paced monologue. In addition, its prescriptive semantic quality was outstanding. Vanessa was extremely concerned to announce all the things that a parent *should* do. Most striking was her use of citations for the points that she made. She explicitly referenced well-known baby-book authorities. She even challenged the worker about these authorities. Did the worker know this book? This author? Did she agree? A glance around the room quickly revealed two tall stacks of library books; Vanessa had about 20 books on caring for babies and raising children!

In spite of all of this accumulated information, Vanessa was not able to (a) identify contradictions among the various authorities although the prescriptions that she quoted were often incompatible, and (b) consider and adapt the advice in the light of her situation (her personality, her beliefs, her babies' needs, the context of twins, etc.). That is, she was not able to reflect on the advice and integrate it with other information about herself, her children, and her context to render it helpful.

Instead, her urgent need to do the right thing (a procedural motivation), combined with the intensely arousing effect of having two infants screaming at once (imaged memory) and the difficulty of calming them both, especially as her own arousal was increasing, catapulted Vanessa into action. She grabbed a broom and pressed. Two babies fell suddenly silent at once.

In the aftermath, Vanessa was probably left with both cognitive discrepancy and somatic relief. She 'resolved' the cognitive discrepancy semantically; she got books, studied, and focused on the right rules for raising babies. But, affectively, she was relieved; affectively, she *felt* she had done the right thing because the crying had stopped. It did not feel like abuse, she had not intended abuse. In her mind, she had not abused her babies.

Once in a mothers' group, Vanessa excelled. She was in her element, having women to talk to and the opportunity to show off her knowledge. More importantly, she wanted others, especially the group leader, to approve of her performance. Vanessa was compulsively concerned with performing well. Given that she used an A4– strategy, focusing on her failure would increase her agitated efforts to do the right thing. Under the condition of disapproval, the probability of enabling her to think about her situation in a reflective manner would drop and that would interfere with changing in her psychological process. To change psychologically, Vanessa needed to reach a comfortable and alert state. For that, she needed to feel good about herself.

If the worker had focused on the injury, Vanessa would have withdrawn, possibly refusing service. We know how that would have ended. If the worker assigned Vanessa to a program of informational instruction, Vanessa would have learned well. On a test of the material, she would have had the answers. Vanessa was ideal for parent education if we assess the outcomes by written tests. If changed behavior with her children, especially when they are all distressed, is the goal, at the completion of the course Vanessa would still be unprepared to care for her infants safely.

In this case, the group leader capitalized on Vanessa's gregariousness, using it both to the group's advantage socially and to support Vanessa's sense of competence in verifiable ways. That is, simply telling Vanessa that she was 'good' would not convince her that she was valued. Using her competence made the praise meaningful. Approval and acceptance on terms that she valued permitted Vanessa to relax.

Learning to reflect is not easy. Indeed, it takes all of childhood to accomplish it. It certainly is not easy if one must begin in adulthood and begin by reflecting on one's own dangerously reprehensible behavior. The group leader stayed completely off the topic of the broomstick or Vanessa's competence as a mother; that was a child-protection issue, not a therapeutic one. Instead, the group members looked at videos of themselves. The videos were taken at the beginning of each meeting, as the group members were arriving, and consisted of one-minute long, play interactions of each mother with her child. Reviewing these videos permitted the group leader to individualize the intervention for each mother while fostering other mothers' observational learning.

The group leader invited Vanessa to comment on the desirable things that other mothers did (while largely overlooking Vanessa's own interactions). Vanessa loved being a 'coteacher', the group accepted it because it was framed positively and overseen by the leader, and Vanessa learned to observe interaction with concrete (event specific) reflection. In particular, she was coached to notice how babies showed what they liked and to identify what other mothers had done just before their babies calmed. Vanessa wasn't given any prescriptive semantic guides; instead, she was encouraged to discover them herself through her accumulated observations. This gave her the data upon which she could reflect. Without accurate data, reflection must be incomplete and can be misleading.

In addition, the group leader imagined that Vanessa would try out at home what she had observed other mothers do successfully. Because she was not asked directly to do that, Vanessa did not frame it as a task which she then should perform well. Instead, new ways of interacting with her babies could be explored, i.e., played with, in privacy. By simply looking at Vanessa's videos each week, the group leader could gauge Vanessa's progress - without having to comment and, thus, risking changing Vanessa's focus.

There were two central goals of treatment with Vanessa and they were both accomplished: keeping her infants safe and enabling Vanessa to regulate her own behavior through gathering important information and integrating it. Moreover, Vanessa left treatment feeling in charge of what she had accomplished – as indeed, she had been.

How was this accomplished? Several ideas were crucial to enabling the intervention to work for Vanessa and her children. It was most important that the group leader began by assuming that Vanessa wanted the best for her infants. She sought information to support that notion. It wasn't hard to find: Vanessa's urgency to tell how much she cared, the stack of library books, her eagerness to come to the group. Connecting with Vanessa around her semantic intentions and procedural strengths rather than confronting her on her imaged and procedural outcomes and limitations made it possible for Vanessa to use the intervention effectively. Capitalizing on her desire to perform well (the upside of her strategy) gave Vanessa added competence, and keeping that competence slightly deflected from her own parental performance (the downside of her strategy), reduced her anxiety, and promoted reflective processes (which she lacked at the beginning of treatment). Her social competence was used to build new observational, interpersonal, and reflective skills.

What happens, however, when the mother is not socially skilled and eager to excel, as Vanessa was? Another mother from the same group can suggest how that might work.

Denise was identified by child-protection authorities for both abusing and neglecting her children. When the group leader made her first visit to invite Denise to the group, Denise was withdrawn and sullen. She said very little, looked down, and only mumbled in response to questions. Behind her withdrawn appearance, she seemed resistant and resentful. The group leader focused a lot of attention on approving of her beautiful children, chatting with the older ones, and playing with the younger ones. She sought ways to commiserate with Denise about ... well, about anything, housework, husbands, just any of the usual things that irritate in life. Denise didn't refuse, but didn't warm either. The worker set a time to come back, not mentioning the group yet, because Denise would refuse and refusals that must be overcome make the process harder.

Of course, Denise wasn't there for the next visit, but that opened the door to a drop-in visit. The group leader left a note saying she'd try another time when she was in the area. She did and found Denise at home. It was a brief visit, again focusing on the children and establishing rapport. Without prying, the group leader sought information from Denise that she could support or agree with. That meant asking about hopes and plans for the future – the unsullied aspects of life. Slowly, visit after short visit, Denise became less wary, more willing to engage, more familiar with the routine of talking to this lady about her kids and her family. It almost seemed as if Denise were preparing what to tell the group leader when she came next. Appointments were made – and increasingly they were kept.

It was time. Now the invitation to the group could be offered. Denise accepted but very hesitantly. The group leader said she herself would pick Denise up, knowing that coming into a strange place with a strange person to meet more unknown people was just too much for Denise. A transitional attachment figure, working in Denise's ZPD, was needed. Denise wasn't there for the pick-up – of course. The group leader left a cheerful note and dropped by again two days before the next weekly meeting. This happened a few times and then one day Denise was ready and came in.

The videos were taken. Denise's was terrible! Really terrible. So terrible that professionals laugh when shown the video at professional meetings. Denise sat silently behind her daughter (who was so overdressed that she looked like a wedding cake) and dangled toys in front of her eyes. Then just as her baby mobilized a reach, Denise, who couldn't see the reach, zipped the toy away and zipped a different one in from the other side. The baby's empty hand fell, then she began another reach on the other side and – zip! the toy was gone. As this was repeated again and again, the reaches became less and less eager and eventually the baby's head and arms slumped. She no longer wanted to look at the toys she couldn't have. During this process, Denise was becoming increasingly frantic, offering toys faster and faster as she tried desperately to get her daughter to perform.

What a way to begin! And they hadn't even begun. The leader hovered reassuringly and walked with Denise to the meeting room, seating her near herself (as a good attachment figure would!). The task that day for the already established group (who knew each other and the routine well) was to view their own videos from that morning and check 'yes' or 'no' on a piece of paper (that they would keep and not hand in) whether they (a) faced their baby, (b) talked to their baby, and (c) patted or cuddled their baby. This was a 'private', self-rating task (Crittenden 1991). Everyone except Denise had done at least one of these three things. Then the meeting went on to other topics. At the end, as they were going to the car, Denise said in a low voice, '*I didn't do anything right*'. Usually there is something else good to point to, but this time there was nothing. The interaction was really terrible! The leader took Denise home, talking as encouragingly as possible. Then she dropped by two days before the next meeting to remind Denise that she'd pick her up. But she didn't expect Denise to return. Such a shame! So much effort, so much slow building of trust and it was all lost because of an unexpected outcome. Life seems to have these moments.

It also has surprises. On the meeting day, Denise was ready. Her daughter was dressed up cute as a button (and not like a cake!). In the car, Denise said, *'I've been practicing all week'*. In the video, she sat facing her baby. She spoke to her baby. And she 'pat/cuddled' her baby on her back – twice. OK, it sounded like beating a drum as the thump echoed through the baby's rib cage. OK, it was tossed without warning into the play. But it was a 'pat/cuddle' and her baby knew that. She looked up and smiled full and big and happily at her mother. Nothing makes a mother feel more like protecting her child to the ends of the earth than a smile.

So what worked with Denise? Most of all, having a sensitively responsive transitional attachment figure (the group leader) who engaged with Denise in *her* ZPD. It would have been easy to come in with a list of Denise's incompetencies and failures and a list of goals that would correct these (and that described good parenting.) Denise would have to agree to the plan, but inside herself, she would feel that it was a betrayal of herself. She wasn't a bad mother – or at least she didn't mean to be that. She had hopes and dreams and plans – like all good mothers. But she wasn't there yet.

The group leader took the time in the initial home visits to let Denise get to know her. She observed what Denise valued (her children) and she openly valued the children too. She was patient. Vanessa was fast-paced; Denise was slow (depression and a sense of futility can slow anyone). The group leader let Denise set the pace and didn't suggest new things until they were likely to turn out successfully. She stayed upbeat and supportive regarding Denise's (semantic) hopes. I don't mean that she was always smiling and cheerful while Denise was sad (that would have left Denise feeling misunderstood). Instead, the leader conveyed that she was always optimistic that Denise could become what she wanted to be: a good mother. More than anything, the group leader sought to connect with Denise as the young woman she was around becoming the mother she wanted to be at the pace she could manage.

When Denise felt that her perspective was understood and valued and that things were being managed with her preferences and abilities in mind, she could take a few chances, as in coming to the meeting. Of course, it took a few tries before she managed it, but the group leader never shamed her or threatened her. Instead, she conveyed that she understood that meeting new people was hard. Again, Denise felt understood – and normal (i.e., not like a 'case'). Once at the meeting, the leader, imagining Denise's feelings, stayed comfortingly close. She wanted to keep Denise's spirits up, but she didn't lie about what Denise had observed about her own interaction. Nor did she confirm it. She let Denise's evaluation stand and supported Denise as a person.

When Denise returned the next week, telling the group leader in the car that she had practiced, she provided clear evidence of the power of a transitional attachment relationship to support her. She actively wanted to succeed for her attachment figure. The basis of success had been made very clear: face, talk, pat/cuddle. She could do it! The task was really a fantastic one because while Denise wanted to please her new attachment figure, the process was one that pleased her baby, so the *baby* gave the reinforcement to Denise. That improved the relationship between Denise and her baby. (This is a reminder that being a good attachment figure means not getting in the way when things are going well enough. In this case, the group leader needed to approve of Denise's changed behavior, but not so strongly as to tie Denise to her or to trump the baby's pleasure.)

Before setting this example aside, we should consider why Denise wasn't offered individual treatment. Surely, coming to a group was a challenge and some individual connection was needed or she never would have gotten to the group. So why not take the more direct route and offer individual treatment? Although it isn't clear that individual work was really a better choice (because observing other mother–infant dyads was very helpful to Denise and because she needed social skills and friends), the question never came up. Why not? Because individual work is expensive and there were no funds to cover it. The trick was to conduct a group so as to meet 10–15 mothers' individual needs. Forcing Vanessa and Denise into an identical program would have met neither mother's needs. Creating an individualized group program was helpful to both.

I often tell audiences that the psychotherapist must become the bridge between the patient's dangerous reality and our safer one. Being a bridge means having one foot on each side of what seems like a chasm of difference so as to link the two. Once the patient sees (or feels) that the therapist understands, then together they can begin the dangerous journey back across the chasm. The critical features of this metaphor are taking the patient's perspective from the start, functioning as a transitional attachment figure in the patient's ZPD, and organizing around the notions of danger and keeping the danger just manageable as skills are developed.

To conclude, abusive parents' semantic appraisal of situations and of themselves (when explored under safe conditions) is usually consistent with approved parenting practices, whereas their procedural and imaged behaviors, which are known implicitly, are often at odds with their explicit intentions. Moreover, most abusive parents are highly motivated to be good parents and able to make at least superficial changes quite quickly. Given time, safety, and a trusted guide, these parents can learn new skills and reach appropriate conclusions, but under the pressure of perceived threat, they act dangerously on preconscious DRs. This is true whether the threat comes from the child's actions (as with Luke) or feelings elicited by the child (both Luke and the twins, albeit differently), or from professionals (whether they intend threat or not.)

This suggests two possible processes leading to physical abuse. First, if some aspect of the situation generates arousal, the parent is likely to curtail processing and act on a familiar procedure. The more often this recurs, the more primed that response will be, until we see it as habitual and the parent barely 'sees' it at all. This fits both Vanessa's and Denise's experience. Second, there may be an intrusion of unresolved trauma; this is the more likely explanation if the behavior is inconsistent with the parents' ordinary behavior. The intrusion can be an instance (as with Luke's father and Vanessa) or it can be a set of circumstances that set off a long and complex response that endangers the child. The latter is exemplified by a case of 'factitious illness by proxy' (i.e., formerly Munchausen's syndrome by proxy (Kozlowska *et al.* 2006). This is what was operating in the case of Luke's father. In one study, using the DMM on mothers' AAIs, 50 per cent of mothers with children in care for child abuse had unresolved traumas (Seefeldt 1997).

Immigrant populations

Errors of overestimating danger are relevant to immigrant populations, especially when parents have moved from relatively dangerous to relatively safe countries. Such parents use child-rearing strategies that were accepted and even essential to safety in the country in which they were learned, but which seem unnecessarily strict or dangerous by the standards of the new country. In addition, they experience a variety of threats in their new country: lack of family and friends, unfamiliarity with the new culture, sometimes not knowing the language, and sometimes being ethnically different from the dominant population. These threats cause immigrants to use their traditional protective strategy even more frequently and intensively – even when needing these strategies was part of the reason for leaving the original country. The effect can be that they use their implicitly known strategies more intensively and more pervasively than do parents in their home culture. Finally, many immigrants have fled from traumatizing situations. This leaves them vulnerable to the distortions of perception associated with psychological trauma. Without explicit consideration of these three conditions, misapplication of parenting strategies is likely to occur.

Outcomes for children

Two outcomes are important, one involving shaping of the maturing brain to fit the child's actual life context and the other involving relationships and behavior. These two, of course, are related.

Neurologically, the brain organizes using experience-dependent and experience-expectant processes (Glaser 2000). Experience-dependent processes result from spontaneous input from the environment and use that input to generate synapses that are hypothesized to represent the event and facilitate the contingent response and its relation to the self. The production of synapses shapes the growing brain as part of a transactional process between the dependent and expectant processes. The residual synapses maintained through their continued activity after the initial 'pruning' of the excess of synapses present at birth in the experience-expectant process, provide the basis on which the dependent process then further shapes the growing brain. In cases of child abuse, the input is injury and pain, and the shaping occurs around the contingences that the child can control. What initiated the sequence? Inhibit that in the future; i.e., Type A inhibition. What could change the sequence? Do that more in the future; i.e., Type A compulsion. What signals preceded the sequence? Be vigilant regarding these and when they occur, inhibit and act as needed to lessen the danger; i.e., Type A vigilance and anxiety. This process of learning from abusive input shapes the brain to overidentify potential threat and to generate excessive self-protective responses, some of which will not be needed, i.e., when the threat was expected, but not actual. The effects of such shaping affect both behavior and children's relationships, both attuning children to their unique developmental contexts (a short-term advantage) and shaping their relationships to fit their expectations (a long-term disadvantage in that the child 'selects' contexts that meet expectation, thus unknowingly selecting dangerous relationships and contexts). This is structural coupling between organism and environment (Maturana and Varela 1987).

When the abuse can be predicted but not controlled, it would be expected that the arousal component would be generated, but not compulsive responses. We would expect to see this as general agitation in an inhibited, noncoercive child. If the abuse could be neither predicted, nor controlled, but could be systematically elicited by displayed negative affect, a depressed Type A strategy would be expected.

In terms of relationships, children of authoritarian parents both know that what they do is important to their parents and try to avoid parental attention. They adapt to fit their parent's representation. Children's feelings of being competent depend upon parental satisfaction with their behavior or upon their finding alternate attachment figures who support their development. Some (over)achieve and become very successful. More, however, remain locked in anger, fear, and failure, carrying this into their child-rearing. Most do not become abusive parents themselves (Kolko 1996; Zigler and Aber 1981), although an important minority of these becomes overly permissive (by using a 'reversal strategy' that, like a pendulum, overshoots the balanced middle).

Conclusions

Clusters 1 and 2 are similar in the completeness of information processing. Parents in both clusters process information through the implicit memory systems and as far as explicit, conscious, semantic and connotative transformations, but they have very limited access to reflective integration. In addition, both groups of parents often fail to do what they know they should do and intended to do. Their reasons, however, are different. Parents in cluster 1 tend to have strong personal needs that often override signals from or about their children in the DRs that actually motivate behavior.

These signals are often somatic and are usually represented in imaged ways (as opposed to being represented in verbal, semantic ways that could more easily be examined consciously).

Parents in cluster 2 tend to organize on the basis of cognitive, temporal contingencies and to hold strong, conformist, and relatively absolute semantic guidelines to behavior. However, when they implement the behavior, they are vulnerable to setting such high standards of performance for both themselves and their children that they almost guarantee failure, with ensuing frustration. In addition, many parents in cluster 2 are responsive to their children's imaged signals of negative affect, but the response is one that terminates their own engagement and leaves the child unprotected and uncomforted.

Note

1 Respect is important because respectful behavior signals to parents that children are attending seriously to what parents are telling them about the right things to do, especially when the parents are not present to protect their children.

Chapter 10

Parents whose own needs skew their perceptions: Distortions that emphasize parental self-comfort

Understanding parents' behavior requires knowing (a) how far their processing of incoming information progressed (from perception through attribution and selection of a response to reflection), (b) what incoming information was given priority (cognition, affect, or both), and (c) the extent to which the information was transformed (from true through omitted-and-distorted to falsified).

As described in the previous chapter, parents in clusters 1 and 2 understand what their children need, both in specific moments and in general, and are able to identify appropriate responses. Too often, however, their own motivations interfere with acting in their children's best interest. Nevertheless, when the children make themselves perceptually more prominent in the parent's mind than the parent's self-representation, they effectively capture their parent's attention. Reframed in terms of DRs that contain both self and nonself components, the DRs of parents in clusters 1 and 2 emphasize the self-relevant portion of the representation at the expense of the nonself portion, that is, the child portion. The child representation, however, is not greatly distorted; instead it gives a relatively accurate picture of the child and his or her needs. According to which DR regulates parental behavior, the outcomes can be protective or threatening to children.

Clusters 3 and 4 have in common that parents both place too great emphasis on their own need for comfort and protection, and use that information to shape the representation of their children. That is, children's signals are *distorted* to fit parents' self-representations. The outcome varies from one parent–child dyad to another, but all are characterized by children being seen through the lens of their parents' needs and desires. For example, children's coy signals of wanting attention may be misunderstood as flirtatiously sexual bids. If the child's response to parental sexual touch is mixed pleasure at the attention and displeasure or confusion at the sexual aspects of the touch, parents in cluster 3 may fail to perceive the discrepant part of the information.

The transformations can occur both at the level of perception, where discrepant signals may not be perceived, and at the level of attributing meaning, where the child's context may not be used to suggest the most likely meaning of the child's behavior. Put another way, the parents in clusters 3 and 4 have such intense self-protective needs that they misconstrue signals from their children as fitting their own needs and expectations (i.e., they filter their perceptions by their needs or desires and they misattribute the meaning from their past experience in other contexts).

Were the parents more alert to discrepancy, they might notice the difference between their semantic beliefs and their behavior, but, more than parents in clusters 1 and 2, parents in clusters 3 and 4 keep information apart (i.e., they disassociate that which should be associated). Clusters 3 and 4 form a transition from parents largely without psychiatric disorder to those with serious disorder (cluster 5 and 6).

It should be remembered, however, that symptom-based diagnoses or behavioral groupings do *not* map directly onto the functional patterns described here. Traditional diagnoses or offender acts are offered in the same way that types of maltreatment were offered: to give the reader a general sense of what is being described. However, there is no implication that people with the diagnoses are all similar in the functional terms used here, nor that they all use the sorts of parenting strategies described here. Instead, it may be that the differences between functional formulation and symptom-based diagnosis could explain some of the complexity and imprecision of the relation between parent and child symptoms and diagnoses (Marmorstein and Iacono 2004).

Cluster 3: Parents who transform desire for comfort into sexual desire and respond to children's needs with sexualized behavior (thus sometimes sexually mistreating their children)

Two sorts of problems are considered: incest and spousification. The former tends to involves fathers and the latter, mothers.

Incest

Two decades of research seeking profiles of men who sexually abuse their own children (incest) have largely failed to identify such profiles (Murphy and Smith 1996; Veneziano and Veneziano 2002). Similarly, treatment seems ineffective (Crighton and Towl 2007; Shine *et al*. 2002). Part of the problem may be the excessive reliance on self-report assessments to identify character traits. If sexual offenders split descriptive and prescriptive semantic generalizations, self-report measures may emphasize prescriptive generalizations. Put another way, men who sexually abuse may respond to self-report measures with information about either how they think they *should* be (Ward and Beech 2006) or, alternatively, with excessively negative self-descriptions (tied to feeling they have failed to meet the prescriptive beliefs that they hold). Further, the traits that are measured may not reflect the crucial features that differentiate offenders from nonoffenders. Possibly the problem lies in two assumptions regarding the motivations of men who sexually abuse their own children: (a) that sexual abuse is about sex or power, and (b) that men who sexually abuse their children are predators who intentionally entrap children. If these assumptions are in error, research and treatment based on them are unlikely to be successful.

A different perspective, one drawn from current information processing and developmental history, is offered here. This perspective was introduced in the vignette of David; here it is described in terms of existing research. Because most research on sexual abuse is on men convicted of sexual offences, I will primarily refer to 'fathers'. Whether the process is similar for sexually abusing mothers is not known. Indeed, it is not even clear whether the same behavior is considered abusive when used by men and women. We do know, however, that the chemistry of sexual arousal is different for adult males and females (Hughes et al. 2007; Wilson and Hill 2007).

First, desire for comfort transformed into sexual desire is hypothesized to be the motivating affect in many sexually abusing fathers. Semantically, these fathers are hypothesized to intend to reverse the isolating and threatening experiences that typified their own childhoods. That is, affectionate behavior, including sexualized affection, may be abusers' expression of desire for comfort and closeness as well as their offer of comfort and affection to their children. One study has found that incest offenders had experienced a lack of nurturance and empathy compared with nonoffenders, were not different from nonoffenders in their ability to empathize, and tended to rely on children to meet their needs for nurture (i.e., role reversal; Cremer 1996). The power of touch on the lips and genitals (compared with other parts of the body) to elicit arousal and behavior (Eibl-Eibesfeldt 1970; Fisher 1992) may help to explain why men who desire to connect to their children (as their fathers did not connect to them), and who lack normative experience and interpersonal skills, use such intense, sexualized forms of giving and receiving comfort and establishing interpersonal contingencies through reflexive responses.

Second, the developmental pathway to incest may be a series of age-salient experiences that accrue over childhood and adolescence and that culminate in a form of attachment characterized by dismissing the self, focusing on others' needs, and expressing affection in sexualized ways. It should be noted that this perspective, drawn from DMM discourse analysis of offenders' AAIs, is very different from the power and aggression focus of most theory on sexual offending (Ward et al. 2006)

Third, to ensure that their children will not experience the isolation and humiliation that they experienced as children, these fathers may try to take their children's perspective. That is, fathers who sexually abuse their children may be unusually attuned to their children's signals of anxiety or desire for comfort. If, in addition, they attend carefully to feedback from the child, i.e., to signals that the child is becoming more comfortable or relaxed, the effect will be that the child shapes the adult's behavior. Because the child is his own son or daughter, this closeness is likely to be satisfying for both father and child. In the literature, this is called 'grooming' the child; here a different set of motivations is imputed to the same behavior.

Adequate developmental studies of men who sexually abuse do not yet exist (possibly because the emphasis has been on *identifying* men who sexually abuse as opposed to *understanding* their developmental experience and adult needs). AAIs of men who sexually abuse, however, suggest a developmental pathway to their current functioning (Crittenden 2000; Haapasalo *et al.* 1999).

These include

(1) lack of family intimacy and comfort (psychological maltreatment); (2) bullying attacks by fathers or stepfathers (i.e., physical abuse); (3) witnessing violence to their mothers (i.e., abuse to their protective attachment figure); (4) mocking and shame for seeking comfort (i.e., psychological abuse); (5) abandonment, lack of supervision, and separation (i.e., physical neglect); (6) feeling singled out or marked for mistreatment; (7) display of relatively few acting-out problems and, instead, internalizing problems; (8) exclusion from symmetrical peer attachments (best friends and peer groups); (9) inclusion as victims in peer bullying (i.e., peer abuse); (10) precocious sexual activity (Bumpy and Hansen 1997; Duane *et al.* 2003; Garlick *et al.* 1996; Hunter *et al.* 2003; Levant and Bass 1991; O'Halloran *et al.* 2002; Salter *et al.* 2003; Smallbone and Dadds 1998, 2000; Starzyk and Marshall 2003). The great majority of men who sexually abuse their own children were not themselves sexually abused although most were abused psychologically or physically, or both (Murphy and Smith 1996). In addition, many have sexual role problems (O'Connor 1991).

Shame is particularly important with regard to sexual abuse. It is an emotion (rather than a pure affect) in that it combines affect with recall of the event(s) that elicited the feeling. Thus, it is integrative and more complex than either affect or cognition alone. In addition, it is self-relevant: one feels shame for his or her 'self'. Usually, the feeling of shame is intense, unpleasant, and somatic: one feels shame in one's gut as a nauseous urge to rid the self of the shameful thing (i.e., the somatic component is derived from disgust; Rozin and Fallon 1987). Finally, shame is experienced on a gradient from (a) feeling ashamed of an action (that is not inherently a part of oneself), to (b) feeling oneself to be unacceptable when one *acts* in a particular way, (c) feeling oneself unacceptable when one *feels* a certain way, (d) feeling oneself unacceptable *as a whole* and under all conditions because one is inherently bad. When the thing to be gotten rid of is the self, shame can lead to intense conflict between living and dying.

Men who engage in incestuous sexual activity with their children have usually been shamed for feeling vulnerable and desiring comfort when they were small children and for being bullied as school-aged children. In most cases, they actively try to avoid shaming their own children – while themselves continuing to feel shame for their vulnerability. Feeling ashamed, they keep their behavior secret, but do not directly shame their children. Nevertheless, the children perceive the need to hide what they do, and this can engender shame in the children.

Their AAIs show that many sexually abusive men idealize their intimidated mothers and dismiss their aggressive fathers. That is, they identify with victims in ways that suggest a desire to protect and care for vulnerable, picked-on, and uncomforted people. They do not, however, organize vengefully against their fathers (or father substitutes); i.e., they do not employ a coercive Type C strategy. It is proposed that the compulsive patterns of attachment (Types A3–8) that involve inhibition of their own desires and negative feelings in favor of meeting others' expectations and soothing their feelings can account for these observations. Further, this is consistent with abusers having internalizing problems, an external locus of control, and low expressed anger (Beck-Sander 1995; Fisher *et al.* 1998; Marsa *et al.* 2004).

This brief review suggests a series of developmental risks whose cumulative effect increases the probability of a boy becoming a man who sexually abuses his children. Paradoxically, these risks are not directly tied to sexuality; rather, they consist of lack of comfort until adolescence when sexual desire may initiate the first satisfying experience of closeness and comfort. It should be stated clearly that this focus on the development of fathers who engage in sexualized behavior with their children is not meant to diminish our concern for their children. It is meant to provide a more accurate picture of the men in the hope that *all* participants in such troublesome family experiences can be helped. Further, a clear understanding of the developmental process is essential if such problems – and the suffering that they bring to all family members – are to be prevented.

Parental behavior

Most sexual abuse by fathers is touching, not sexual intercourse; moreover, very little involves violence (Herman 1992; Russell 1986; Trickett *et al.* 2001); to the contrary, incestuous sexual offenders tend to be more passive than other men (O'Connor 1991). Similarly, families in which there is sexual abuse are rarely the source of the report of sexual abuse. Instead, they usually support the father and prefer to remain together with him. In particular, the wives of incestuously abusing men generally support their husbands (Carter 1993), although the reasons for this may include partner abuse or economic limitations. This can force child-protection authorities to remove the usually unwilling, victimized child from the family. Again, the family's cohesion and the man's selection of a passively supportive wife (like his idealized mother) are consistent with the hypothesis of overinvolvement proposed here. A particularly inexplicable finding, in the light of the sexual predator hypothesis, is that penile erection to child stimuli does not differentiate men who sexually abuse from other men (Murphy and Smith 1996). This is, however, consistent with the hypothesis offered here that the abusers' sexualized behavior is intended to comfort and engage children rather than to satisfy adults' sexual desire or establish power and dominance. (It should be noted, however, that incarcerated men may try to 'fake good', i.e., avoid arousal, in order to increase the probability that they will be seen as safe enough to be released. This possible effect has not, however, been tested.)

When accused of sexually abusing their children, most men deny doing so (Barbaree 1991; Maletzky 1991). As with physical abuse, this may indicate a difference in semantic meanings. Did they touch the child? Yes. Did they 'abuse' the child? No – because they intended to comfort the child. The point is that labels tied to outcomes (i.e., moral/legal prescriptive labels) may not fit parents' intent. The relation between intention and action, however, may be quite complex.

Higher rates of all types of mistreatment, including sexual abuse, are found among nonbiological parents (Daly and Wilson 1996). This may be because nonbiological parents or parent substitutes, e.g., stepparents, childcare workers, professionals, and religious caregivers, are less inclined than biological parents to define the child as an extension of self. Further, the children may attempt to make themselves attractive to the new father figure; if doing so includes using coy behavior, it might contribute to stepfathers misconstruing the meaning of their behavior. In sum, stepfathers may be more likely to act on their adult desires. In addition, stepchildren can threaten or dilute stepparents' reproductive success. That is, desire for comfort may motivate many biologically related men who sexually abuse, but be a less prominent motivation among nonbiological parental figures. As a consequence, nonbiological abusers will be more likely to complete the sexual act and to use threat, coercion, and even violence to accomplish that. The essential aspect of the risk, however, is the parent's distorted DRs.

Parents' DRs

Like all fields of study, the literature on incestuous child sexual abuse began with simple descriptive data, then progressed to linear, single-factor hypotheses regarding attributes that could differentiate abusers from nonabusers. More recently, profiles have been sought. What may be needed now is an understanding of the functional meaning of incestuous fathers' behavior, one that would permit us to see the interpersonal organization and function of the parents' representations. It is proposed that the compulsive patterns of attachment (Types A3–8) combined with unresolved and dismissed trauma around seeing their mothers harmed, being shamed and rejected, and being bullied can account for much of the data. In addition, such an hypothesis can enable us to reframe incestuous behavior in ways that match families' understanding more closely. The advantage would be that, if we had a more accurate understanding of parents' DRs, we might be able to establish therapeutic relationships more easily and focus treatment more accurately.

Sexually abusive fathers' motivation may reflect a series of transformations of information. Procedurally, they may try to reverse experienced dominance hierarchies by creating more nearly symmetrical parent–child relationships. This can create risk that children will be treated like adults. That is, they may bring the child up to the adult level, thus transforming their experience of humiliating vulnerability and rejection into excessively attentive and sexualized caregiving. In addition, abusive fathers' experience with closeness and intimacy may be tied to sexual relationships after puberty; if so, then sexualized affection becomes the source of their procedural and imaged DRs of affection. Semantically, they may organize around ensuring that their children do not experience the isolation, lack of comfort, shame, or domination by a threatening father that they experienced in their childhood. Because this is a semantic *reversal* strategy, it is not undergirded by procedures and images drawn from their own childhood experience. Moreover, like other parents using compulsive strategies, incestuous parents may adapt their behavior to the child (cf. showing 'emotional congruence'; Beckett 1994), but in these cases, they may misconstrue the meaning of children's coy, attention-seeking behavior (because of their own imaged experience with flirtation). In all cases, there is a notable lack of integration in the process of generating behavior and an absence of reflection after the event.

Regardless of whether the adult's response is based on empathic caregiving or is tinged with sexual desire, the adult's behavior is likely to consist of behaviors that are common to both the attachment and sexual behavior systems, such as caressing, hugging, kissing and reassuring. This suggests a means by which disparate affects can be substituted for one another. Nevertheless, there are semantic dictates against sexual acts with children and they are well known and accepted by sexual offenders. This probably leads to a second transformation in which comforting/sexual action is rationalized as being both something else, e.g., affection, and justified by worthy motives: she wanted it, I was only comforting him, we were only being close and affectionate. A third transformation is displacement of the source of the dispositions. Because parental behavior should be based primarily on the needs of the progeny, in sexual abuse, parents' need for comfort and intimacy may be denied and displaced onto children. As one man who sexually abused children said, '*I would have loved to have someone touch me like that*'. Finally, sexually abusive adults already experience shame for their normal feelings and hide their comfort-desiring behavior. Adding actually shameful acts that also must be hidden changes their psychological state very little. That is, the alarm bells of conscience (i.e., semantic DRs combined with somatic imaged feelings of shame) and the practice of hiding shameful behavior are already so familiar and so broadly applied that adding new eliciting conditions changes little or nothing for the adult. The warning system fails because it has been activated excessively, and thus does not distinguish risk from nonrisk. This array of (a) substitutions (of one feeling for a similar one, of a good deed for a taboo, and of altruistic motivation for self-motivation), (b) distortions (excessive fearfulness, shamefulness, and concealment of feelings and behavior), and (c) displacements (of self-interest to interest in children) may combine in the sexually abusive adult to promote the fusion of affectionate and sexual behavior with children.

Punishment is unlikely to correct the mental processes leading to such distorted DRs, and even treatment must be managed carefully and compassionately. It is sadly ironic that treatment of sexual offenders often emphasizes their taking children's perspectives by empathizing with their victims and taking responsibility for their moral transgressions (Frenken 1994; O'Connor 1991; Scavo and Buchanan 1989; US DHHS and Faller 1993). This may both misconstrue their intentions and also reify their already distorted self-denying, victim-glorifying strategy. If so, our treatments may function to increase the probability of future offending, and thus to make sexual abuse appear impervious to treatment.

The crucial hypotheses offered regarding sexually abusive parental behavior are as follows:

1 Its roots are in normal comfort seeking that is punished and then inhibited in childhood, first accepted in romantic relationships, and, in that form, applied to one's own children.

2 Incestuous parents have themselves been seriously victimized, psychologically, physically, and occasionally sexually, over long periods of time.

3 Fathers who sexually abuse act on the confluence of personal motivations to seek comfort and to protect and comfort their children and child signals that elicit sexualized affection.

David (from Part 1) is typical. It might be worth noting that David's wife was a passive, but well-meaning woman who was mildly depressed. Even after the sexual abuse by David of their daughter was revealed, she trusted David and did not want him to leave the family. Consequently, the court placed their daughter in protective custody. When she was returned home, a 'Strange Situation', classified by the Preschool Assessment of Attachment (PAA), indicated that she was a cheery, agitated, compulsive caregiver to her mother. Thus, although David's wife was not sexually abusive, she, like David, was motivated by a desire for comfort. She, however, turned to David for comfort and gave too little care to her children.

In some cases of incestuous child sexual abuse, the parent's childhood experience has been more dangerous than David's and the resulting distortions are greater and more dangerous to children. Such a case is described in Chapter 11.

Child outcomes

Sexual abuse has an array of serious and long-term effects on children. Children who are sexually abused are not necessarily a random draw from the population. Instead they are often more vulnerable in the sense that they live in environments characterized by nonprotection that are conducive to exploitation. Quite often, mothers of abused children were abused themselves (Dixon *et al.* 2005) and re-create, albeit inadvertently, environments in which abuse is allowed to persist. Via avenues of caregiver distress (including psychiatric problems, PTSD, and attachment disruptions), alcohol and substance usage, and interpersonal and family violence, children born to mothers who were victims of childhood abuse are at high risk of a host of deleterious outcomes including involvement in child protection (Noll *et al.* in press). These caregiver characteristics may serve to interfere with accurate appraisals of environmental threat, preclude recognition of potential danger to offspring, and impair the judgment necessary for appropriate escape or action (Kihyun *et al.* 2007). Expressing desire for comfort and fear as coy behavior may constitute a contribution by children to their abuse, albeit one over which they have neither control nor responsibility.

However, when the abuse is part of an enduring relationship (as in incest), it changes the child. Child and parent adapt to one another – as do mothers and babies and lovers. Thus, over time, sexually abused children may become complicitous victims who may experience intense and confusing affectional bonds to their parents (Herman 1992; Russell 1986). The child's inadvertent contribution may include signaling in ways that initiate intimacy, reinforcing the parent's attention, and participating in keeping the intimacy private. An obvious risk is overattribution of responsibility by the children to themselves. Further, as the child approaches puberty, the extent of complicity increases, as do the risks of sexualized behavior outside the family (Noll, Trickett, *et al.* 2003). In addition, there are physiological, emotional, and intellectual effects that extend into late adolescence and adulthood (Noll, Horowitz *et al.* 2003; Noll, Trickett, *et al.* 2003; Trickett *et al.* 2001). A particular concern is that changes in the child's behavior may attract other, more endangering abusers and romantic partners.

The child's complicity, the duration of the abuse, and the presence of strong and reciprocal affectional bonds between parent and child make incestuous abuse more damaging and its treatment more complex than in extrafamilial abuse or random and isolated stranger attacks (Fischer and McDonald 1998). In familial cases, the mixed feelings of love and confusion/distress, as well as the attachment to the father, who is both protective and abusive, must be acknowledged and addressed. Failure to do so may harm children psychologically as well as harming their relationships. In single-instance, nonfamilial cases, there is no form of relationship or complicity between victim and perpetrator and the culpability is indisputably that of the perpetrator.

Spousification

Spousification refers to treating one's child as if he or she were one's spouse. That is, it is more that just treating the child as a peer adult or asking him or her to grow up rapidly and assume some adult responsibilities; 'spousification' or 'child-as-mate' includes the spousal attributes of sexualized attachment (Goglia *et al.* 1992; Jacobvitz *et al.* 1999; Kerig *et al.* 1993; Walsh 1979). Spousification can occur as early as infancy (Sroufe and Ward 1980) and extend into adulthood. Mothers are more likely to treat a young son as if he were a spouse than fathers are their daughters (Burton 2007).

The fact that spousification of children occurs more often among single than married parents (Brown 2004) may merely reflect that more women are custodial single parents than are men. Alternatively, it may reflect differences in how men and women conceptualize adult roles. Specifically, women who spousify their sons may feel they need the protection of a male, but fear adult males and prefer their less threatening sons, whereas, with their daughters, they may establish a role-reversing, caregiving relationship. Further, it is possible, but to date unknown, that cultural differences, including religious beliefs, would affect what parents deemed appropriate with their children. Another unknown is whether we accept in women behavior with children that we would not accept in men, for example, mouth-to-mouth kissing, tender cupping of a child's buttocks, or touching of children's genitals.

Spousifying parents usually lack adult partners or have very distant or rejecting partners; possibly in replacement for this lack, they treat one of their children as a spouse. In this case, parent and child are like peers, and the child is brought up to an adult position. Often the relationship has sexualized features, but not necessarily sexually abusive ones. One way to think about this is that it is the maternal parallel of child sexual abuse, but it reduces the emphasis on sexual behavior and increases that on the adult role of the child for the mother. Because the child fills two roles (child and partner), spousification can have an even more substantial impact on children than sexual abuse. Two examples are offered, one of a toddler and one of a young man.

Candace was an exceptionally beautiful, softly spoken young woman who had a directness and warmth that was unusual among women known to child protection. She had five children, all of whom had been removed from her care for neglect. The three older children had been adopted whereas Robert and his brother had been born later and were still in foster care. They had been removed after Robert fell out of a second-story window. Candace had lived alone since her boyfriend, the father of these two young boys, had left after a dispute that had turned violent. Candace had suffered bruises and a fractured rib. The incident described here occurred during supervised contact with the two boys.

Sixteen-month-old Robert was lying across Candace's lap, facing down, as she tenderly 'slapped' his bottom. She turned him over and their bodies twisted in a gentle chase, as she tried to come close and he shifted, always smiling, in ways that avoided closeness. Robert's mouth was open wide, as were his unfocused eyes. He laughed in a gurgling, overexcited way. When Candace put his back against her chest and gave him a toy, he calmed a bit, focused on it, and reached for it. Then as she prepared to lift him toward her face, his body went limp except for his upper body that was turned out and away from her face. As she lifted him, her face became bright and engaging and she made whispering sounds; Robert mirrored her expression, but with glazed eyes. Then she kissed him and he pulled back, protruding his belly (in the classic disarming manner). She pulled him closer, saying, 'Where are you going?' and shaking him gently. His eyes were wary and glazed; he had a toy in his mouth. She nuzzled him and he twisted his head back and away, eyes still unfocused. She kissed him again, saying, 'Robert, Robert!', in a high-pitched, urgent voice. He opened his mouth very big as if smiling and looked blankly past her. The 'smile' died as suddenly as it had come, and he looked empty and fearful. Candace's voice became concerned, 'Robert, Robert ...?' All the while, his body was entirely in her gentle control. 'Robert ... Robert,' Candace almost pleaded. He half-looked, with a half-smile, but twisted away at the same time. 'Robert ... give me some sugar ...' She repeated this 4–5 times, once looking down with forlorn sadness, but coming back with an inviting smile. By now, he was held high over her head, tipped a bit toward his mother's upturned face. 'Robert ... give Mama some sugar ...' As she lowered him toward her face, as if to kiss him, his body became very still, his back arched away from her, and his eyes became big and round with a glittering, unfocused look. Suddenly, Candace mock-bit his arm, lingering as she sucked a bit on him. He remained glazed, eyes focused in the empty distance. He raised his arm to block himself from being pulled in closer. Candace then lifted him high overhead, with his body dropping down from her hands. With his face hanging above hers, she lifted and dropped him several times, each time landing his mouth on hers while she made growling sounds. Then she lowered him and nuzzled his cheek and ear. He remained distant and pliable, seeing nothing and resisting nothing, but also not satisfying her need for affection. It ended when Candace turned him away from her face and gently put him on the floor, leading him away.

Statements from her Parent's Interview can help us to understand how she arrived at needing so much affection that she treated her toddler son more like a romantic adult partner than a child.

What was your childhood like?

It's hard for me to say 'cause I was being placed in different homes and I was transferred from my foster mother to my mother and then from my mother to my father. My mother and I was living here, my father was living a long way away. So me being transferred from foster home to mother and father, three different places. Till I got on my own and I got on my own at 16. That's when I got married. It was a lot of changes. ... To me, it changes your feelings with the moves. Have to get used to the surroundings that you're in. Have to get used to new people and that's kind of scary.

[later] Were you a good child?

No. I was a mischievous child 'cause my father used to always tell me and I know I used to stay, I can't remember what age I was, but I used to stay into trouble. Run away from home, play hooky from school, and I think that came from being placed from one place to another. ... I remember I would feel different each time, like when I was with the foster parent, I wanted to be with my momma. But when they shipped – we was sent – to our mother and then my father came and got us from her and took us to the city and then my mother got real sick and we came back home to here and she died and then I got married. I got married before she died. I was 16 when I got married and I just stayed here.

[later] How much influence do you think you'll have over how he'll turn out?

I hope my life don't affect his, not as he's growing up. I want him to grow up to be the person he wants to be. 'Cause that's mostly the way I really grew up. I grew up the way I wanted to. Not because of what my parents taught me or anything. I just grew up on my own. That's the way I feel.

Did you like that?

It doesn't really bother me much now 'cause I'm taking care of myself, but then I was feeling uncared for. I just felt like my parents didn't care for me. I was 14 or 15. I used to stay out all night long and that wasn't an age that a child should be staying out. Nobody cared, they didn't sent nobody to look for me. I really felt they didn't care then.

The outstanding features of Candace's discourse are (a) her speaking of herself as an object sent (shipped!) from one place to another, (b) her factual and affectless mention of her mother's death, (c) the omission of personal pronouns (*I, my, me*) in crucial places, and (d) the absence of any affect in this crisp tale of being unloved and uncared for even when in danger and left to fend for herself. The discourse places her firmly in Type A, probably A5–6. In addition, she has unresolved trauma and loss of her mother, both in a dismissed form (of acting as if these events were of no consequence now). Overriding everything is a quiet depression. It holds almost all her feelings in check.

The exception is sexuality. Sexual behavior got her married at a time when she needed a home, had no parents, and couldn't yet support herself. Hidden in her statement that young girls shouldn't be out late at night is the sexual mistreatment and rape that she suffered from early adolescence until the present. Candace both knew what sex could offer her (and she dressed to take advantage of it) and feared the anger and violence of disappointed or jealous men.

Like incestuously sexually abusing men, Candace uses sexual behavior in place of affectionate, maternal behavior and does so because she needs someone close to her. Her son has the same sort of mixed feelings that sexually abused children do. The two major differences are that (a) she isn't sexually or genitally engaged with him, and (b) she needs his affection whereas most fathers who sexually abuse seek to give affection. Candace's affection in the interaction and her words in the interview seem sad to the observer, but she herself doesn't refer to sadness. It is sad that she doesn't want to influence her son's development, fearing it could only be for the worse. Once Candace's history and psychological organization are understood, it becomes hard to be angry with her. The difficulty becomes meeting her needs so that she can reorganize her relationship with her son so as to meet his needs.

Later Candace will have another baby, by a man with a close relationship to his mother. For a while they will live together as a family of four people, and Candace will be as happy as she has ever been. When the boyfriend leaves, Candace will stay on with her de facto mother-in-law/acquired mother. This time Candace will keep and raise her child.

Albert's mother Maryia (from Part 1) provides a similar situation, 20 years further along and with a less felicitous outcome. She, too, is a single woman who is left with a son from a one-night stand. She builds her life around her son. Unlike Candace, she skirts child protection, but never actually attracts investigation, far less removal. Albert grows up in her cocoon. Because he needs her and has no alternatives, he accepts his mother's closeness, including her need to sleep in his bed. Like Candace, Maryia doesn't sexually abuse her son; instead, she treats him like her partner, her other half. If he grows up and finds a young woman to love, her life, as she has lived it to now, will become empty both of people and of her single reason to exist. The bind for them both, now that Albert's role as a pseudo-spouse has lasted for two decades, is terrible. Unlike Candace, she is not young and beautiful anymore. She gave her youth to a man for one night and to his son until her middle age. Where does such a woman turn now? Like Candace, she has a strong Type A organization that prevents her from even identifying the dilemma that she creates for her son.

It is important to note that sexual abusers' and spousifying parents' semantic representations reflect normative beliefs about what is appropriate with children. However, like many people, they emphasize prescriptive generalizations over descriptive ones, i.e., 'Do as I say, not as I do'. This difference between types of semantic attributions involves splitting (i.e., failing to integrate) descriptive observations of the self with semantic prescription to the self. Such splitting is, however, quite normative. It is common among parents as well as among professionals and parent educators who intervene in cases of parenting problems; for example, physicians are largely described as being compulsive, i.e., Type A (cf. Holmes 1997; Wilkinson 2003). That is, none of these groups expects the learner (child or parent learner) to evaluate the behavior of the guide in terms of whether they are carrying out the intervention by doing what they are advising.

Child outcomes

Much less is known about the effects of spousification on children than the effects of sexual abuse. There are hints, however, that being spousified is more seriously negative than simply having a caregiving relationship to a depressed or withdrawn parent (Haley 1980). Specifically, maternal depression predicted mothers' engagement in a boundary violating relationship with their children, but differently for boys and girls (Burton 2007). For boys, spousification predicted higher levels of self-reported depression. For girls, a confidante relationship with their mother predicted lower levels of self-reported depression (Burton 2007). The difference may be that the role-reversing function of compulsive caregiving left girls able to develop as children in other contexts, whereas the sexualized involvement of mothers with their sons both isolated them in shame and, as with Albert, blocked their transition to adolescent and adult roles.

Professionals' DRs and behavior

Disconnection among types of information and various representations typifies parents in clusters 1–4. The public is well aware of cases of child abuse and neglect, and moral disapprobation of them is high, without regard or even awareness of other aspects of abusers' lives and developmental history. Social-work and mental-health professionals, however, focus on protecting children, as opposed to punishing parents. The question is whether explicit policies for protecting their children actually dispose professionals' behavior or whether more punitive motivations, often written into funding priorities, do so. The issue arises because placement decisions are sometimes at odds with their probable outcomes.

For example, parents are labeled in pejorative ways ('abuser') as is their behavior. Moreover, in an attempt to change their behavior, they are threatened with negative consequences, including loss of custody of the children. This, of course, is to protect the children from the danger of sexual maltreatment that the parents present. Nevertheless, the intention to protect the children is inconsistent with the data on the effects of out-of-home placement on children and parents.

Although foster care does protect and benefit some children (Horwitz *et al.* 2001; Taussig *et al.* 2001), many other children:

1 suffer maltreatment at the hands of their nonparental carers (Fanshel *et al.* 1990; Pecora *et al.* 2006);
2 perceive themselves to be sufficiently unloved or endangered by their caregivers that they run away (2–5 per cent of US foster children run away every year, Nesmith 2002; US DHHS 2006b);
3 begin a process of changing homes that will culminate in 20–35 per cent of them living in an average of five placements each (England National Statistics 2005; Pecora *et al.* 2006);
4 reach adulthood with 35–40 per cent living in a nonfamily setting as opposed to a foster home (Child Welfare League of America n.d.; Courtney and Barth 1996; Keller *et al.* 2007).

There may be negative effects of child removal on parents as well. For parents, loss of custody produces awareness that their children are not ultimately their own and that they can be taken away. Once parents recognize this, they may never feel secure with their children again – regardless of their parenting skills or custodial status. This is likely to be true for most parents, but is especially true for parents who were not secure in their own childhoods, nor in their relationships with their children before the children were removed. Although there are no empirical data to support these conclusions, there are data showing that loss of potential children through infertility and the death of children, both born and unborn, has long-term effects on both parents and the parents' other children (Kupper 1995; Meyers *et al.* 1995; Pepe and Byrne 1991; Schwab 1997; Wash and McGoldrick 2004). Why would it not be similar for parents whose children were removed? If parents' ability to feel secure with their children is harmed, their ability to be a good parent may also be reduced. Ironically, this would be an outcome of our efforts to protect children and improve parenting. It is curious that we have not investigated this effect so as to take it into account when making placement decisions.

Out-of-home placements occur at a higher rate than professionals deem appropriate (Freundlich *et al.* 2006; Goldstein *et al.* 1973), and decisions regarding permanent placement occur far too slowly, again according to professionals themselves (Chestand and Heymann 1973; Stein *et al.* 1977). Indeed, almost all jurisdictions have regulations intended to speed permanency decisions (CWLA 2003). This suggests that professionals remove children on relatively *slim* evidence, are reluctant to return them without *certainty* of safety, and *lack* evidence that the parents are truly incompetent or dangerous (i.e., the evidence necessary for permanent termination of parental rights). If that standard cannot be met in large numbers of cases, one must consider whether, among professionals (and the community that they represent), there might not be elements of unrealistic hope (Beckett *et al.* 2007), punitiveness toward nonprotective parents, or funding priorities whereby foster care, with its unlimited funding, is a more cost-effective solution from a budgetary perspective.

Chapter 11

Parents whose own needs skew their perceptions: The absence of parental protection

Parents in cluster 4 fail to protect their children and, in the cases that I have seen, more often have psychiatric disorder than do parents who maltreat their children. The disorders tend to be midrange in severity (e.g., depression, substance abuse, anxiety disorders, PTSD) and to reflect parents' anxiety (or hopelessness, in the case of depression) regarding their own safety and comfort.

Parental psychiatric disorder is among the most powerful indicators of risk of child disorder, including both acting-out sorts of problems and role-reversing care of the troubled parent, i.e., A3 compulsive caregiving (Falkov 1996; Fombonne *et al.* 2001; Howard 2000). Depending upon the study, 60–80 per cent of mothers with psychiatric disorder ultimately lose custody of their children (Göpfert *et al.* 2004). Moreover, when the child has symptoms, the mother's psychiatric state is related to poorer outcomes in both child treatment and parenting treatment (Kazdin and Wassel 2000). Although that might be explained by genetic contribution, the data suggest otherwise (Barnes and Stein 2000; Murray and Cooper 2003). For example, parents with psychiatric disorder are more likely to show maladaptive parenting than those without, and this, in turn, is related to children's disorder, but when maladaptive parenting behavior was not shown, the relation between parental and child disorder did not hold (Johnson *et al.* 2001). Based on a meta-analysis of treatment studies, it appears that treatment of maternal depression is related to improvements in child symptoms and functioning, except in cases of postnatal depression (Gunlicks and Weissman 2008). Finally, the evidence indicates that psychiatric personnel rarely consider the effect of their patients' condition on their children even though more than 50 per cent of psychiatrically distressed women are mothers (Göpfert *et al.* 2004). This in spite of the fact that professionals were alerted to this problem four decades ago and frequently thereafter (Hawes and Cottrell 1999; Rutter 1966).

In some cases, the child is the identified patient, and the parents gravitate to parent support groups. In all cases, the parents are so self-focused that they lose sight of their children (without intending them harm). The children then must find a strategy that improves their chances of receiving parental attention. Usually, this means shaping their development around the holes and gaps in their parents' functioning (Crittenden 2000c). When parents' needs are intense, but inexplicitly expressed, the effect on children can be both more pernicious and less visible than when there is competition for parental attention, physical abuse, or sexual abuse (as in Chapters 8–10).

In information-processing terms, cluster 4 parents' representation of the child is (a) absent (not perceived) at crucial moments or (b) does not lead to an attribution that the child needs parental attention. In the former case, the parents' representation of themselves takes priority when both parent and child need attention. In the latter case, the parents fail to discern the child's need for protection and comfort. For example, a child's aggressive behavior may be misunderstood as the child rejecting or hating the parent when the child was actually trying to elicit more attention. In this case, the perception is accurate, but the attribution of meaning is shaped by the parent's negative self-representation. In a few cases, the parents may understand what is needed with reasonable accuracy, but not believe that any action on their part could be effective. This is consistent with severe and pervasive depression. In contrast to parents in clusters 1–3 who have a clear DR of the child, but who select or implement inappropriate behavior, parents in cluster 4 barely perceive their children.

There is a very wide range of parent and child behavior associated with parents' efforts to protect and comfort themselves (Stanger *et al.* 1999). Children may organize around the parent's desires (i.e., a false self); this response causes children to be seen as mature and resilient and does not often elicit professional attention. Nevertheless, it is detrimental to children's long-term adaptation because children must yield awareness of their own feelings and motivations. Alternatively, children may act out, provoke, or take risks to gain parental attention; this response is more likely to elicit professional attention (Hay and Pawlby 2003). Because child characteristics have little or no impact on parental behavior, children using either form of response (caregiving or oppositional) have difficulties with self-identity that can lead to depression. The importance to children of all ages being included in parental representations is clear in elevated rates of malnutrition (Rahman *et al.* 2004) and hospitalization (Guttmann *et al.* 2004) of children of depressed mothers. It is probable that the psychological consequences of not being crucial in parents' lives can become as extreme as forming a basis for suicidal thoughts and action.

Cluster 4: Parents who fail to perceive children's signals or to attribute a need to protect the children to the signals (thus sometimes physically and psychologically neglecting their children)

Four patterns suggest the nature of parents' psychological functioning. They are ordered from clear interpersonal contingencies to complex and largely obscured contingencies.

1 non-caregiving parental relationships;
2 unpredictable and extreme changes in mood and caregiving;
3 triangulation of the child into the marital relationship;
4 disorientation among incompatible representations that then motivate contradictory behavior.

Non-caregiving parental behavior

Some parents are so overwhelmed by their own distress that they cannot perceive their children's needs, and thus cannot function as protective figures for their children. In moments of conflicting need, they generally protect themselves, even at the expense of their children. Very withdrawn (depressed, traumatized, or sorrowing) parents are an example. In moments of distress, they 'shut down', i.e., fail to process incoming information that would lead to protecting their child. Some children are able to establish a relationship with withdrawn parents by caring for the parent as if the parent were the child (i.e., compulsive caregiving; Bowlby 1973; Crittenden 1992c). In role-reversing relationships, the parent–child hierarchy is preserved, but the child takes the adult role (Byng-Hall, 2002, 2008). In other cases, the parents feel so threatened that there is simply no place in their priorities for one or more of the children. These children are psychologically abandoned by the parent. Often sets of siblings show an array of different responses to the family environment (Jean-Gilles and Crittenden 1990). In the example below, Donnie's older daughter probably used a compulsive caregiving strategy. The younger girl may not have found a way to reach her mother.

> Donnie was the mother of two girls, Beth (4 years old) and Amanda (2 years old). Investigation of reports of neglect indicated that Donnie failed to prepare meals, to clean her children or the house, or to dress the girls appropriately for winter weather. When the girls were ill or injured, she failed to provide even the most basic medical care. She left dangerous knives scattered on the counters, the stove on and unattended, and the girls outside for hours at a time without supervision. The children roamed the neighborhood, scavenging for food and attention.
>
> When confronted, Donnie had little to say except that she loved her children. The professionals investigating the complaints found her withdrawn and suspicious, a woman of few words and fewer actions. Observations of the children showed Beth hovering attentively over her silent, sad mother, using a probable compulsive caregiving strategy (A3), and Amanda out of control.
>
> Donnie's children were placed in foster care and a treatment plan was drawn up. Donnie obediently attended the designated meetings, including a parent education course, but she made no behavioral changes. She seemed 'too thick' and unable to learn. Once she said she didn't like one of the workers, and later, when a new location for

contact was selected (one with a play area in hopes she wouldn't use all the visit for feeding the children), she protested that a fast-food play area would generate disputes about eating sugary foods. Both these preferences were overruled, partly because the staff concluded that Donnie was being obstructive. After six months in care, a decision about permanent placement loomed. Questions arose about Donnie's attachment and an AAI was sought.

The AAI provided three major pieces of information. First, Donnie spoke in monosyllables, asked about the questions before answering, and answered very, very slowly. Still she answered almost every question, dutifully and in a monotone. Was this suspicion and an attempt to withhold information (consistent with using an obstructive C5 strategy), or was Donnie afraid to answer without knowing precisely what was wanted (consistent with using a compulsively compliant A4 strategy)?

Second, Donnie idealized her parents semantically, but could not recall episodes to support what she said. Instead, she came close to fabricating impossible episodes, for example, implying that her mother took her to hospital when she was injured at school, but omitting to state that her mother had no transportation. Taken together, it appeared that, in her childhood, Donnie had been pervasively neglected physically, emotionally, and medically. Was her idealization of her parents delusional (A7)? In addition, she had been intermittently abused when her father was drunk; the injuries went untreated. Donnie had learned to obey (compulsive compliance, A4) and had taken care of her own needs and that seemed right to her (compulsive self-reliance, A6).

Third, Donnie was silent and without affect until she was asked about loss. Suddenly, she spoke in long, rapid sentences, gulping back tears and occasionally breaking into sobs. Her uncle had died when she was 11, then her father had died, then Elisabeth had been taken to hospital and … The story became very confusing, with jumps back and forth in time and changes of person. It seemed that Elisabeth had died, but it was unclear of what. Then Donnie's husband had disappeared, but then it seemed that nothing was more important to Donnie than taking care of Beth now. For almost five minutes, nothing made sense in the rush of words and tears.

The history clarified that Donnie had had three children. The firstborn, Elisabeth, had died before the next two were born. The second born was named Beth, after the deceased Elisabeth, but this was unclear and confused in the AAI. Two years later Amanda was born.

When the discourse was analyzed by the DMM method, Donnie's interview was assigned to unresolved loss (in a disorganized form) of the first Elisabeth, unresolved trauma (in a dismissed form) from physical abuse by her father, and all forms of neglect, with a strategy of compulsive compliance (A4) and partial delusional idealization (A7), all of which was in a depressed state. The little that Donnie said was expressed in prescriptive semantic terms, stripped of any images or evocative language. Donnie was quietly adamant that she would not let her children be hit or hurt as she had been. She said nothing, however, about neglect, seeming unaware that she herself had been neglected.

The conclusion drawn was that Donnie was deeply depressed after a pervasively neglected childhood in which she could only stoically accept what happened, but was unable to change anything for the better. Further, she was now grief-stricken from loss (of her first child, father, and uncle), abandonment (by her husband) and placement in care of her remaining two children. Indeed, she was so heartbroken and so unable to articulate her thoughts that the losses had become confused. The confusion was made greater by her near-delusional attempt to resurrect the dead Elisabeth by naming her next child Elisabeth.

Parental DRs

In terms of information processing, Donnie functioned compulsively out of inhibitory procedural routines, e.g., repeatedly checking that she was doing the right thing, and prescriptive semantic guidelines, e.g., always articulating community values. Affectively, she was empty, without self-awareness, and unable to address her unspeakable losses. Of course, she did not integrate, not even to construct episodes (which would have conflicted with her semantic generalizations). Without a sense of temporal efficacy and an awareness of her feelings, there was nothing for Donnie to integrate.

On the other hand, analysis of the AAI made it clear that Donnie had strengths as a mother. She had decided to protect her children from abuse and had done so successfully. She was committed to her children – enough to tolerate the ignominy of the child-protection investigation, imposed services, and supervised contact. In addition, she held values regarding families and respect for authority of which we all could approve. Realistically, however, she and the professionals had been unable to transform these strengths into even minimally competent parenting. The children were left to find their own way to elicit the caregiving they needed. Beth, being both older and the substitute for her dead sister, used the compulsive caregiving strategy with some success. Amanda found nothing; she had no pull on her depressed mother. Given Donnie's strengths and her terrible losses, the issue became how to work with her to enable her to care adequately for the children who were so precious to her.

Effects on the children of maternal depression and withdrawal

As noted in Chapter 8, the brain has evolved to shape itself around experience-dependent and experience-expectant input (Glaser 2000). In the case of neglect, it is the absence of caregiver behavior that is crucial. The brain expects certain kinds of input and uses the input to stimulate further maturation. When that input is absent, the maturation fails to occur. In cases of child neglect, normal parental caregiving and protection fail to occur. This absence of what is expected interferes with the production of synapses. To understand the significance of this process, consider that in rats one day of maternal deprivation was sufficient to decrease brain-derived neurotropic factor in the hippocampus and initiate preprogrammed cell death (Zhang *et al.* 1997). Although the results aren't quite so dramatic in humans, where one day in the life of a newborn rat is equivalent to approximately six months of maternal deprivation in human infants (Glaser 2000: 99), it does make clear that sustained neglect has far more detrimental consequences to children than child abuse (Crittenden 1993, 1998, 1999b).

On the other hand, when the child finds a way to elicit some caregiving, even minimal caregiving, the outcome is behaviorally a compulsive caregiving strategy (A3) or, sometimes, when the neglect is less tied to avoiding children's negative affect, a coercively aggressive strategy (C3). In these situations, children have elicited the experience-expectant input that is needed to propel maturation of the brain and then used the experience-dependent process, tied to the sequential conditions of the caregiver's response to their own behavior, to shape synaptic representation of contingencies. Both of these outcomes, while skewed, are advantageous as compared with severe maternal deprivation (Rutter 2006d).

As with all of the high numeral patterns in the DMM, it is not the designated behavior that is the problem, but rather its compulsive or obsessive application to all aspects of the parent–child relationship. In the case of compulsive caregiving, the child both gives care to the parent when it is beyond the range of what the child can manage developmentally and is uncomfortable receiving care. Beth offered caregiving to her mother as a way to be represented in her mother's DR, but it was insufficient to elicit protection and comfort, and Beth refused what care her mother offered. Her sister Amanda lacked both the advantages of an imagined connection to her deceased sister through sharing a name and the functional connection of caregiving. Without these, she had no way to access her mother. She was one child too many in this emotionally impoverished family. Amanda ran wild.

Children using a strategy of compulsive caregiving shape themselves to meet parental needs – without entering the parents' perception as people who themselves need protection and comfort. Instead, the child is given importance and reality only to the extent that he or she increases the parent's comfort or safety. This carries both advantages, in the form of competence, responsibility, pride, and a sense of having some control over what happens to oneself, and disadvantages, especially in the transition to adulthood, as adolescents begin to establish personal identity. For compulsive caregivers, this identity is defined by others' expectations.

Alternatively, some children refuse the caring role or are refused by the parents; in either case, the child's feeling is likely to be increased anxiety and anger. This may be displayed behaviorally as a range of attention-getting, protection-eliciting, and aggressive behaviors that are often diagnosed as conduct problems, oppositional behavior, risk-taking, etc. Underlying this behavior is a desperate anger that can so dominate behavior that potential caregivers are both misled about the child's actual feelings and needs and afraid of the child. The strategy, in other words, can backfire for the child in ways that lead the child to self-destructive behavior that cannot be limited by either child or parent.

A particular risk for the younger siblings of successful role-reversing children is that, once the protective function is fulfilled by one child, the others may have fewer possibilities for organizing a successful strategy.

In the most severe cases, the parents, individually or as a couple, feel so threatened themselves that there is simply no place in the marriage for the children. In these cases, there may be no child strategy that can penetrate the self-focus of the parent(s). Such children are at risk of psychological withdrawal, escape into a world of fantasy, and depression. In extreme cases, there may be risk of suicidal thought, threats and action.

Unpredictable and changing dangerous parental behavior

A second group of parents displays unpredictable and dangerous changes in contingencies and arousal, such as parents with bipolar disorder or those who abuse substances. The changes can be between negative and positive affect, one negative affect and another, low and high arousal, submissiveness and vindictiveness, sober and not sober, or awareness of the child and lack of awareness. Such changes place excessive demands upon children to adapt to the parent's state. Children from such families sometimes become 'codependent' or 'enablers' as they try to accommodate their parents' changing states. For example, when the parent is aroused and angry, the child may behave with compliance or submission, but when the parent is frightened or anxious, the child may take charge and manage the household, siblings (as a 'parental' child), and even the parent (i.e., role reversal).

Maggie Drucker had been known to child protection since Josh was an infant and had been discovered by the visiting nurse to be underweight, bruised, and developmentally delayed. Even now, when Josh was in his fourth year at school, Maggie's weekend binges and explosions of vindictive anger were legendary.

Maggie and Josh lived alone in a rural area, but Maggie's mother, Rosie, lived nearby and functioned as a member of the household. Even compared with the other impoverished households in the area, Maggie's stood out as bleak and forbidding. Indeed, her demeanor was so dark and threatening that few professionals dared to visit her at home. This made the results of her Parent's Interview all the more striking.

When Maggie, Josh, and Rosie entered the interview room, Rosie was anxiously polite and cheerful, Josh was inhibited and watchful, and Maggie glowered. The interviewer invited Josh to play while she talked with his mother and grandmother, asking Maggie to keep an eye on him. Josh slipped gratefully into a corner, held a toy as if playing with it, and watched the adults with a half-turned face. After hesitating, as if she might flee, Maggie sat sullenly at the table with her mother and the interviewer. The interviewer gave an explanation of what they would do, then asked:

How was *your* childhood?
It was all right.
Were you a good child?
Good and bad.
Could you tell me a bit more …?
I don't remember. I don't remember that good.

And Maggie shut down.

   In sales, they say that you have 30 seconds on a cold call to establish a relationship. The 30 seconds was up and Maggie was gone. More questions followed, each blocked by monosyllabic responses or *Don't remember. I got a bad memory.* The impact on the interviewer was dramatic. First, she pulled her clipboard closer, then put it upright on her knees, and then upright on the table, blocking the space between Maggie and herself. Maggie gave no sign of noticing; she was closed and she stayed closed. In desperation, the interviewer turned to Rosie, who responded with an eager rescue, chatting helpfully in response to every question. Maggie was forgotten in the interviewer's relief in finding a socially acceptable response. She lowered her clipboard. Maggie, however, had both admitted defeat and rejected everyone; she had dropped her head onto her folded arms on the table! Josh watched warily. A few moments after his mother put her head down, he came over, silently and carefully. Gently, he placed his hand on her back.

Maggie?
What do you want? [said sharply from behind her barricaded arms]
You sick?
Yes, I am.
Uh … Mag, come here.
[Silence]
Mag, are you sick, Mag?
What?
You sick?
Yes, I'm sick. Now go sit down.

Josh went and sat, but he remained watchful. The interview continued. They discussed disciplining Josh (*I beat him. That's all.*) Asked how she and her mother handled disputes, Maggie turned to Josh, saying, *You're getting on my nerves. Glad when I leave.*

As the interview closed, Maggie was asked what made her feel especially good about Josh.

Nothing.
The question was rephrased.
Nothing. Nothing.
You're a little angry at him now. Are you glad you're a parent?
Not really.
Why not?
I don't know. I got no answer for that.
That's it for the interview, etc.
Good. I'm ready to go. Get up, Josh, no more toys, you ain't playing with no more toys today. Come on. We're getting ready to go home, child.

What a terrible conclusion! It fit everything that was known about Maggie, but it didn't fit Maggie. I rushed to meet Maggie in the anteroom. No mother should go home feeling like Maggie felt now. I took my 30 seconds and used it to offer sympathy (*That was hard!*), but Maggie brushed it away. So I tried a little joke; Maggie almost smiled. Feeling I'd made the breakthrough, I leaned in confidentially and said, *Now, Maggie, I heard you say you didn't want to be a parent, but I see how much Josh matters to you … doesn't he?* Maggie nodded. *So, tell me, do you like being a parent?* Suddenly, Maggie changed. She wanted two children, a boy and a girl, she … I stopped her, saying the videotape didn't have this version of her. Could we go back in and correct that video so we'd know how she really felt? She came in and, while not morphing into Miss Congeniality, she said, *I love raising kids and I always did want to be a parent 'cause I wanted two kids, a boy and girl.* I asked whether she'd choose the same father and whether she'd want him to live with her. *No, I wouldn't. By myself.* How come? *Men, I don't know. I can't get along with them too good. I can't get along with Josh's father. We couldn't get along. That's why we're not living together now. He comes around, sees Josh, I speak to him. We get along good now. I've got my mother. She helps me.* Then Maggie's reliance on her mother to cook some extra when Maggie felt too bad to cook or to take Josh for a few days when Maggie felt really bad came up. *I can count on her.* What followed were paragraph-long discussions of how she and her mother worked together, what their daily life was like, what Josh liked.

Why couldn't this Maggie be seen by more professionals? She was limited as a mother, for sure, but briefly she was engaged in telling her perspective and thinking about herself in her major relationships. Why could she do that with one professional and not another – indeed, not with the majority?

Parents' DRs

Maggie's DRs were about what could go wrong and stopping things from getting worse. She blamed herself and she blamed Josh. But she could be sweet-talked and she could warm up. Still, the other person had to declare their love first. The risk had to be theirs – and, if they were scared of her (as our interviewer was), she simply shut them out with scorn. It was as if she were saying that life was hard, and, if you couldn't take it, git! Even though he was only a boy, Josh knew all of that already: you had to love his mama, even though sometimes even that wasn't enough, and you had to respect her anger, whether you deserved it or not, and you daren't be so scared that you waited for her to come to you – because she wasn't coming. You had to go to her. And all bets were off when she went on a drunk. Then Grandma was your protection.

Strategically, Maggie was depressed, had unresolved traumas mostly tied to men who beat her and left her, as her father did to her mother, as Josh's father did to her. She counted on herself; she didn't expect much. Even her mother's cheerful cooperation denied Maggie's reality. We'd call her compulsive self-reliant (A6), with an opening for sweet-talk and resentful anger (C5-6). Her representation of Josh, when she was aware of him, was tied to her own needs for comfort and for deflecting anger from other, more powerful people.

Effects on children of highly variable maternal behavior

As an infant and small child, Josh couldn't shift rapidly enough to match his mother's moods. He couldn't see the changes coming and he couldn't find the strategies with which to protect himself. He was abused and he was neglected. But as he matured, he learned what worked. Don't draw attention to yourself, be as quiet as possible, look serious, be concerned about her, but don't, under any conditions, be sullen. An array of compulsive strategies worked best with his mama, and by the time he was 9 years old he knew them all.

Children from mood-dysfunctional families sometimes become 'codependent' or 'enablers' as they try to accommodate their parents' changing needs for protection and comfort. That is, the children's self-protection functions to makes the parents' strategy work and, in so doing, it removes the discrepancies between the parents' DR and external reality. This makes it more difficult for the parents to perceive the inappropriateness of their behavior and thought processes. It can have the same effect on professionals.

Triangulating parental behavior

Triangulating parents try to protect the children *from* problems in the marriage or, in more severe cases, engage children in protection *of* the marriage. 'Triangulation' refers to a particular distortion of parent and child subsystem boundaries (Minuchin 1974). In triangulated relationships, the children perceive themselves as having a direct relationship with the parent, whereas, in actuality, the parents' interest is tied to how the children function to preserve the spousal relationship. Changes in parents' perceived threat can have a powerful impact on the parents' behavior, often in the form of emotion-based action (Hein and Miele 2003). When the threat is not tied to, nor visible to, the children, but is acted out with the children as if they had caused the parents' behavior, children become very confused about their causal contribution to relationships.

Monia and her husband had five children. Early on, the family lived in two rooms and a kitchen with Monia, her husband, and their second born, a daughter, sleeping in one bed. They kept this sleeping arrangement during the period when the younger three children were conceived. From time to time, however, when things got really difficult, the children lived with Monia's mother.

Monia worked as a nurse and her husband was a sailor. When he was away, usually for weeks at a time, Monia had all the children to cope with by herself and, at times, she felt quite frantic and deserted. Although she wanted her children to be kind and gentle, often the house was filled with the bedlam of squabbling brats all clawing for her attention. Sometimes she had to punish them to get any control at all. She found that if they all had to watch the punishment, they could be shamed into being quiet for a while. As her parents had done with her, she pulled their pants down, laid them across her knees, and swatted them (but not so hard as to injure them). But when her husband was in port, he could fly off the handle and punish them very severely.

In addition, he was often violent to Monia, fearing that she had not been faithful in his absence. In fact, he eventually stopped sailing in order to monitor her activities more closely. One night, they had a huge fight in which Monia was almost killed. The police intervened and had him committed to a psychiatric hospital. According to her, the court then imposed divorce on the couple. All of this was against Monia's will, as she relayed it, although it wasn't clear why.

Monia told people that he needed her support because he was mentally ill, and she encouraged the children to forgive him even though she could see that they were terrified of him. Throughout, she seemed proud, but it was the sort of lonely pride that pushed people away. She tried to keep up appearances and seemed especially worried to keep the children quiet and out of sight because of what the neighbors would think.

After her husband's commitment, Monia became desperate. She continued to visit her husband at the hospital and didn't think she could carry on alone. In this context, her oldest child, a boy, helped her, functioning as the man of the house even though he had barely reached puberty. Nevertheless, as she had done when her husband traveled, she frequently disappeared for hours at a time or sometimes even overnight. Several years later, one of her daughters, after developing an eating disorder and then leaving the country for a year, revealed that her brother had sexually abused her.

Monia never admitted to having the affairs she was accused of by her husband, but her behavior suggested that she felt at least as guilty about his violence as she felt frightened of it. Indeed, if one noticed how little she could tolerate being alone, how freely men looked at her, and how often she and the children were apart, one might seriously question whether all five of the children were her husband's. Once that thought was entertained, it quickly became plausible that her anger, disappearances, and concern that the neighbors would see something might all be about keeping her sexual life secret. Her apparent seeking of men, in turn, was tied to her inability to feel safe alone. Moreover, she appeared to use the comfort of children's bodies (as do some men) and sexual activity with men to comfort herself.

Parents DRs
Monia operated out of somatic images that sent her looking for closeness and procedures for hiding what she did. Fear lay near the surface, right next to loneliness and desire. The problems were to keep the children and neighbors at bay and unaware of things happening so close. For Monia, that meant secrecy and hard discipline – with no thought to how her children felt or what they needed. Only when they could harm her or, in the case of her oldest boy, when he could care for her or fulfill her obligations, did she have a DR of them. None of this was put into words; indeed, this was a family of exceptionally few words and equally strong feelings that were often in conflict with one another. Fear, guilt, anger, and desire swirled through the home, but had no verbal place with a mother who said everyone should be 'kind' and 'good'. Nothing added up, but still it went on with the children being pulled into activities that were not childlike, sent away without explanation, beaten for offenses they couldn't identify, and ultimately left with rage as undirected and inarticulate as their mother's feelings.

Effects on the children
The two central issues for the children in triangulated relationships are (a) forming accurate understanding of self-relevant causation, i.e., knowing what they elicit from their parents versus when their behavior is irrelevant to outcomes, and (b) developing a sense of themselves as important in their own right, i.e., developing self-esteem. When children are 'protected' from awareness of problems in the marriage, they are prevented from knowing the conditions that motivate parental behavior. When children are engaged to protect the marriage, the triangulated relationships use children contingently in ways that children cannot understand while also preventing them from seeing the actual causes of parental behavior.

There may be a gender effect in triangulated relationships with mothers triangulating daughters into the marital relationship and daughters responding with passive-aggressive strategies, e.g., eating disorders and drug abuse. Fathers and sons may more often use directly aggressive strategies such as extreme risk-taking and antisocial behavior. In either case, triangulated relationships deflect appropriate anger because the causal conditions are clouded (Bosco *et al.* 2003). Children who have elicited attachment behavior through simulating the spousal role often become conflicted both about their parents and potentially about peer relationships.

In addition, cross-generational relationships may be established in which the child both colludes with the opposite gender parent to demean or expel the other (sometimes in a fantasy of replacing the rejected parent) and attempts to seduce that parent, often with sexualized behavior. The chosen parent, both out of relief at finding a way to be close to the child and for self-serving reasons, usually fails to establish appropriate parent–child boundaries.

This weakens the marriage further and leaves children, especially adolescent children, angry, confused, and unable to extricate themselves from their childhood family and unprepared for adulthood relationships. The outcomes are various forms of the coercive strategy: in childhood, psychosomatic distress and passive risk-taking; in adolescence, severe disorders such as eating and conduct disorders; in the transition to adulthood, full-fledged personality disorders, i.e., stuck forms of passive resistance, depression and suicidality.

Disoriented parental behavior

Disoriented individuals confuse DRs from different sources, treating them all as self-relevant in the present and compatible when, in fact, they are in conflict. Overlooking these discrepancies leads to unstable and incoherent behavior.

Disorientation occurs infrequently, but is almost always associated with severe problems in the children, such as ADHD, Asperger's syndrome, and autism. It is most often seen together with A/C combinations where the specific subpatterns of A and C are relatively normative, i.e., A1–4/C1–4. Because disorientation in parents does not produce dramatic and visible effects (as, for example, depression does), it generally is overlooked, and only the highly troubled child's deviance is noticed. For example, Benjamin's mother sought consultation a year after Benjamin had been diagnosed with ADHD and treated with medication; she wanted the medication discontinued and psychotherapy offered to both of them because, according to her, Benjamin's problems were related to her marital difficulties. The AAI of the mother and the SAA of Benjamin found both to be disoriented with A/C strategies and assorted unresolved traumas. Therefore, a recommendation was made that was consistent with the mother's request; it was denied and Benjamin remained on medication (Crittenden and Kulbotton 2007). In cases of disorientation, including both Benjamin's mother and Gerd (below), the parents' behavior could best be described as 'all over the place', but not extreme.

Often disoriented parents are seen as merely very talkative, aroused, and arousing. Initially, most seem quite engaging. Many urgently seek resolution to amorphous, entangling problems, and often these involve worthy causes. Nevertheless, at some point, listeners become overwhelmed and want to conclude the endless discussion. At that point, they discover that these individuals resist disengaging. They don't respond to signals that one has had enough; instead, they intensify their efforts to keep the conversation going, speaking faster and adding chapters to their saga of troubles. Aspects of the disoriented person's behavior are incompatible; e.g., asking for help while not listening to the response. They seem unable to accomplish their stated goals. For example, one potential adoptive mother at the last minute refused two different matches offered to her. Another woman had inexplicable panic attacks, one was in treatment for inability to experience sexual arousal, another was the mother of a convicted sexual abuser, and yet another was considering surgery to change his gender. Gerd will serve as an example of the group.

> Gerd was the mother in an intact family with three school-age boys. The 11-year-old was referred for psychological evaluation by Gerd because of her concerns regarding his personality, specifically his being a loner with outbursts of aggression directed toward her. Gerd reported that he had had early eating problems, and, at the time of the referral, she thought he was autistic. Considerable inconclusive work with the boy led the professionals to wonder whether Gerd displayed the Munchausen's syndrome by proxy. To explore that hypothesis, Gerd was given an AAI. At that time, the boy was no longer in treatment. He was doing well in school and his behavior was considered normal, with only mild learning difficulty.
>
> Gerd's AAI began clearly enough with her birth, their moves, and then the birth of two brothers ... *Paul who's 32 and I've another who's 22. But ... um ... his name? He's called Andy. We're not that ... we're not very close, you know.* Suddenly, the younger brother stood out, marked by dysfluency in the discourse. In addition, Gerd's inability to spontaneously use his name and the rhetorical question to herself asking for it alerted the coder to the possibility of disorientation. That was followed by a switch to the recent divorce of her parents after 35 years of marriage that came as a total shock because they were the *'ideal couple'*, according to Gerd. One wonders how 'ideal' and 'divorce' can be in the same sentence; what had Gerd failed to notice? Then there was a very fragmented section about Gerd and her younger brother Andy, given in response to a question about their ages (which in fact had already been given, but the interviewer had forgotten in the confusion of Gerd's way of speaking): *I'm 35, but with like being ...*

there's a few years between me and Andy – I sort of was, you know, made to be the 'mummy' if you like – you know, getting up on a night – seeing [incomprehensible] to enjoy it – hiding in my bedroom. I'd be the one that ... Gerd went on to say that the family lost contact with Andy when he left home at 16. We wonder why Paul wasn't mentioned (the age of both boys was queried), what happened in the bedroom that she saw, enjoyed, and hid, but could not speak articulately about. Themes of beds, irregularities in her sexual development, the silence around sexuality, and closeness with her father were scattered in unconnected ways throughout the transcript. She talked in other places about secrets and said, 'I know it's awful what happened'. But we don't know what happened and Gerd didn't tell. One considers long-term sexual abuse by her father and even whether he fathered her out-of-wedlock baby when she was 16 years old. One considers whether she sexually abused Andy when she was a parental child to him. Nothing is conclusive.

At times, Gerd's discourse is very Type A:

Do you remember a particular incident when you were upset as a child?
Um ... well, I was upset when I got an iron bar stuck in me head.
What? An iron bar?
Yeh, stuck in the back of me head, you go running in and blood everywhere and me mom just passes out on the floor.
She passed out on the floor?
Yeh, 'cos she can't stand the sight of blood. I had to get round to the neighbors with this iron bar stuck in me head.
How did that happen?
We were playing out on the green and this boy threw the iron bar up into the air and I looked, knowing it was going to come. To save me eyes, I put my head down for it to go into.
Did it stick in?
Yeh.
How big?
Quite long. The neighbors got it out and I remember a lot of blood, and they were more bothered about me mom passing out, but I never really did get to hospital and me dad came home – I remember him saying that I should of gone for stitches, blah ...

This is chilling because Gerd seemed to lack feelings (even pain is missing!) or arousal for herself. She distanced herself as 'you', and she focused on her mother's reaction (a displacement). The only key to arousal was in the present-tense verbs used for her mother. We assign an unresolved trauma that is displaced onto her mother for this incident.

In the next lines, her discourse is very Type C and disoriented as well:

When you were upset, say, emotionally, what would you do?
I'd probably go to me bedroom – again – my mom wasn't one who'd say, 'Sit down, what's the matter?' She wasn't one to recognize that there was something wrong – whether she'd turned a blank eye or whatever – I don't know, but, you know, to me, I can sense there's problems – there's something wrong – and I tend to look a bit more – whether it's knowing that my mom didn't to me and I wish ... it would have been nice to have a close relationship and say, 'I can see you're upset, let's sit down and talk about it', but she never did.
Do you remember any specific incident that happened?
Um ... I got called a lot of names at school and I think that developed if I could have spoken. I did run away from school a few times and again through problems, but, you know, I suppose again – maybe it was a bit attention-seeking, I'd got in with the bad crowds – I was that honest I phoned up the headmistress and tell her.

Gerd spoke with a run-on structure, a bit blaming ('*She made me what I am.*' Later: '*I never forget.*'), and with direct quotes – all of which are Type C indicators. But she was neither pervasively angry nor dismissing of other people. She has the Type C markers, but not the strategy. Instead she has many markers of disorientation:

1 reorienting self-speech;
2 repeated comments on herself being the source ('*As I said*' – usually when she hasn't said!);
3 misspoken phrases that state the opposite of what we think she meant to say (e.g., *I think that* [would not have] *developed if I could have spoken.*);
4 slipping from one generation to another;
5 mixing of topics (e.g., mother not asking about what might be wrong, which seems better tied to the possible sexual abuse references; '*not knowing what's happening to* **your** *body*' and '*what should've been happening to* **me** *body*' [emphasis added]).

That is, things are out of place, scattered through her speech in ways that hint at meanings, but make nothing clear.

Gerd is aroused and dismissing at once. She keeps shifting her perspective until we can know nothing and expect that she, too, knows little with certainty about her developmental years. Indeed, she said exactly that: *I've sat down and thought about it at home and there's not a lot really, whether I've blanked it a lot or not, there's not a lot I can remember of childhood as such at home ...*

But her final words were: *I mean it was always up front, you know, em ... we always knew where we stood erm ... nothing went on, you know, that we didn't know about, really, erm, you know, everything was, we, we was always out in the open and you know but ... er ... as I say, it's just a shame it wasn't between my mom, me and my mom a bit more open towards each other maybe.* But we find nothing open and clear. We don't know where anyone stood. We only know there was a lot of loose, shifting danger and possibility of danger. We can't even say with certainty what strategy Gerd used!

It is little wonder then that Gerd's son doesn't know how to act and can't relate to her. She's a blurry, moving target. Our conclusion is that she needs desperately to find a perspective on her experience that she can use consistently: dismissing it, or becoming preoccupied and angry, taking her own perspective (very difficult if she was both abused and herself sexually abused her brother), or taking someone else's perspective. It only seems clear that taking all perspectives at once and mixing them together is confusing and distressing to both Gerd and her children.

Parents' DRs

Disoriented parents confuse the representations from different sources (including 'borrowed' parental perspectives, their own perspectives at different periods of their life, and their children's perspectives), thus motivating incongruent and often self-defeating behavior. In information-processing terms, they lack source memory. As a consequence of their ineffectiveness, they are anxious, but without an evident focus for their agitation. Their affective states are unstable and not tied closely to current conditions because they are generated by a shifting array of incompatible DRs from different periods in their life, different people, and, particularly, dismissed childhood traumas. Each DR by itself is reasonable, but, combined, they leave parents out of sync with daily life, puzzled about contingencies, and unable to discern the effects of their behavior on others. Even more important, they leave the parent without a 'self', without a perspective regarding who they are and what they desire. Lacking this, they find it difficult to connect with other people. In this confusion of arousal-without-perspective, children's physical needs are met with unfocused overconcern while the children themselves are often not treated as social and psychological beings.

Effects on children

As noted in Chapter 8, the brain has evolved to shape itself around experience-dependent and experience-expectant processes (Glaser 2000). In the case of neglect, it is the absence of caregiver behavior that is crucial. The brain expects certain kinds of input and uses the input to stimulate further maturation. When that input is absent, the maturation fails to occur. In cases of child neglect, normal parental caregiving and protection fail to occur. When nothing the child does makes a difference, learning cannot occur.

On the other hand, when the child finds a way to elicit some caregiving, even minimal caregiving, the outcome is behaviorally a compulsive caregiving strategy (A3) or sometimes, when the neglect is less tied to avoiding children's negative affect, a coercively aggressive strategy (C3). In these situations, the child has elicited the input that is needed to propel maturation of the brain. This then activates synapses and keeps them from dying away (being 'pruned') in the second year of life. Both of these outcomes, while skewed, are advantageous as compared with severe maternal deprivation (Rutter 2006d).

Children of disoriented parents cannot soothe the parent, nor will the parent fight with them, nor are they used by the parent. Indeed, they cannot elicit contingent responses from the parents at all. Even explosive coercive displays do not engage the parent. Trying to coerce a disoriented parent is like trying to wrestle with fog. That is, nothing the child does connects them to the parent. Instead, the children are treated with benign irrelevance, rather like the way one absently pats a pet. Lack of contingency and shared affect drives humans crazy. These children retreat to internal worlds of self-generated contingencies and private affective states that increase their isolation. Such children use failed forms of both Types A and C strategies and often have autistic characteristics. Without contingent and affectively attuned responses, children lack the basic inputs needed for development. Ironically, disoriented parents who lack DRs of their children often devote immense effort to advocating the very issues that trouble their invisible children.

In all four subgroups of cluster 4, the triggers to parental action are hypothesized to be primarily within and about the parent. Unlike incestuous abusers (cluster 3), these parents take *too little* account of the information from or about the child, who, therefore, is largely missing, as a unique person, from the parent's DRs. In addition, parents distort their self-representation, such that the self appears vulnerable, childlike, and blameless, while overestimating the child's competence or power. Often this is expressed semantically as statements regarding children's maturity (in the case of role-reversing children) or resistance to caregiving and guidance (in the case of oppositional or withdrawn children). In a sad irony of misunderstanding, the parents' effort to protect the child from the parents' experience denies the child essential information about causal relations, thus greatly harming the child's development. In addition, as the child's efforts to be cared for become more distorted, both parents and professionals become convinced that the child is either highly competent and resilient or irreparably damaged.

In sum, the parents in cluster 4 fail to represent their children as *children*, i.e., people who need protection and comfort. The errors of thought that underlie this misperception differ among the four subgroups, but have in common (a) failing to resolve past loss or trauma, and sometimes (b) structuring adult relationships in ways that create current risk.

Across the course of this chapter, the DR of the child in the parent's mind has moved from being hardly present to inextricably intertwined in the parent's needs in inexplicit ways. When a DR of the child is absent, the child knows, suffers, and seeks a solution by which he or she can be meaningfully attached to the parent. When the child is pulled into the parent's world for parental purposes, the child does not understand, has conflicting feelings, and fights a shadow battle that can't be won, but neither can it be lost. It can only go on, holding the child in place, unless the child opts for isolation or death.

Although children in this cluster cannot easily discern them, especially at young ages, there are still real conditions in the family that influence parental behavior. By understanding the parents' needs, we can reconceptualize the children's needs, and the situation changes for the child 'magically'. This is less true of clusters 5 and 6.

Chapter 12

Distortions that substitute erroneous information for accurate information and that miscontrue children as being threatened

Parents who fear danger in irrational ways combine many of the distortions described in previous chapters and add to them one crucial transformation. Because they rely on erroneous information generated during exposure to danger (usually in early childhood), these parents are confused about the current presence and source of danger. Because the threat is not real, it cannot be disarmed; consequently, the parents' efforts to protect themselves and their children cannot relieve their perception of threat. Such parents take repeated extreme and irrational protective measures, (e.g., repetitive actions, excessive cleansing, bizarre forms of punishment) on behalf of themselves and their children. These procedures and the images that often elicit them operate outside conscious and reflective awareness. In many cases, the parents' self-protective response is so primed that it occurs in widely disparate situations. The semantic basis for these procedural actions is often erroneous belief in either the parents' inherently bad (or evil) nature or their continuing vulnerability to others' vengefulness. Although these beliefs are irrational, in childhood they may have created the perception, however slim, that the procedures could control the danger.

An example, albeit an extreme one, is the Jonestown massacre, a mass suicide directed by the Rev. Jim Jones on the belief that his religious community, the People's Temple in Guyana, would be attacked imminently by enemies and everyone would be killed in an 'undignified' manner. That belief was partly based on fact, i.e., the community was being investigated for child abuse and neglect, but it was exaggerated delusionally out of proportion. The result was that 913 children, parents, and other adults (of the approximately 1,100 community members) died on November 18, 1978. How did so many adults share a delusion that caused them to kill their children and commit suicide themselves?

There appear to be two crucial effects of the erroneous transformations of information that define the self (or all humans) as bad and others as vengeful. First, a delusional representation of their child may fill the void left by the absent accurate representation of the child (as observed in cluster 4 parents). Second, erroneous conclusions about the immediacy and pervasiveness of danger may forestall further processing, and that may both impede the correction of erroneous information and make possible the generation of additional erroneous information (Freeman *et al.* 2007).

Such behavior and beliefs appear to be the developmental outcome of a childhood history of (a) serious and repeated exposure to danger (Üçok and Bikmaz 2007; Whitfield *et al.* 2005), (b) very serious neglect, even to the point of not having any consistent attachment figure (Enns *et al.* 2002; O'Conner *et al.* 2003), often combined with (c) gratuitous and uncontrollable abuse by caregivers (Breier *et al.* 1987; Read 1998) who also (d) provide at least some comfort. The last two observations fit evidence drawn from AAIs of PTSD patients, non-PTSD patients, and nonpatients (Crittenden and Heller 2008). Many of the adults with PTSD had no committed and constant caregiver in the early months and years of life to provide structure or offer comfort when they could not yet manage this themselves; this is associated with higher probabilities of a trauma response (Perry *et al.* 1991). In these circumstances (items a–d above), infants and young children have so little influence over their own well-being that superstitious behavior and self-negating beliefs may create the perception of control.

In adulthood, the parents' fears are at least semidelusional (in that they are self-generated and violate boundaries of time and space), and their attempts at self- and child-protection are often desperate and dangerous (Freeman *et al.* 2007; Salmon *et al.* 2003). Among the cases that I have seen, many, but not all, of these parents have severe psychiatric diagnoses that include such conditions as severe personality disorder, bipolar disorder, schizophrenia, and major or psychotic depression (keeping in mind that these diagnoses are not necessarily stable, mutually exclusive, or defined functionally). This is consistent with the literature on nonpsychotic delusions (Altman *et al.* 1997). Common to the diagnoses are dramatic shifts in mood and arousal that alternate between depression and excitement. In addition, it is likely that essentially all of these adults have unresolved traumas or losses from early life (Perry *et al.* 1991; Read 1998; Whitfield *et al.* 2005).

Cluster 5: Parents who misconstrue powerful forces as threatening both themselves and their children (thus sometimes severely injuring or killing their children)

There is a wide array of organizations of delusionally threatened parents. They have in common that rigid procedural schemas learned when they were in danger are released in certain sensory contexts (imaged memory). In addition, however, they add an irrational overlay of semantic understandings that function to justify or explain what otherwise would have to appear (to the parent) aberrant or dangerous. That is, erroneous information generates dangerous forms of 'protection' that then are explained with delusion-like prescriptive generalizations. A few are described here, but the list is not exhaustive. They include parents who:

1 shame children for normal feelings and behavior through semantic belief systems (including religious beliefs) that denigrate feelings and/or find humans to be inherently sinful (for example, diapering older children, putting derogatory signs on children);
2 engage in compulsive rituals (intended to protect the self or child) while neglecting basic life needs of the child;
3 apply semantic rules that forbid essential protective action (for example, using faith-based rituals instead of medical treatment);
4 apply semantic rules that require punishment in ways that threaten children's survival (such as confinement, extreme fasting, physical restraint or punishment, etc.).

Kate exemplifies a mother who was shamed as a child and used compulsive rituals that endangered her child (Crittenden 2005b).

> Thirty-eight-year-old Kate lived alone. Her 2-year-old son was in foster care awaiting adoption following an incident in which Kate, believing she was poisonous and infecting others, including her son, had put bleach in his bath water to cleanse *him* of *her* contamination. Although the child was not harmed, Kate worried that this might escalate. Therefore, she voluntarily placed him in foster care with plans for adoption.
>
> Kate suffered from severe depression, delusional states, and self-cutting and was diagnosed with bipolar depression and comorbid borderline personality disorder. She had had a decade of behavioral and cognitive-behavioral therapy, particularly for agoraphobia and anorexia. Recently, she had been hospitalized for self-harm. She was on antipsychotic medication, tranquilizers, and antidepressants, but did not always take the prescribed medications.

To understand Kate's behavior as a mother, we need to know her history.

> When she was one month old, Kate was placed in a children's home by her psychotic mother. Her drug-abusing father had already disappeared. From 4-6 years of age, Kate lived in a foster home, but was returned to the children's home when her foster parents' marriage broke down. Kate's first cutting incident occurred at age 9 when she accidentally cut herself and was surprised to find that it felt good. From this incident, she may have erroneously learned that cutting brought both comfort and professionals who became concerned and caring. Beginning at age 9 and continuing until she was 17 years old, Kate had a relationship with one of the young male staff members in the children's home; Mick was both affectionate and kind and also engaged with her sexually. In Kate's words, this relationship was one of the best things in her otherwise lonely life in the institution. At 16, one of the adolescents in the children's home found out about her

sexual contact with Mick, considered it abusive, and informed the police. Nothing came of it for lack of evidence.

Kate later married the adolescent who made the complaint. They had one child (already an adult at the time of these events) and eventually divorced. Kate remarried and gave birth to a boy, who, at the time of the AAI, was 2 years old. Soon after the birth, her second husband died. Thereafter, Kate had dreams about macabre experiences with babies including 'chopping them up'. She believed she was poisonous and infecting others, including her son.

Around the time of the AAI, Kate had regular contact with her son and recognized that he was happy in his foster family. However, she feared losing contact with him completely and became increasingly depressed. In the past, promiscuous sexual activity had counteracted her chronic depression by arousing her, but it no longer interested her. Kate needed something very strong, very arousing to counteract her depressively low arousal. Kate heard voices that told her to cut herself, something she had not done since adolescence.

Pain induces very high arousal, higher even than anxiety or sexual arousal (Peyron *et al.* 1999). Failure to respond with affective arousal to pain severely jeopardizes survival (Diatchenko *et al.* 2007; Hendry 1999) and, in rats, has been shown to be associated with maternal separation early in life (Weaver *et al.* 2006). Thus, cutting may function to reverse the effects of depression on arousal. This, by itself, feels 'good' when previously one did not feel anything. It is, in a distorted way, proof of an 'affective' self – and thus to be treasured by someone who feels little else. Moreover, very high pain and very high positive affect are cogenerated; that is, the neurological signals are often brought online together (Doidge 2007).

After cutting herself, Kate contacted neighbors, who took her to hospital, and professionals again cared for her. The aftermath of cutting, however, was a sudden decrease in arousal, accompanied by intense tiredness, disillusionment with herself, awareness of having failed yet again, and an even greater sense of futility than before. After returning home, Kate would isolate herself, then feel lonely and depressed – and the cycle began again.

Clearly, Kate could not find the balance in arousal that is necessary for life. The central construct in the DMM is danger. Kate had faced danger in the past, but now she imposed it upon herself and her child. The issues to understand are (a) how her processing of information led to recurrent alternation of depression with delusional and injurious behavior and (b) how this cycle can be changed.

Kate's DR

Kate's AAI was classified as: Dp Ul(dp)$_{\text{All AFs}}$ Utr(dp)$_{\text{SA}}$ A+(4, 6b, 8) [ina: desire for pain]. That is, Kate used a depressed form of three compulsive strategies: compulsive compliance (A4), compulsive self-reliance (A6b, isolated type), and externally assembled self (A8). Put more generally, (a) cognitively, Kate believed she must do as others told her to do and relied on professionals to both stabilize her and give her life meaning, all without intimacy; (b) affectively, she had hardly any access to feelings. The depression expressed her experience-based belief that her own actions made no difference in what happened, i.e., learned helplessness (Abramson *et al.* 1978; Klein *et al.* 1976; Peterson *et al.* 1993; Seligman 1975), and was displayed as excessively low arousal.

In addition, she had unresolved loss of all attachment figures (mother, father, foster parents, Mick, two husbands, and now her son) in a depressed form. These losses left Kate feeling empty and suggested the futility of engaging in intimate relationships.

Kate's AAI also indicated lack of resolution of the trauma of sexual abuse by Mick in a depressed form. One of the 'best' things in Kate's youth, her relationship with Mick, was defined by others as bad; because Kate depended on others for her self-definition, she was left with even less access to the rousing and pleasant feelings associated with sex.

Finally, Kate had intrusions of forbidden negative affect [ina]. In the past, these were excitingly promiscuous and dangerous sexual encounters, but now, desire for pain (expressed as cutting) fulfilled the function of generating arousal. The repeated instances of cutting functioned, however briefly, to increase her arousal, to cause others to express extreme distress, and to attract others, especially professionals, to care for her. That is, cutting was multiply determined in that it met many of Kate's needs at once.

Kate's two modifiers functioned in a coordinated way. The 'Dp' indicated that Kate's compulsive Type A strategy was in a depressed, nonstrategic form. It marked Kate's loss of self-relevance and relevance to other people; very little motivated Kate or had personal meaning for her. Her arousal was dangerously low. Her son was one exception, but she conceptualized herself as bad for him and had accepted that she could not raise him. The professionals on whom she relied approved of this decision (indeed, they had suggested it), but it increased her depression by reducing both the meaningfulness of her life and the external stimulation she received.

A functional formulation

Kate's cutting created an extreme fluctuation in her arousal by counteracting depression with pain. For Kate, the normal process of context-dependent 'fluctuation' was better described as a desperate oscillation between life-threateningly dangerous extremes. That is, dangerous as cutting is, it can function to reverse equally dangerous low arousal, and thus to approximate, in a very crude way, the variation in arousal that is essential to life. The sight of blood in particular had a possibly innate function of generating arousal in both the bleeding person (through imaged memory) and others who see the blood (through integrative empathy) (Godinho *et al.* 2006; Marks 1987). Kate's oscillation between depression and delusions, leading to cutting, may have served an essential intrapersonal, biophysiological function as well as an interpersonal, care-eliciting function.

In addition, however, cutting had a macrosystem function in that it gave Kate access to professional caregivers in institutional settings. These, of course, had been her secure base since infancy. Being physically cared for in stable circumstances by people with no personal interest in her and who required nothing from her fit Kate's expectations very well. Cutting achieved this. It gave Kate contact with the class of people who represented comfort for her and made safety available to her.

Given these three hypothesized functions of cutting, it is unlikely that Kate would stop unless the functions of regulating arousal and engaging with other people were fulfilled in some other way.

Kate's delusions can be interpreted functionally as well. They (and not she herself) told her to do what authorities told her not to do. That is, she needed to defy the 'orders' of powerful people in order not to slip from depression toward catatonia and death (i.e., increasingly low arousal). But she was an A4 and could not willfully defy orders. So someone more powerful must give orders that overrode those of the professionals. It would help if the source of her orders could never be challenged. Indeed, it would be even better if the source could facilitate her having contact with other people, especially the professionals whom she trusted and felt comfortable with. Transformation of her thoughts into delusions, which were erroneously attributed by Kate to a source outside herself, accomplished all of this. Like most people with delusions, Kate had a history of traumatic experiences that could elicit delusional associations (Üçok and Bikmaz 2007). In the delusion process, the perceptual DR of her child faded from view to be replaced by her fear-induced representation.

Kate's idea of being poisonous was consistent with her strategy in the sense that the self was perceived as bad and was blamed for all negative outcomes. Further, her decision to give her son up for adoption came from her fear that her threat to her child might escalate. Given that Kate could not regulate affect safely, this was both a realistic concern and a dreadful sacrifice, one that could only deepen her depression, reduce her motivation, and reduce her access to essential incoming affective stimuli. Thus, her behavior that was aimed at 'doing the right thing' for her son also might have reduced her ability to manage herself.

To summarize, Kate's processing of incoming information reached only preconscious levels before it instigated behavioral responses. That is, she perceived danger in images and sequences and, because her past experiences of danger were truly self- and life-threatening, her fears shaped her DR of her child in ways that did not closely resemble the boy. The combination of recalled experience and feelings with her now transformed DR of her son catapulted her into a self-protective response. All this occurred before she could consider the situation consciously or verbally. Moreover, at the preconscious level, she had erroneous information, but because it was not made verbal, she could not examine and correct it. In other words, her 'start-point' information derailed her information processing such that her outcome behavior was unrelated to conditions that other people could perceive.

These points are important because the behavioral treatment she had received focused on stopping the outcome behavior (cutting, poisonous baths, etc.) and the cognitive-behavioral treatment focused on semantic generalizations regarding behavioral rules. Both of these interventions are aimed at endpoints in information processing. It might be necessary, for parents like Kate, for treatment to focus the intervention on the sequence that leads to perception of danger – because once that perception occurs, it may be nearly impossible to stop the self-protective process. That is, a focus on outcomes and consequences may miss the point at which the process goes awry.

Parental behavior

Many adults who have delusions faced frequent, severe, and unpredictable childhood threats, leading the child to associate some ordinary conditions with threat. For example, being alone or going out alone are normal and usually safe conditions, spilling or soiling are ordinary, not knowing what will happen next occurs frequently without dangerous consequences, etc. For adults who have been abandoned, had numerous placements in care, been punished for drawing attention to themselves, or been left uncertain that basic life needs would be met, these ordinary conditions may instigate extreme self-protective behavior. That is, there was once actual threat, but the adult has not discriminated between threatening and non-threatening aspects of the past situation; all are responded to as if they were threatening. Moreover, because the threat is identified preconsciously, the rationale for behavior cannot easily be discovered by, nor communicated adequately to, others, thus making it difficult to correct.

John was convicted and imprisoned for physical child abuse. In his AAI, he tells the facts of his childhood and adult behavior in considerable detail and to the best of his understanding. The DMM discourse analysis opens a second level of understanding. The interview began as usual with a question about his childhood family:

What? Will I start now?
Yeah ... wherever you like.
Erm ... I was born in ... in 1961 ... erm I don't know much about that, erm, we lived in ... a kind of ... I don't, it wasn't a B&B or nothing like that, it was just a fuckin' boarding house ... and ... like, the old man, he got a house after a few years living in this place ... and I went to nursery, and I done

a runner on my first day. I done a runner back home from my first, on my first day, and I didn't like it. I fuckin' hated it in fact.
How old were you then?
I was about 5 or something like that … I can't remember much about my childhood, but what I do remember was total shit, all the beatings, all the shoutings … [John tells an event] And … I don't know if it's I can't remember or if it's all fuckin' blanked out, but it wasn't a happy childhood, to be truthful.

John began by seeking clarification or possibly permission to speak. Is he compulsive compliant (A4?). Then he used *fuckin'*, which is completely forbidden (taboo) in a formal interview with a professional. He used it an incredible 217 times in his AAI. He referred to his father in a derogatory manner – and did so throughout. As he did here, John showed a pattern of repeated phrases. Most have been removed here; they functioned to lower his arousal. Because he used professional language, i.e., 'blanked it out', to explain himself, we wonder to what extent he will rely on others for his understanding of himself. If it is almost entirely, we might consider him to have an externally assembled self (A8). Finally, he nominalizes the acts of beating and shouting, thus making them less arousing, more distant. All of this suggests Type A in spite of John's being very aroused and angry; i.e., we'd usually expect Type C for such anger.

In the next section, John said his mother also *did a runner* because *of all the beatings she used to get and what the old man was doing to me and my sister.* This is important not only for the physical abuse, but even more because something unstated happens to both him *and* his sister. Then he idealized his grandmother in a contradictory manner: *she was fuckin' totally brilliant.* Because we learn that he hardly ever saw her, we treat this as delusional idealization (A7) constructed out of John's need for a comforting figure.

When he is 11, John is sent to boarding school: *'Cos the old man was working shifts. I went to school with various bruises all over my body, and I was telling the school that I'd fell over … knowing that I was lying … knowing that I was lying to protect him.* He protects his abusive father because he is John's only attachment figure. The repetitive speech, this time with variation, functions to wind John up at a moment when, otherwise he might have felt vulnerable: *He, he used to beat me with a belt … he used to beat me with the buckle … he used to fuckin' punch me … and I totally hated him for it. On some occasions, I wished he was dead.*

John recalled an incident: *I got into a fight, I went in crying … I said, 'Dad, I've been into a fight.' He fuckin' shouted at me … for going in crying. He says, 'Right, get outside and fuckin' give him a good hiding. Otherwise don't come into the house no more 'cos I'll fuckin' kill ya. Then I'll kill his old man … for letting his son beat you up.' Then I had to go outside and literally beat this kid up … bashed his head off the pavement … I literally bashed his head off the pavement because ... all the fear I was feeling about going back home to him. I was more scared of him than I was of anybody else, and that's the way I've always been even until now.*

John's pattern of discourse was short, declarative sentences with prominent active verbs and speech that moved the plot forward. The use of the present tense suggests unresolved trauma, as does his continuing fear of his deceased father.

Asked about his relationship with his father, John said, *He was a total bastard! I can give you a billion fuckin' words about him! I feel as though he hated me ... he wasn't protecting me ... he used to beat up on me ... and he deprived me of things ... He deprived me of a fuckin' childhood.* John's anger was palpable, but not directed at the interviewer. Over the course of the interview, we will need to decide whether or not this is a coercive, very threatening use of a Type C strategy or something else.

John described going to bed as a child:

I was frightened. In one way I was glad to be in bed 'cos I wasn't around him ... and yet I was frightened of being in bed because I knew I had no run-away place ... 'cos he used to come up and fuckin' bring his belt up to me and batter me. Nearly every night ... I wasn't safe ... I wasn't ... I don't think I felt safe ... being around him 'cos I knew what was coming every single time ... I mean like, if I was downstairs, I was able to run out the front door or something like that. My escape route was, if he was gonna come upstairs, was to jump out the fuckin' window, but I never even done that ... I just had to lie there and cower in the bed and just watch him fuckin' punching me ... and watch him fuckin' ... erm, raise his belt to me.
You used to watch him punch you?
Well I just ... I had no choice but to let him do it, just cower there, just like a little fuckin' ... just like a little ... I don't know.

John claimed he was physically abused, but the intense image of cowering and watching fits sexual abuse better. The location of the event in bed fits sexual abuse better than physical beatings. The pauses (...) suggest other phrases that were not said. The interviewer suggested that he was 'just very frightened' ... and John echoed it: *Just very frightened indeed yeah, I hated him ... And I wished, on some occasions, I could have killed him ... and wished, on other occasions, he was fuckin' dead ... and other occasions, I just wished he'd go out and never come back ... 'cos every time he went out, I knew what was coming. When he came back, he beat up on me, and yet he wouldn't do like that to my sister ... he wouldn't do things like that to my sister ...*

Though the whole AAI, John echoed the interviewer's words and conclusions, suggesting the source of his understanding might be professionals, not himself.

The difference between himself and his sister is repeated and is important:

No ... as far as I know, he never even shouted at her or nothing ... and then when I was 15 ... I seen why he wasn't hitting her ... I seen why he wasn't shouting at her ... she was getting punished in other ways, I think ... I seen him sexually abuse her when I was 15 ...

Here are the first clearly erroneous conclusions: (a) if you are sexually abused, then you aren't physically abused, and (b) both kinds of abuse are punishments.

He was on top of her ... [angrily] He even had the fuckin' cheek to say 'What's wrong?' 'You know, you, what's fuckin' wrong, I just seen you, bastard!' ... and you know what he done? He tried to put his arms around me... I said, 'Fuck off, I don't want it!'

John told the exchange as dialogue, thus emphasizing its living quality. Then he said his father put his arms around him. This sounds both comforting and also potentially sexual, but not aggressive. Why would the father do this if he had never done so before? Moreover, it is told as if it were a familiar act that his father might think he wanted, not a shocking act. The evidence that John might have been sexually abused is increasing. Then:

I run with my sister behind me, and I told her to get the fuck away from me 'cos I felt she was letting him down ... she was fully clothed and that, but yet he was still on top of her. He was rubbing on her ... [sob] ... he was rubbing on her... like a bastard ... as though he was having sex with her ... and yet they were fully clothed ... but yet he was still rubbing on her ... and I took it out on her ... I shouted at her for letting him do it.

We now have two bits of the act: rubbing and hugging. These two images are very powerful – as if John had experienced them himself. John had repeatedly described his (absent) grandmother as holding him. Did he like comfort? (Don't we all?)

John made two more errors: (c) she was letting *him* down and (d) his sister was responsible for letting her father rub on her. These are erroneous conclusions, but more than that, his speech suggests concern with both their clothed state and their shared involvement. The repetitions indicate that he can't get past the image, but its meaning to him is unclear. Was John possibly jealous? Was he upset because he wasn't special anymore? Then he wondered now whether this was the first or the last time, suggesting he had known, but possibly not seen, before.

Then he said: *I wish I was dead.* This and his sobbing simply make no sense unless he was both a victim of sexual abuse and also felt guilty about it. Had his private pleasure been exposed? The interviewer tried to change topic, but John couldn't. He continued, saying that he asked his father why he did it and got no answer, and that he then left home and began abusing alcohol.

Discussing being hurt, John asserted that everyone (peers, teachers) was scared of him; aggression seemed to buffer his underlying fear, but it also left him isolated and in danger. In this situation, he turned to professionals: *Social workers ... nowadays they are crawling out of the fuckin' woodwork ... but back then I don't think there was enough of them.* This is more evidence that John treats professionals as his protectors and his source of information (A8). For example, he explained that when he was aggressive to boys, *I seen the old man ... I seen all the times that the old man beated up on me ... and seen this lad ... as the old man.* John said this frequently such that it sounded rehearsed, like a formula explanation, possibly given to him by a well-meaning professional, but not something that was marked in the discourse as meaningful to John. He frequently commented on his behavior and motives; we must decide whether he generated these reflective insights or 'borrowed' them from therapists and whether we think they are accurate. In any case, they demonstrate an analytical stance with regard to himself; that is, he sided with professionals in thinking about himself as an object to be described and explained.

Instead, his discussion of hitting his wife because she threatened to leave him is filled with the changes in arousal (dropping), misplaced tenses (present), and self-protective reversals of meaning that he might be expected to feel for a traumatic event.

Whenever I shouted at her or threatened to leave her ... she says, 'You're not leaving me, you bastard!' I said, 'I am, watch me' ... so she'd throw me up the wall, slam my fuckin' head off the wall. Then when I hit her the first time ... then I stopped ... then I stopped. I threatened to kill her ... on many occasions. I threatened to kill other people.

In spite of his glib explanations, John seems puzzled about his own behavior. Did she really throw him against the wall? Or did *she* threaten to abandon him and he threw her against the wall? Did his fear of abandonment transform his self-representation from victim to aggressor, as his father had taught him? Indeed, he was unable to continue responding to the interviewer after he said that he had received the divorce papers. This suggests that *she* divorced him.

Although he never admits to sexual abuse by his father, he does admit to abuse by a female teacher: *she come in and kissed me good night ... then she slid her hands down the blankets and touched me ... it only happened once ...* When he started this discussion, he said she came in (to his room), but he ended by saying, *I never stayed in her accommodation again ... in the housemaster's accommodation, but other pupils did.* Now we understand that he went to her: he sought comfort, but cannot admit to himself that he did. But still he did not admit to sexual contact with his father.

For loss, John said: *Yeah, I lost my sister ... Through me throwing her away ...*

There are two errors of thought here: (e) his sister isn't dead and (f), he takes all the responsibility, leaving none to her or their father. This makes him feel less powerless, but is inaccurate.

Asked about how he raises his children, John first said he wants to protect his children as his father did not (a reversal strategy), then: *Well, I thought I was disciplining them so I'd hit them ... I'd hit them ... I'd bend them over across the settee, I'd hold them down and I'd hit them with a belt, I'd hit them with a slipper, I'd hit them with my hand ... And I'd sometimes ... knock them flying ... by hitting them with my hand. I wouldn't just hit them across the legs, I'd hit them across the face as well ... knock them sprawling across room. It never stopped until I got locked up ... that's when it did stop ... 'cos they got taken away.. five of them got taken away.*

Now we see a possible effect of the erroneous attribution that physical abuse protects one from sexual abuse enacted. John might physically punish his children in a superstitious effort to protect them from sexual abuse. When asked whether he understood that what he did was wrong, he switched to borrowed legal/moral terms, speaking of 'assaulting' them and referring to himself as an 'abuser'. The language is completely different from that when he told the story spontaneously (above.) It suggests that John has accepted the professionals' explanation of what he did. After the AAI (and possibly in response to it), John chose to continue his treatment, which was entirely voluntary, and to deal with the issues of sexual abuse.

A particularly poignant section occurred around his father's death when he said:

You know what I hated most about him dying? I never got no answers to my questions. The interviewer assumed this was about abuse of his sister, but John said: *'Why did he abuse me as well ... why did you have to do it? Why did you fuckin' treat us in the way you did? Why did you beat up on me? Why did you send me to school with different bruises? Why couldn't you be a loving father?'* John combined himself with his sister, spoke directly to his deceased father (you), and ended with his desire for comfort. We conclude that they both were sexually abused and that John (a) is intensely confused about aggression, affection, power, and vulnerability, and (b) brings this into the present.

John then said that he no longer hurts people even though he hears voices telling him to do it: *I sometimes hear voices* (angry whisper) *'Hit him … Hit him … He fuckin' deserves it, you bastard. Hit him' … and you know what? These same voices tell me to harm myself as well … and I listen to them … and I do it.*

Asked if he wanted to add anything more, John said:

I just want the anger to stop … and the voices to fuckin' stop and the … thinking to stop. I just want some sort of medication to help me to stop … just a quick fix if you like … and I feel as though I'm not getting the help … I don't think I'm getting the fuckin' help. I've been fuckin' … been asking for help for years … Jail doesn't work from me.. Jail does not work for fuckin' me! I am trying to do it differently, but the anger is still there, the resentments are still there, fuckin' the hate.. and the hurt are still there. It spills up from childhood. I'm a 41-year-old fuckin' man now, for Christ sake, why am I still feeling things like this? Why do I still feel that I need to hurt people as well?

John cuts himself. He is confused about what happened, who is to blame, and why it happened. He doesn't know how he feels. If John were sexually abused and if he both welcomed the comfort that all children need and also dreaded the sexuality of his father's needs, then we could understand (a) his reaction to his sister, (b) his need to focus on aggression (to cover vulnerability) and punishment (to protect from sexual abuse), and (c) his belief that he is solely responsible (because he wanted it and, therefore, must be punished – by cutting or suicide). To change his behavior, John must correct his erroneous beliefs. To do this, John must understand himself in his terms, not professionals'.

Functional formulation

When the majority of John's angry, violent speech is removed and all his sad, regretful, vulnerable moments are retained, we can see – and feel – John's need for comfort, his distress at how he found it, his vulnerability, and his lack of understanding at all that has happened. John hides this from both himself and us with violent acts and violent speech that arouse him and protect him from the lows – in which he harms himself. Nevertheless, the 217 intrusions of *fuckin'* inject the taboo of sexualized comfort throughout the AAI, thus representing its prominence in his mind. *Fuckin'* is an unconnected image, however, and until it is connected to himself and his development, it seems unlikely that John will be able to control either it or his superstitious protective strategy of pre-emptive aggression.

To conclude, we note that John is neither deceptive, nor manipulative. He is very angry, but is not using a Type C strategy. Instead he inhibits all the vulnerable affects and defends himself with aggression. But he tells us this directly and with shame. He splits good and bad, attributing the bad to himself. John, in other words, is both angry and violent and also uses a temporally ordered Type A strategy of taking responsibility for his contributions to negative outcomes and also other people's. He uses a compulsive Type A strategy.

We could summarize his strategy as: dp Utr(p)$_{PA}$ (b,p,dpl)$_{CSA}$ (dl&dx)$_{PA/ASA}$ l(p)$_{GM}$ (p,ds)$_F$ A4,6,7$_{GM}$,8 [ina]. This looks complex, but is merely a shorthand way of saying John is (a) partially depressed, with (b) unresolved trauma, in a preoccupied state around his childhood physical abuse; in a blocked, preoccupied and displaced (onto his sister) state regarding his sexual abuse by his father; and in a delusional and disorganized state regarding his sexual abuse in adulthood of his own children, all tied (c) to a compulsive Type A strategy that has elements of compliance, self-reliance, delusional idealization, and external reference, with (d) intrusions of forbidden negative affect, i.e., the sexual abuse and the aggression that is John's attempt to forestall both the sexual abuse and his awareness of needing comfort. Of course, it might be easier just to say that John is 'unresolved' or 'disorganized', but such a condensation (a) loses the unique personal history that lies in the DMM classification and (b) fails to identify the psychological processes that have gone amiss and need correction. Most importantly, it drains the meaning from John's attempts to protect himself.

Once John's motivations and strategy are understood, his father's can be imagined as well. If John can come to see that his father's behavior, like his own, expressed his love and desire to protect his son (albeit in a distorted manner), John might be able both to experience himself as having been loved as a boy (after all, his father didn't 'run') and to live in the future safely – for himself, his wife, and his children. This could finally transform what was tragedy into sadness with hope.

Once we understand John's motivations and strategy, it becomes possible to move from what John did (a legal issue) to how it happened (a psychological issue) to how can we change it (the treatment issue). One might think – as the professionals working with John thought – that John needed to inhibit negative affect. Instead, the DMM analysis suggests that John needs access to desire for comfort and fear and to see his anger, once it is reduced in proportion by the enlargement of the other negative affects, as reasonable, but not necessarily the representation he should act on.

Unlike David, John is both sexually involved with his children and violent to them, the women he loves, his father, other males, and random people. If we compare him to nonviolent sexual abusers, we find several important developmental experiences. Unlike David, John did not have a present mother to idealize; he appropriated his grandmother for this purpose, but he experienced no relationship with her that could enable him to feel some comfort as a child. Consequently, there was nothing real to shape his relationships with adult women. In addition, he was attacked, repeatedly and harshly, by his father. He was probably also sexually abused by his father – and he probably liked the affectionate part of it. His father encouraged him to fight back, and eventually he became a feared bully – thus being excluded from the precocious sexual affection that men like David find. Finally, in an out-of-home placement (where there were no attachment figures), John was bullied by many males and sexually abused by adults and peers alike. The combination of more severe and pervasive threat, less comfort, less access to attachment figures, and more access to strangers has left John with massive psychological errors. These appear as maladaptive behavior that endangers his children, his partner, and himself. A very basic confusion is that if you are strong, you can't be vulnerable. Another is that if you liked the sexual contact in any way, you are responsible for it. Both of these irrational absolutes remove the complexity from very complex experiences.

Picking up on the point made about Kate and the information processing that resulted in cutting, interventions that emphasize social standards (prescriptive semantic generalizations) such as John experienced might be aimed too late in the processing sequence that disposes behavior. There are two costs of such misaimed treatment. First, it won't correct the problem, as noted for Kate. And second, it could make individuals feel worse – because they can't live up to 'borrowed' standards that they accept as desirable. Not knowing why they repeatedly fail to make the standard can only make them feel worse, potentially increasing their comfort-seeking and dangerously maladaptive behavior.

The issue is really whether, for individuals whose dangerous behavior is generated by preconscious processes, a 'top-down' (beginning from the integrative goal) or 'bottom-up' (beginning from preconscious 'releasing' stimuli) intervention is needed. The latter requires the effort to understand the unique distortions that each individual parent generates. It would necessarily be time-consuming and expensive. The question is whether it would be effective – because treatments for parents such as Kate and John are generally ineffective now.

Compared with parents in cluster 3 who distort and substitute affectionate feelings, parents in cluster 5 focus almost exclusively on the bad aspects of themselves and their children. Many display repetitive compulsive behavior that is inexplicable in terms of current conditions. They tend to rocket between extremely low arousal (e.g., depression, excessive sleep or tiredness, and suicidality) and excessively high arousal (e.g., inappropriate sexuality, self-injury, and manic states). Their behavior includes preoccupation with illusory self-protective schema in agitated states and isolating withdrawal in depressed states such that children's basic care may be overlooked. Their inappropriate parental behavior includes neglect of children during depressed states, exposure of the children to bizarre and dangerous behavior and individuals in aroused states, and excessive reliance on others (such as cult members) for authority and directives, including dangerously inappropriate application of rules, e.g., Jonestown. In addition, these parents have a tendency to see their progeny as an extension of self (and, therefore, marred or vulnerable as is the self). As a consequence, the children may experience (a) isolating withdrawal during which their basic needs are not met; (b) humiliation; (c) severe, cruel, and abusive punishment for normal child behavior; and, sometimes, (d) ritualistic cleaning and/or abuse. Mothers, more often than fathers, carry out these very dangerous forms of caretaking (Kelley 1996), and often the actions involve intense religiosity.

In adulthood, parents in this cluster have severe problems with intimate relationships including both isolation from normal social support and inordinate reliance on strangers and organizations. This exposes them to risks of physical intimacy with potentially dangerous people (for example, promiscuous sex) and excessive reliance on delusional people (e.g., religious cults). They are particularly vulnerable to authorities that prophesy dire outcomes and require painful sorts of propitiation because these are consonant with their childhood experience.

The death of Victoria Climbié illustrates many of these problems at their worst. Following her death in the UK, a Crown Inquest was held; the information that follows is drawn from the official report (Laming 2003).

At 8 years of age, Victoria was entrusted by her parents in the Ivory Coast to her great-aunt, who brought her first to France and then to the UK to give her the advantage of a European education. In both countries, she was enrolled in school, but frequently absent because of incontinence and illness. In the UK, she was admitted to hospital and brought to the attention of social services several times. Nevertheless, the medical staff all found her engaging, 'a ray of sunshine' (p. 11), and as having 'the most beautiful smile that lit up a room' (p. 11). Her demeanor and verbal denials of abuse were such that the physical evidence of her injured and wasting body was disregarded; protective services were never instituted. In the words of the great-aunt's boyfriend (with whom Victoria and her great-aunt lived), 'You could beat her and she wouldn't cry ... she could take the beatings and pain like anything' (p. 11).[1]

To protect Victoria from her boyfriend, the great-aunt asked Victoria's childminder to care for her on a permanent basis; this did not occur. In addition, on at least two occasions, her great-aunt reported to child protection that Victoria was being sexually abused by the boyfriend; an investigation was not undertaken. The great-aunt also consulted church authorities several times, saying that Victoria was a 'wicked girl' (p. 28) and 'possessed by an evil spirit' (pp. 42, 45); the boyfriend called her 'Satan' (p. 44).

Out of all of these pleas for help from the great aunt, only the church responded. The pastor offered prayers 'for deliverance from witchcraft, bad luck and everything bad or evil' (p. 46). In the end, Victoria died of organ failure consequent to at least 128 injuries and severe neglect, including sleeping each night enclosed in a black plastic bag containing her urine and feces. Her great-aunt and the boyfriend were convicted of murder.

What were they thinking of?! How could the great-aunt offer to educate Victoria, ask for help, warn of sexual abuse, and seek spiritual guidance, and still participate in criminal abuse and neglect? How could Victoria be so appealing to nonfamily members, including strangers when she was hospitalized, and also be viewed by her family as an incontinent evil spirit who needed isolation and punishment? The photos of Victoria are haunting. The one at the front of the Crown Inquiry Report shows her dressed well, even with matching hair ribbons, and having a huge smile, very bright but unfocused eyes, and her arms stuck stiffly to the sides of her body. Her bright, unseeing eyes are disturbing.

In the words of the report 'some important tell-tale sign has been missed' (p. 11).

The signs of interest are, ironically, already present in the report, but their meaning goes unnoticed. Specifically, the discrepancy between events and Victoria's affect openly amazed many people, but was not considered a warning sign. Even the Inquiry Report itself does not suggest that this little girl, who 'twirled' in the hospital corridors (p. 11), might be suffering at that moment and hiding her true feelings of fear and pain under the guise of false positive affect and intense inhibition.

But how could a little girl, taken from her family, living first in France, then in the UK, be understood as happy, even joyful – especially when in hospital? Why would strangers see happiness whereas her great-aunt and the boyfriend saw a wicked, devil-possessed incontinent monster? Is it possible that Victoria used the extreme compulsive behavior that other maltreated and orphaned children display? That is, was she compulsively compliant with her caregivers (inhibiting even expression of pain) and promiscuously friendly with strangers? Both displays are based on fear as a motivating internal state, fear of abuse in the first case and fear of abandonment in the latter. Under such terrible threats, it may be that only Victoria's body could tell the truth. Was she so scared that she urinated without control? Was she literally 'scared shitless'? Could these two symptoms, incontinence and encopresis, help us to understand both Victoria's inner state and also the disgust and outrage that may have motivated her great-aunt and the boyfriend?

When we try to understand the great-aunt, we are faced with the contrast between her good intentions (educate a poor African relative) and strong religious beliefs, on the one hand, and, on the other hand, heinous abuse of a child. Such splits between semantic beliefs and behavior can be understood psychologically if the great-aunt, too, felt overwhelmingly frightened and had been traumatized. Her extreme religiosity suggests an intense need to do the right thing – as defined by external authority. The boyfriend's behavior fits a recognizable stepparent role in physical and sexual abuse, but we can only surmise what his meaning to the great-aunt might have been.

The pity, in this case, is that no one responded helpfully when the great-aunt sought help from appropriate sources (the childminders, social services and hospitals). Instead, only the church responded – and that response confirmed her highly distorted beliefs. The church's response, both verbally and in carrying out an exorcism, gave guidance and comfort to the great-aunt that could only reify her beliefs while convincing Victoria that she, in fact, deserved the treatment she was receiving at home. The effect of the church, in other words, might have been to reduce the probability that Victoria would complain or reveal what had happened to her. How, indeed, could a 'good girl' confess to such shameful behavior and its necessary and justified consequences? Wouldn't a child who used a Type A strategy seek to hide such shame and also to protect her only protectors? After all, her own parents had given her to the great-aunt.

The extreme religiosity of the great-aunt suggests a feeling of powerlessness in the face of very substantial threat. Was the relationship between the great-aunt and her boyfriend marked by both desperate need on the great-aunt's part and concurrently fear of her protector, the boyfriend? Unfortunately, almost nothing is known about these substitute parents, beyond the evidence of their crimes against Victoria.

A similar case in Blackstock, Canada, throws light on the parents' experience. For 13 years, an aunt, who adopted her deceased sister's two orphaned sons, caged and tethered them, diapering and beating them to control their soiling and disruptively 'unmanageable' behavior. At school, the boys were withdrawn, obedient, and academically accomplished; after school, even into their teens, they returned home to the cage, diapers, and beatings.

As always, understanding the adopting aunt's behavior requires understanding her developmental history. As a child, she had been so severely abused by her father that she sustained permanent physical injuries that caused her physical pain even in adulthood. The abuse continued in her marriage to a man whose anger so frightened her that she engaged in compulsively protective rituals (both truly protective and irrationally protective). In adulthood, she was diagnosed with (a) PTSD (i.e., a psychological disorder of dismissing from awareness some aspects of past threat while excessively retaining other aspects) and (b) chronic physical pain from past injuries (Wente 2004). The role of current pain (a somatically imaged representation of fear and the consequences of infractions) in keeping past threat perceptually present is important as is her daily experience of fear of her husband. The adopting aunt's DR is likely to be one of unresolved trauma within a compulsive compliant Type A strategy. In this case, her own fear of being punished if the boys were bad may have motivated extreme self- and child-protective behavior that endangered her adopted children.

Equally confirming of the rationale offered here is the response of the boys. Once rescued and given psychological treatment, the two adolescent boys were able in court to forgive their adoptive mother (Wente 2004). That suggests that the boys were more responsive to her perspective than to their own, as would be the case if they, too, used compulsively Type A strategies.

Outcomes for children

The outcomes for children of these very serious forms of inadequate parenting consist of more symptoms, more serious symptoms, and often more ambiguous or misleading symptoms (e.g., success in school) than more ordinary physical abuse, neglect, or sexual abuse (Burke 2003; Waterman *et al.* 1993; Young *et al.* 1991). When children cannot make meaning of parents' endangering behavior, they feel confused and very threatened. Children need adequate (for their age and intelligence) explanations for what parents do. That is, they need DRs in each relevant memory system that can enable them to predict, in self-relevant ways, what their attachment figure is likely to do and how that may affect them. Further, when parents define children as flawed, children find it almost impossible to develop a responsible, empathic, and integrated self-representation. It should be noted, however, that when parents' behavior becomes blatantly irrational (especially when other adults clarify that the parent is mentally ill), children are able to define the parent as crazy or mentally ill and to protect themselves psychologically. This, however, is not a full resolution of the problem because it does not address (a) children's lack of safety and comfort, (b) the role reversing quality of asking children to empathize with and forgive inappropriate parental behavior when no one has first understood their perspective, and (c) the void in the construction of self left by parents who cannot organize caregiving behavior around children's signals.

Parents' DRs

It is unfortunate that the child-maltreatment literature is almost exclusively concerned with what parents did and the effects on children, and is often content to think of parents as 'perpetrators' or 'offenders'. The literature on mentally ill adults, on the other hand, sees the same individuals not as parents, but rather as victims of disease conditions. One of the goals of the theory offered in this book is to tie developmental processes together across generations around the issue of protection of self and progeny in a manner that permits us to think productively about such motivation – without having to dehumanize the parents or to construct a different psychology, an abnormal psychology, for them. The outcome could be better coordination between child protection, child psychology, and psychiatry, and adult psychology and psychiatry in which issues of morality and punishment are set aside to allow understanding of the history of needs, experiences, and strategic attempts at solution by both children and their parents.

Parents whose early development was compromised (e.g., Kate and John) may face the problems of both psychological distortions and learned, but now maladaptive organic/somatic functioning (i.e., peripheral nervous system accommodations of both input and output). These implicitly learned accommodations to both very severe neglect and very severe abuse may make adaptation to more normal contexts difficult. Further, even when minimally acceptable adaptation has occurred, the risk of failure to adapt physiologically to change is greater than for most people. Variations that other people could accommodate might exceed the range of possibility for people whose past experience has generated extreme forms of accommodation. For example, Kate, together with her husband, was able to raise her first daughter without needing professional help, even though doing so required that her daughter become a compulsive caregiver to Kate. Later, however, when Kate was left to raise her son alone, she was unable to do so. The gross evidence of this was her bathing her son in bleach to cleanse him, triggering his removal. In addition, however, Kate was unable to regulate her own state of arousal in ways that protected her survival; she flipped from extremely lethargic (depressed) to excessively excited (cutting); i.e., she was unable to regulate basic biological processes in a life-preserving manner. John faced similar issues, albeit in a less extreme manner (his survival was less at risk than Kate's). Both needed outside assistance, not only with conscious problem-solving functions, nor even with bringing implicit procedural and imaged functioning to awareness where it could be regulated consciously, but also with managing biological arousal, i.e., the array of peripheral functions that adapted them to their immediate context. There are areas in the frontal lobes that are devoted to both somatic awareness and affect regulation, as well as integration of memory systems; this facilitates anticipation of what might happen in the near future, i.e., 'mental time travel' (Siegel 1999).

A particular characteristic of the thought patterns (i.e., the psychological functioning) of this cluster of parents is the splitting of contradictory DRs. Splitting, as used here, is a psychological process for simplifying complex information. When a situation or person has complex or contradictory qualities (for example, most people are both loving and also angry, threatening, withdrawn, etc.), the mind can 'split' the qualities into internally consistent components, assigning each to different people or situations. Individuals using a Type A strategy tend to split good and bad, assigning good to the (idealized) other and bad to the (denigrated) self. This smoothes interpersonal negotiations, but does so by distorting semantic information. Individuals using a Type C strategy tend to split within negative affect, displaying either the invulnerable feelings (anger) or the vulnerable ones (fear and desire for comfort) while inhibiting display of the other. This clarifies the disposition to act, but does so on the basis of distorting affective information (in this case, somatic images). Memory systems can also be split such that a person uses information from one memory system and discards or discounts information from another. Individuals using a Type A strategy tend to favor 'cognitive' memory systems, whereas individuals using a Type C strategy tend to favor affective memory systems. Integration is antithetic to splitting; neither Type A nor Type C is associated with integration.

The basis for these distortions appears to be the parents' history of inexplicable and unrelenting exposure to danger, without the advantage of parental protection and comfort. Procedurally, parents respond with both obedience and intense arousal. The parents' images include both unconnected trauma-related images and also intensely arousing images (often tied to sex and pain). Semantically, the parents split good and bad, with some parents assigning the bad to the self (and child) and others assigning it to others (sometimes including the child). Recalled episodes are reduced to traumatic events and near delusional episodes of escape or protection.

It is important to recognize that the conditions that trigger dangerous parental behavior do not include an accurate representation of the child. Instead, that representation is highly distorted and infused with personal, idiosyncratic meaning. Three sorts of distortions seem possible: belief that all children have the triggering condition and thus all warrant the treatment given to the parent's child (i.e., it is normal and proper), belief that the parent transmitted the condition to the child (either genetically or socially/ behaviorally), or belief that the child has some unique aspect that takes on threatening meaning for the parent. This characteristic may be real (but distorted in the parent's mind) or delusional. For example, the child may be marked in a way that the parent associates with threat, such as being red-headed in some cultures. Similarly, the child may be associated with a feared or hated person. Alternately, the eliciting condition may have nothing to do with characteristics of the child, but rather with child's role in the family. For example, the conception of the child may present problems (e.g., rape, stepchild, forced pregnancy). It should be noted that the characteristics and roles are given a threatening meaning by the parent; that is, the child is not abnormal.

The term 'delusion', as used here, refers simply to information that is generated by the mind, but not attributed to that source. To the contrary, it is attributed to some external source. In addition, however, the original source may be external – for example, something one read, something one's mother said, etc. Delusions are, in other words, an error of source memory. The misattribution of source limits the individual's opportunity to consider the validity of the delusional information.

In sum, these parents act with intention, believing they are doing the right thing. Their responses range from irrationally reasoned (for example, on the false premise that physical abuse confers protection from sexual abuse), to reliance on external authority (for example, religious scriptures), to privately accessible instructions that cannot be challenged by others (for example, delusional voices). Long periods between instances of danger tend to reinforce the compulsive rituals whereas intermittent danger confirms the need for the 'protective' measures. That is, because the ritual is irrational, it is performed when nothing bad was going to happen. When nothing bad does happen, the individual erroneously attributes that to the 'protective' ritual. But when occasionally something bad does happen, that reinforces the need for the ritual. Thus, errors are rarely corrected and risk escalates. Needless to say, under conditions of perceived threat (such as a violent spouse who is easily angered by children's childish behavior), integration is nearly impossible; therefore, less fully evaluated DRs regulate behavior.

211

It should be made clear that parents in all the clusters described above love their children and express it in ways that children recognize. Were this not the case, it would be much easier for children to understand and adapt to their parents' endangering behavior. The complexity of parents' DRs is, in other words, a problem for their children.

Notes

1 It is worth keeping in mind that failure to respond to pain with affective arousal is associated with early death (Hendry 1999). Although this finding was based on genetic anomalies, the effect (failure to take self-protective action) is the same in cases like Victoria's where the inhibition of response to pain is almost certainly learned.

Chapter 13

Distortions that substitute deadly delusional information for accurate information misconstruing the child as being the threat

Parents in cluster 6 know what is right and what is wrong, and they know what is dangerous to their children. Yet, still they do the wrong and dangerous thing. They kill their children, knowingly and intentionally. The following is the conclusion of Dr Park Dietz, who gave expert opinion on the state of mind of one woman who systematically drowned her five children. His conclusion probably applies to all or almost all parents who intentionally kill their children.

> I conclude with reasonable medical certainty that Mrs. Yates, at the time of drowning each child, knew that her actions were wrong in the eyes of the law, wrong in the eyes of society, and wrong in the eyes of God. She may nonetheless have believed that the killings were in the best interests of the children and that the ends (saving the children) justified the means (wrongly and illegally killing them). (Dietz 2002: 103)

How can we explain that?

This is a book about knowing. What we know, how we know it, and how we employ that knowledge, especially in cases of conflicting knowledge. Empirical studies indicate that the mind can 'know' in more than one way at one time. The construct of memory systems permits us to define some of these ways, each of which may yield a different representation of how to act. Particular arrays of conflicting DRs might explain Dr Dietz's conclusion.

In information processing terminology, Dr Dietz assessed whether Mrs Andrea Yates' understanding of prescriptive semantic generalizations included knowing that killing one's child is wrong. He determined that she knew this. But that does not mean that Mrs Yates acted on the basis of her prescriptive semantic DR. If she acted on some other disposition, then the second statement could also be true: Mrs Yates could have believed that she was acting protectively. This chapter explores conditions under which incompatible DRs can coexist and how lethal action can be taken intentionally by a parent who (mis)believes that it is protective.

Specifically, it is proposed that mothers' fear regarding their own survival becomes tied to their children in such a way that the mothers believe either that the children jeopardize the mother's survival or that the children are doomed to suffering from which she must protect them. If the discrepancy between self-protective and child-protective (i.e., prescriptive semantic) DRs appears irreconcilable, delusions may resolve the discrepancy. In either case, the mother's beliefs are derived from personal experience, leading to transformations of information that, at the time of the killing, coalesce in a delusional DR. Thus, the probability of killing one's children might depend upon a confluence of DRs indicating immediate threat that could be resolved for both mother and child by killing the child(ren).

Cluster 6: Parents who implicitly believe that their children threaten their own survival (thus sometimes deliberately killing their children)

This chapter is the most speculative in this book. Little research exists and sound research designs are impossible to implement. Nevertheless, it has been proposed that parents who intentionally kill their children differ greatly from parents whose motivation is to protect the child, protect the self, or correct/purify the child (Gelles 1991). The DMM, on the other hand, proposes that all humans use the same biopsychological processes in an attempt to adapt to their circumstances. Other investigators find a social/cultural basis for parental homicide of children (Meyer *et al.* 2001). They propose that mothers sometimes kill their children because they are overstretched by a society that doesn't support motherhood sufficiently. That is, lack of social support, poor coping skills, and low economic status leave some women unable to care for their children. Under these conditions, they sometimes kill their children. Certainly, there is evidence that many mothers who killed their children had experienced recent failed relationships (42 per cent; Meyer *et al.* 2001), separation and divorce (Bianchi and Spain 1996; Nelson 1989), and recent immigration (Meyer *et al.* 2001). More than half had attempted suicide themselves, either earlier or as a part of the murder of their children (Meyer *et al.* 2001). Although these factors surely contribute in many cases, they are too general; the overwhelming number of women in such conditions do not harm their children in any way, nor is every woman who kills her children in such circumstances. Some other explanation is needed.

It should be noted that some parents who kill their children have severe psychiatric diagnoses, including bipolar disorder, borderline personality disorder, psychotic depression, schizophrenia, and/or psychopathy (Howard and Simon 2003), although, of course, the majority of parents with such diagnoses do not murder their children. Framed in DMM terms, the diagnoses suggest that these parents have experienced at least childhood threat, instances of unresolved trauma, and ongoing threat, all with a strategy that fails to protect (i.e., a nonstrategic self-protective strategy). Others, however, are undiagnosed and do not easily fit within current diagnostic systems, but may meet the DMM criteria for nonstrategic self-protective strategies.

It is proposed here that once (a) unique developmental processes have been accounted for and combined with (b) adult experience and (c) the parent's immediate context, parents who kill their children intentionally can be understood in the same way as parents who intend to protect their children and succeed in doing so. That is, the difference may not be in intent to harm, but rather in the parent's false, erroneous, and delusional understanding of what is needed to reduce the danger to themselves and their children. Specifically, conflict between protecting their children and protecting themselves from their children may be crucial to understanding the deadly behavior of cluster 6 parents. Delusional DRs are offered as one way of reconciling incompatible representations.

The common denominator among parents who kill their own children may be their paired beliefs that (a) the children threaten their parents' survival and (b) such severe danger is imminent that death is preferable. In addition, it may be (c) that mothers who kill their children intentionally do not fully differentiate themselves from their children. The basis for these understandings and the action they dispose to appear to be both accurately and erroneously rooted in past and present circumstances. That is, the information that the women use to organize their behavior reflects many transformations of information from truly predictive through omitted-and-distorted, erroneous, falsified, and delusional. Further, these transformations are applied to both the child and the self. In the series of chapters that precede this one, the DR of the child has been seen as being progressively diminished and, by Chapter 12, it was taking on delusional qualities not tied to the child's. Parallel to that, however, the parent's self-representation has been changing in increasingly negative ways.

The crucial conditions that lead to murder are probably as follows:

1 a childhood history of misunderstood age-salient threats leading to an unintegrated self-protective strategy with transformations that include false-positive affect or false cognition or both;
2 exposure to one or more traumatizing events that are unresolved;
3 ongoing threat in adulthood to physical, psychological, or reproductive safety;
4 the absence of protection or safe alternatives in both childhood and adulthood;
5 conditions in adulthood that can be confused with childhood conditions, thus eliciting an inappropriate response.

The actual misunderstandings are proposed to be tied to whether the parent has organized by a Type A or Type C strategy. Mothers using a Type A strategy would be expected to hold high and absolute prescriptive standards that they believe they must meet and also believe that they cannot meet. That is, the self must be or do what the self cannot be or do. Type A gives certainties; failure to meet these absolutes can lead to depression. Mothers using a Type C strategy would be expected to feel that they have been mistreated or rejected unjustly and that this has destroyed their life. That is, the self must have what others refuse to give. Type C generates conflict; failure to get what one needs can lead to drastic measures.

Two high-profile cases will be offered to demonstrate how this might function. Andrea Yates, who drowned her five children in the bathtub, is explored as a probable Type A exemplar and Susan Smith, who drowned her two sons in a lake, exemplifies the Type C process. The process by which the distorted information and representations accrued is considered, as is how the representations might have coalesced to produce homicide.

Crucial to understanding the parents' perception of extreme threat associated with the child is the parents' sense of having no protector for themselves and of being abandoned by people who could have supported them (Milgrom and Beatrice 2003). This perception is usually both accurate in childhood and also exaggerated in that, as adults, the women do have alternatives. Usually, however, there is a basis in reality for the perception of abandonment in adulthood, albeit one that is greatly exaggerated (i.e., distorted in its representation). For example, in the few years before she killed her children, Andrea Yates had been hospitalized several times for psychosis, hallucinations, self-harm, and suicide attempts. It is written in her medical record that having more babies was a very severe threat and that her husband insisted on unregulated conception. It is also written that she was observed practicing ways to kill her children (O'Malley 2004). But no medical or social service personnel acted to protect either the children or Mrs Yates. Might she have concluded that the 'protector-of-last-resort', the medical and child protection systems, had declined to protect her? For Susan Smith, divorce from one man and being dumped by another may have left her feeling unprotected.

Type A

Oscillation between depression and intense negative arousal in a compulsive Type A strategy is exemplified by Andrea Yates.

Mrs Yates methodically drowned her five children, ranging in age from 6 months to 7 years, in the family bathtub. In her words:

So after you drew the bath water, what happened?
I put Paul in.
And how old is Paul?
Paul is 3.

OK, and when you put Paul in the bath water, was he face down or face up?
He was face down.
And he struggled with you?
Yes.
How long do you think that struggle happened?
A couple of minutes.
And you were able to forcibly hold him under the water?
Yes.
By the time you brought him out of the water, had he stopped struggling?
Yes.
There was no more movement?
No
And, after you brought him out of the water, what did you do?
I laid him on the bed.
Face up or face down?
Face up.
Did you cover him?
Yes.
Did you cover his entire body?
Yes.
With what?
A sheet.
OK, so after you put Paul on the bed and covered him. Then what happened?
I put Luke in. (Associated Press, Yates confession 2002)

These words are repeated almost without change four more times as Yates describes killing each of her five children. Although we wish the police officer had asked open-ended questions,[1] e.g, 'Tell me about ...', nevertheless, Yates' speech is still striking for the absence of affect and lack of detail to differentiate the children. The systematic, repetitive procedural quality of her actions is chilling (for the reader), but stated entirely without affect. For Yates, killing her children appears to be a procedure, carried out identically and without feeling on each of her children, who were only differentiated by the amount of struggle that they put up before dying. But even her discussions of their struggling and her overcoming them are without affect:

OK, and after Mary had died, um, what did you do with her body?
I left it in there and called Noah in.
OK, did Noah come immediately?
Yes.
And, when Noah walked in the bathroom, did he see Mary in the tub?
Yes.

What did he say?
He said, 'What happened to Mary?'
And what did you say?
I didn't say anything. I just put him in.
Did he try to run from you?
Yes.
Did he get out of the bathroom or were you able to catch him?
I got him.
Noah is 7, is that correct?
Yes.
Did Noah put up the biggest struggle of all?
Yes.
OK, did he go in the water face down or face up?
He was face down.
Um, when you were struggling with Noah, did you have to, did he try to flip over and come up for air at any time?
Yes.
Did he ever make it out of the water long enough to get a gasp of air or anything?
Yes.
How many times?
A couple times.
But you forced him back down into the water?
Yes.
How long do you think that struggle lasted?
Maybe three minutes.
OK, and after Noah was dead, when you brought him out of the water, was there any sign of life from him?
No.
What did you do with his body?
I left it there.

Again, we are struck by the desiccated, emotionally bleak, and repetitive quality of Yates' speech. Without the police officer's contributions, the story itself would be almost completely missing. For Yates, however, the repetition seems to have a calming, reassuring quality that enables her to tell the story and, possibly, enabled her to carry out the sequence of acts without recoiling in horror. There is no evidence of images, semantic generalizations, or reflection. Instead, there is a deactivating connotative quality to the sparse repetition in Yates' language.

Yates' speech is similar to Donnie's in many ways except that Donnie became highly emotional when talking about family deaths, especially the death of her daughter whereas Yates has no affect around killing all five of her children. This comparison makes clear how much more healthy and normal Donnie is, how much we have to build on with Donnie, and it confirms the recommendation that it was sufficiently safe to return Donnie's children to her with supportive services. This comparison demonstrates the importance of negative affect. Yates' lack of negative affect enabled the killing. That is, negative affect, no matter how unpleasant it is, has a highly protective function. Without negative affect, neither Yates, nor her children – nor anyone – can be safe.

Immediately after killing her children, Yates called the police, telling them to come to her home; she made no effort to defend or protect herself. She also called her husband, telling him that he should come home.

Did you say why?
I said it was time.
Did he ask you what you meant by that?
Yes, I didn't say it well.
What did he say when you said it was time, what did he say?
He asked me what was wrong.
And you, how did you respond to that?
I just said it was time.
OK, what did you tell the first officer that got there?
That, that I had drowned the children.
OK, did you tell him why or, or go into it with him in any way?
No.
What happened when Rusty got there?
He was crying.
OK, you had told me earlier that, that you'd been having these thoughts about hurting your children for up to two years. Is that, is that about right?
Yes.
OK, is there anything that happened two years ago that, that made you, that you believe led you to have these thoughts?
I realized that it was time to be punished.
And what do you need to be punished for?
For not being a good mother.
How did you see drowning your five children as a way to be punished? Did you want the criminal justice system to punish you or did you …?
Yes.

We note that, when asked to explain, Yates attributes an error to herself (*I didn't say it well*). Then, in her only display of feeling, she repeats *'that'* in a dysfluence around drowning the children. She also omits herself when she said it *'was time to be punished'*. Is this a Type A omission of self or a slip where she indicates a desire not to be punished? Or was someone else to be punished, such as Rusty? The phrase *'it was time'* has a preordained, ritualistic quality to it. It carries the tones of a biblical prophecy being fulfilled, but without any accompanying affect. Hellfire and damnation are implied as facts, but without feeling. Yates, in fact, claims that she acted to save her children from hell. The final line suggests that when the mental health treatment system fails, the criminal justice system is the ultimate protector of the severely endangered.

After you drew the bath water, what was your intent? What were you about to do?
Drown the children.
OK. Why were you going to drown your children?
15 SECONDS OF SILENCE
Was it, was it in reference to, or was it because the children had done something?
No.
You were not mad at the children?
No.
OK, um, you had thought of this prior to this day?
Yes.
Um, how long have you been having thoughts about wanting, or not wanting to, but drowning your children?
Probably since I realized I have not been a good mother to them.
What makes you say that?
They weren't developing correctly.

The 15 seconds of silence suggests how difficult Yates' own logic is for her to keep in mind – in the face of contradictory DRs. If this had been a therapeutic dialogue, this is the opening to consider Andrea's conflicting perspectives. We note that she measures herself by how her children are developing. Like all parents who organize using a Type A strategy, doing the right thing is defined by procedures and performance. Her children performed badly, so she was a bad mother, so they all would go to hell and her only hope for them was to save them before they were too bad, i.e., to kill them so they could get to heaven before they earned damnation though her actions. This line of thinking demonstrates a relentless, compassionless logic. Pure, deadly Type A.

Yates later explained to Dr Dietz that she believed she was possessed by the devil.
Because I didn't want them tormented by Satan like I was.
Was Satan tormenting you then?
Yes, I believe so.
In what way?
Just the thoughts. Bad thoughts.
Tell me as much about those thoughts as you can.
There was the thoughts about the TVs, and cameras in the house, and afraid

Satan would ruin my children through himself, and that maybe even that I had some Satan in me. I just felt like he was inside giving me directions.
What directions?
About harming the children. (Dietz 2002: 43–4)

This section contains both the delusional idea of Satan directing her and then his being in her and also her desire to protect her children from Satan/herself. Yates 'splits' herself, assigning the bad to Satan and leaving herself with the 'good' desire to protect her children from her bad self – by killing them. Semantically, the splitting of good and bad is consistent with a Type A strategy. The unusual bit (from a Type A perspective) is that Yates claims something good for herself, but to do it, she must delusionalize her 'bad self' as Satan. The style of speech is flat and factual. Mrs Yates speaks about feelings, but without feeling. Even the delusion is astoundingly flat.

When Yates spoke about thinking (both above and in the next section), she was describing the process of reflection. But no matter how long she thought over what she knew, she could not reconcile her DRs. One must not kill. One must raise good children. She could not raise good children. And, possibly, she dreaded having to bear more children, all stuffed, all day long, in the crowded converted bus. Killing would reduce the population; killing them was wrong. Killing them would result in prison; prison might be safe? Up to this point, we can describe Yates thoughts as unproductive rumination that needed access to negative affect to become productive. Was the only resolution that Yates could think of the generation of a delusion, specifically one that fit her husband's religious beliefs? Did the delusional integration finally enable her to take action?

How did he [Satan] give you directions?
Well, eventually I thought of a way out. To drown them.
And how would that be a way out?
A way out?
How would that be a way out?
For the children?
Yes.
They would go to heaven and be safe up there.
This section is interesting for Yeats' confusion about whose 'way out' it is. It seems like her way out (of her home, marriage, and motherhood), but when the question is repeated, she clarifies that it is a way out for the children. If there are two DRs, one to save herself by killing the children and one to justify killing the children to save them from Satan, this is where, in the dysfluence, it shows.
How would that happen?
After I ... if I kill them, they went up to heaven to be with God and be safe.
And you figured that was a way out of what?

It's not a way out. It's just something I was told to do.
Who told you to do that?
Satan.
Satan told you that would send your children to heaven?
No. To kill them.
How did he tell you that?
He just put the thoughts in my head.
Explain your thinking to me.
Well, I didn't want them ruined, and I was afraid, being around him, they would continue to go downhill. And I thought I should save them before that happened.
Well, did you want to save them? Or did Satan want you to do this?
I wanted to save them.

Two important dysfluencies mark this section. First, Yates began by saying, *After I [killed them]*, but she cuts that phrase off and restarts, *If I kill them …* In changing the conjunction, she treats the children as still alive and her decision and action as being still uncertain. Does she, for a moment, indulge herself in wanting her children? Second, Mrs Yates transforms killing into saving, a complete falsification of meaning with a retention of affectless logic. The thoughts are (delusionally) Satan's, whereas the saving is hers. Miraculously, Yates is able to use the delusion to find some goodness in herself (but still there is no feeling: not distress, not guilt, not even happiness.) Instead, Yates focuses on being 'safe'.

Mrs Yates had been previously diagnosed and treated for recurrent postpartum depression that included a suicide attempt, several psychotic episodes, and more than one occasion of self-mutilation. In spite of medical advice against it and because her husband's religious beliefs required it, she continued to have babies at approximately 18-month intervals (O'Malley 2004). Her husband's beliefs also required home schooling of the children such that she was never free of them. Professionals who visited the home had reported that the converted bus in which the family of seven lived was filthy, the children were out of control, and Andrea sat glazed and depressed, often unable to even get up from her seat. In spite of her chronic depression and expanding family, family photos show all members, including Andrea, with huge, toothy smiles, wide enough to crack one's cheeks.

Since the deaths and her incarceration, Andrea has had additional several psychotic episodes and talked about committing suicide.

Startlingly little is known about Andrea Yates' childhood. She was raised in an intact family, was Catholic, and was an excellent student in school. She earned a college degree in nursing and worked as a nurse until her first child was born (Denno 2003; McLellan 2006). Andrea has had an eating disorder throughout her life. It is clear that in high school Andrea was bulimic and had suicidal thoughts. One of her first experiences of depression followed a failed relationship at age 24 (O'Malley 2004). Other than wondering whether she might have had a strategy of compulsive performance that led to high grades or compulsive caregiving in wanting to help others, we really know nothing that can explain her later behavior. More interesting, perhaps, is that we know hardly anything. Once one begins looking, there is almost always some childhood history available. In Andrea's case, recorded life seems to begin after she met her husband, Rusty.

Thereafter, the situation deteriorated rapidly. Because her husband's unusual religious beliefs called for it, children were born in quick succession, and Rusty and Andrea became highly involved in a very small, cult-like form of fundamentalist Christianity. The family set up housekeeping in a bus, and the children, when they became old enough for school, were taught by Andrea at home. In spite of this intensely close environment, Andrea got out only one afternoon a week when Rusty sent her shopping for the family.

Andrea became symptomatic and was diagnosed with postpartum depression, had hallucinations after the birth of Noah, her first child, and began self-mutilating (O'Malley 2004). Andrea had several hospital admissions, one involving ten days in a catatonic state after trying to knife herself (but leaving only scratches on her neck). After her father's death in March 2001, Andrea self-mutilated again, and she was hospitalized twice that spring.

Mrs Yates initially claimed that her childhood family was normal and without psychiatric problems. The latter point, however, is clearly false. Her brother had been diagnosed with bipolar depression and obsessive-compulsive disorder and her sister, another brother, and father with depression. None of her siblings had been psychiatrically hospitalized. Knowing nothing about her family (either behaviorally or genetically), we cannot speculate on what dangers Yates might have experienced growing up – except the obvious ones of lack of response to herself, lack of feelings, and the sense of doom and threat of loss that always accompany the experiential component of severe depression, and all of which are indicators of severe depression (Beck and Gable 2005; Clark *et al.* 1983). In addition, there were drinking problems in both Rusty's and Andrea's families (O'Malley 2004).

Parents' DRs

Yates' discourse is exceptional in its limited representational qualities. She has access to procedural memory, but only in a highly repetitive, schematized form, reminiscent of compulsive, erroneously (superstitiously) protective rituals. She has access to prescriptive semantic memory that carries the tones of religious directives. Her logic is inexorable, flawed, and, without recognition of the flaw, irreversible. She splits good and evil and ultimately protects her 'self' (as a psychological quality) and protects her life (as lived with her husband in a bus defined by enclosure, unrelenting reproduction, and obedience to him and his religious beliefs) by delusionally killing her children to save them from evil and to protect them by sending them to God. We note that only performance matters and that Andrea relies solely upon herself, not seeking help even when she feels most terrible and ruminates on killing her children. These characteristics seem like indicators of an A4 and A6 strategy so exaggerated that the strategy is applied universally and without exception. Any strategy that is applied universally and without exception must be applied maladaptively.

Yates' God, however, appears to be demanding, merciless, and vengeful – all without any feelings that could temper the threat. How could she have come to accept such a God and let her understanding of him define her life and destroy that of her children? Again, we know almost nothing of her childhood family life except that everyone was depressed.

There is, of course, no evidence of integration because there is no affect to create the discrepancy that is essential to initiating integrative processes. To make another comparision, John's anger (*fuckin'*) is a life-saving grace (possibly even literally); anger still makes John uncomfortable – and that gives his therapist something to work with. As with Donnie, anger is useful; it is crucial information. Yates lacks all feeling and that is indeed deadly.

The elements of ritualistic procedures, false positive affect, omitted negative affect, semantic obligation to obey, semantic religiosity, calming connotative language, and nonintegrative belief in the futility of action appear to have coalesced in a delusional DR that enabled a parent to believe that she is evil incarnate and that, to save the souls of her children, she must kill them before she harmed them further. *'It was the seventh deadly sin. My children weren't righteous. They stumbled because I was evil. The way I was raising them, they could never be saved. They were doomed to perish in the fires of hell.'*

Functionally, however, the deaths served to free her from both her existing children and the possibility of having to bear future children (under these conditions). Indeed, the murders would take her away from the man whose religiosity had made her life like hell. Possibly, she might even have thought of the outcome as punishing him. A delusion that can accomplish all these things, while meeting the requirements of all her other DRs, including the inhibition of anger, reflects a highly integrative, highly sophisticated delusion indeed.

What a shame that Yates found no way to access negative affect directly so that she could use its power to keep all seven people in her family safe. What a shame that the medical treatments offered medication to assist her to re-establish the inhibition (that broke out in the psychotic episodes) and confirmed her sense that there was no meaning in her madness. In her case, psychiatric services seemed unable to act either for her safety or her children's. Instead, her prohibition against expression, or even acknowledgment, of negative affect forced protection of self and protection of progeny into such conflict that Andrea's short-term, self-protective action defeated the ultimate function of protecting her genetic future.

Type C

Susan Smith illustrates the opposite pattern of finding oneself to be the harmed person, seeing everything through one's own eyes, and using deception to protect the self – at the expense of her children.

> In 1994, Susan Smith fastened her two preschool-aged boys into the car and let it roll down a slope into a lake where the boys drowned. Ms Smith then called the police, telling them the boys had been kidnapped by a black man and, for 9 days, Susan and her estranged husband gave tearful interviews to the media while the police searched for the supposed kidnapper. Eventually, Ms Smith broke down and told the police where to find the sunken car. Ms Smith was convicted of murder. (Smith 1995)

The elaborate deception and ongoing claims of herself being misused by the legal system suggest strongly that Susan Smith used a Type C strategy (probably C5-6) combined with depression and unresolved trauma and loss.

To understand her behavior, we must know about her context, both at that time and developmentally. The current context was straightforward: Ms Smith was depressed, was estranged from the boys' father, and had received a letter from her current boyfriend breaking off their relationship, in part because he didn't want to raise another man's children (Meyer *et al.* 2001). These are unfortunate and understandably upsetting conditions, but they hardly account for the murder of two children.

Her childhood experience (Rekers 1996) provides a grisly backdrop whose tones and themes may have strongly affected how Susan perceived and attributed meaning to her circumstances in adulthood.

> Susan grew up in a troubled home with an alcoholic father and probable domestic violence. When she was 6 years old, Susan's father committed suicide three weeks after divorcing her mother with infidelity being the central issue. Not only that, he did so by shooting himself between the legs and dying of abdominal injuries. Her mother's remarriage only two weeks after her father's death suggests that her father might have been correct in his assessment of the situation, albeit his response was ill-conceived. At that time, Susan stated that she wanted to go to heaven to be with her 'daddy'. Later she said, *'Daddy could not possibly have loved me or he would not have killed himself.'* Later Susan's adolescent half-brother attempted suicide, as did Susan herself several times, the first time when she was only 10 years old. The crucial issues here are how Susan understood her father's death and how well she was assisted to cope with it. Her mother's rapid remarriage suggests there may have been little comfort or help from her. Without recursive attempts to understand her father's suicide as she matured, Susan (like

all children whose parents die when they are children) is unlikely to have resolved the loss. Unresolved loss and trauma can affect behavior far into the future in harmful ways.

Susan's stepfather admitted to sexually abusing Susan in a relationship from when she was 15 until shortly before the deaths of her sons. Susan herself was known for sexually precocious and promiscuous activity and was chosen as the 'Friendliest Female' at Union High School when she was 17 years old. During their marriage, both she and her husband David traded accusations of adultery, with David later admitting to having had affairs while legally married (Smith 1995).

The issues of seduction, revenge, deception, and sexuality stand out starkly against a background of failed protection. In a desperate and deceptive bid to be protected by a man, Ms Smith may have sacrificed her children to win back her husband or retain her lover.

The following is an annotation, using DMM discourse analysis, of Susan Smith's handwritten confession released by the police on November 22 1994, almost a month after the murder. To understand it, we must keep in mind that Susan's self-interest at that time would have been about conviction and sentencing, not about protecting her sons' lives.

When I left my home on Tuesday, Oct. 25, I was very emotionally distraught. I didn't want to live anymore! I felt like things could never get any worse. When I left home, I was going to ride around a little while and then go to my mom's.

Ms. Smith's episode began as if it were going to be a factual account of what happened, but that is set aside almost immediately for a digression on her feeling state, with a focus on negative affect. A peculiar aspect of her self-focus is the absence of the children in the car. Instead, Susan focuses on danger to herself and her innocent intention to go see her mom.

As I rode and rode and rode, I felt even more anxiety coming upon me about not wanting to live. I felt I couldn't be a good mom anymore, but I didn't want my children to grow up without a mom. I felt I had to end our lives to protect us from any grief or harm.

Ms Smith returned to the episode with repetition of 'rode' that both forestalled the conclusion and built suspense. Then she digressed immediately to her feeling state again. Anxiety, not herself, was the actor. Indeed, Ms Smith was more like a victim of 'anxiety' than a murderer. Again, the focus was on self at risk. She had reached an impasse that made murder of children good *for them*; note the reversal of attributed meaning (i.e., false cognition) here – their murder was good *for her*, as she experienced it. She framed killing as *protection* from grief. To understand this, we must remember that she experienced grief at her father's suicide when she was 6 years old. This, possibly, was what she must protect her sons from. In this context, she claimed the role of benevolent actor/agent. We note the false cognition of accepting responsibility for a good act, one that would save her children from harm. Throughout this section she remains in the digression about her own feeling state.

I had never felt so lonely and so sad in my entire life. I was in love with someone very much, but he didn't love me and never would. I had a very difficult time accepting that. But I had hurt him very much, and I could see why he could never love me.

The self's negative feelings were prominent again. Ms Smith focused on her feeling state and futility (a depression marker). What did she do? There was no evidence of her contribution; she cut that part of the episode off. Moreover, she omitted mentioning that her boyfriend did not want to raise her children, thus misleading others about her true motives (false cognition). Because she had said that her father couldn't love her and kill himself, it might be worth knowing whether she imagined that she had contributed to his death. She was only 6; her conclusions might have been irrational and uncorrected.

When I was at John D. Long Lake, I had never felt so scared and unsure as I did then. I wanted to end my life so bad and was in my car ready to go down that ramp into the water, and I did go part way, but I stopped. I went again and stopped. I then got out of the car and stood by the car a nervous wreck.

Ms Smith returned to the episode of killing her children – but her children were not in the episode! It was all about her. She digressed to discussing her psychological state again. She was wrought with distress. Then she returned to the episode. She built suspense by the connotative way that she told the story, bringing us into the moment. Slow steps in the plot increased the drama (connotative language). She ended a paragraph focused on her negative feelings, with the action suspended.

Why was I feeling this way? Why was everything so bad in my life? I had no answers to these questions. I dropped to the lowest point when I allowed my children to go down that ramp into the water without me.

Now, with questions, Ms Smith involved listeners in explaining her behavior; i.e., she was collusive around apparent integration. She continued the digression to focus on herself as a victim of bad feelings and events (indicative of depression). She went back to the episode; her contribution (agency) was only 'allowing', not doing. The children were the agents who went down the ramp! She focused on her being left behind! (and not on their deaths or her agency). Further, she spoke as if they had deserted her! (Did her father's death echo here?) Parental suicide is very powerful; its effects may even reach into unborn generations (Cain 2006).

I took off running and screaming 'Oh God! Oh God, no! What have I done? Why did you let this happen?'

Now Ms Smith held God responsible for not stopping what she did. Note how she twisted religion to free herself of responsibility. She again digressed from the episode of her children's death to her own emotional and mental state.

I wanted to turn around so bad and go back, but I knew it was too late. I was an absolute mental case! I couldn't believe what I had done.

She claimed good intentions that could not be fulfilled, as if to say, 'Poor me! I was overcome.' After the fact, she took responsibility for doing it, but in telling the episode itself, she omitted her act. Nor did she, at this point, even say what she did. She also omitted her children dying.

I love my children with all my (a picture of a heart). That will never change. I have prayed to them for forgiveness and hope that they will find it in their (a picture of a heart) to forgive me. I never meant to hurt them!! I am sorry for what has happened and I know that I need some help.

This is childishly disarming – as if she were 6. She focused on what the children can do for her! Ah, intentions! Self-focus again: *she* needed help.

I don't think I will ever be able to forgive myself for what I have done. My children, Michael and Alex, are with our Heavenly Father now, and I know that they will never be hurt again. As a mom, that means more than words could ever say.

Ms Smith again focused on her own distress. They are with 'family'. They are safe. Note, again, the transformation of their deaths to a good, safe outcome (i.e., a false cognition). It is as if she wants us to conclude that she was a good mom and should be content about her children. (Again, the focus is on herself and her relief at not needing to worry about her children.)

I knew from day one, the truth would prevail, but I was so scared I didn't know what to do. It was very tough emotionally to sit and watch my family hurt like they did.

Ms Smith used a contradicting conjunction ('but') to shift to her negative feelings that counter the certain cognitive prediction. Then she told us that their pain hurt *her*, which implies a (false cognitive) justification for her action. But which family was she speaking of? It only makes sense if it is her childhood family. Did Susan lose track of time?

It was time to bring a peace of mind to everyone including myself. My children deserve to have the best, and now they will.

She said that she had to end her distress, a focus on her perspective and motivations again. She twisted her role from that of killer to savior of her children!

I broke down on Thursday, Nov. 3, and told Sheriff Howard Wells the truth. It wasn't easy, but after the truth was out, I felt like the world was lifted off my shoulders. I know now that it is going to be a tough and long road ahead of me.

She made no mention of her dead children. Again, her focus was on herself. The false cognitive implication was that she will (unjustly and as a victim) pay the price for their peace.

At this very moment, I don't feel I will be able to handle what's coming, but I have prayed to God that he give me the strength to survive each day and to face those times and situations in my life that will be extremely painful.

Ms Smith returned to the basic issue of safety and survival again of herself with no mention of the children She focused on the cost to herself and her negative feelings.

I have put my total faith in God, and he will take care of me.

She appealed to an authority higher than any of us (thus, taking power from human legal systems), suggesting that they, like God, should find her innocent. There was no reference to her own responsibility.

[Signed] Susan V. Smith
[Dated] 11/3/94 5:05 p.m.
The confession was signed by an FBI agent and a State Law Enforcement Division agent (Smith 1994)

The reasons that Susan killed her sons and at other times tried to kill herself are difficult to understand, especially if one looks only at the present. Certainly, her explanations make little sense and are contradictory. These explanations, however, are drawn from semantic memory, and several are given after the murders. For example, after the killing, Susan stated that she was a bad mother and that she did not want to leave her children behind in case she killed herself.

Because representations always combine the present state of the self (especially the safety of the self) with aspects of the past, they cannot fully reflect the state of mind at the time of the killing. For Susan, there are probably at least two past points in time that influenced her behavior: the period around her father's death and the death of her boys. Her own and her brother's suicide attempts may also have influenced her state of mind. Further, Susan's DRs are vulnerable to all the biases of semantic memory, including especially the desire of the self not to be convicted of murder or sentenced to death.

Parents' DRs

The discourse analysis, combined with her family history, strongly suggests that Susan used a C5-6 strategy of sexual seduction and false cognition, combined with unresolved trauma and loss tied to her father, brother, and stepfather, all in a context of depression. It should be made clear that the deception is both self-deception and deception of others, but that it was carried out with awareness of the values (of religion) and prejudices (against black men) of her audience. Inclusion of these functioned to make her false story appear more credible than the evidence would support. The function is self-serving. Killing her boys removes an impediment to remarriage. It almost appears, however, that Susan does not really care whether it is her lover or her ex-husband who accepts her as long as a man accepts and protects her – as her father did not.

The Yates and Smith cases differ from those in cluster 5 in that they are not predicated upon a semantic parenting strategy that was systematically implemented over a long period of time. To the contrary, the dangerous behavior of cluster 6 parents is unique to one or a few specific occasions in which some aspect of short-term, immediate protection overwhelms long-term, ultimate goals. Moreover, these parents know they are doing the wrong thing. Depending upon their underlying strategic organization, they try to deceive others about it (Type C) or willingly submit to punishment (Type A).

The risk of such behavior is continuously present in the sense that parents in cluster 6 have ongoing distortions of thought, feeling, and behavior, but they do not have a steadily implemented rationale for their actions. In addition, all appear to have been exposed to self-threatening danger as children and other dangers in adulthood. However, at the moment of killing, they act on some immediate and unpredictable threat, albeit self-perceived, that triggers their fatal behavior. Knowing the nature of that threat could help to protect both parents and their children.

Possibly, for Andrea Yates, the danger increased as her youngest child approached six months of age – the time when she should soon become pregnant with the next child.

For Susan Smith, it appears to have required rejection by both her husband and her boyfriend, as well as designation by the boyfriend, of the children as the impediment to their relationship. Without that, Susan might have chosen some other action to express her fear of abandonment, such as an attack upon the boyfriend or suicide.

Like Victoria Climbié's death, the deaths of Yates' children are partly attributable to professionals' failure to act so as to protect the children. Yates had been known to both child protection and mental health authorities, had been hospitalized, had attempted suicide, and had been seen carrying a knife and filling a bathtub, both of which everyone considered indicative of her intending to murder her children. Professionals have noted in the record that the children were in grave danger (Deitz 2002). Nevertheless, the children were not removed. Moreover, Yates was not prevented from killing them.

Preventing Susan Smith's action is a bit more difficult. Nevertheless, someone should have looked in on the family after the father's suicide, especially given the gruesome way in which it was carried out. When her mother remarried quickly, it became even clearer that the children would not be adequately cared for by their remaining parent. A professional needed to be there. Finally, Susan's precocious and excessively sexual behavior was a signal that her development was not progressing well. Indeed, it seems that her mother was aware of the sexual abuse by her husband and failed to protect her daughter over a period of several years. Once she left school and married, it was too late. Unless she sought help, none would find her. Then it was left to chance how the unresolved traumas and losses would affect her life and the lives of her family.

In neither of these cases, however, does there appear to be a single factor operating in isolation that explains the fateful actions of a single moment. Instead, it appears that the risk slowly accumulated, without being predestined, across decades until the psychological distortions came together in a moment of dreadful misattributions and purposeful action.

Understanding parents who intentionally kill their children

Mothers who intentionally kill their children perceive themselves to be psychologically abandoned by all possible supportive people. For example, in cases of infanticide, the mother almost always experienced the pain and fear of childbirth completely alone (Crittenden and Craig 1990). Their DRs, in other words, represent their desperation and hopelessness (Milgrom and Beatrice 2003). Both Yates and Smith were deluded about the reasons for their own behavior. Susan Smith was actively deceptive about her actions, whereas Andrea Yates needed delusions to be able to act.

Strangely, parental mental illness is rarely included as a form of maltreatment of children. Indeed, it is often considered an explanation or extenuating circumstance that excuses the parent from charges of child maltreatment. More startling, the professionals who treat adults rarely express more than passing interest in the welfare of their patients' children. Nor do child therapists routinely consider seriously enough the probability of disorder in the parents (Chronis et al. 2003; Schultz and Shaw 2003).

Nevertheless, children of parents with behavioral or psychiatric disorder must cope with an environment in which the parents' dispositional state is highly variable, often misleading or inscrutable, and crucial to the children's physical and psychological safety. Understanding how such parents organize their parental behavior could be very helpful in offering preventive, supportive, and ameliorative treatment to the children.

Meyer et al. (2001: 93) conclude, 'Ultimately, the "mad versus bad" dichotomy fails to accurately classify these mothers because it does not take into account the varying contextual, legal, and psychological factors which contributed to their emotional states and decision to kill their children.' In this chapter, we explored notions of self- and child protection and the distorted DRs that might underlie choosing to kill one's child.

When there isn't time for moral/legal deliberation, biology talks. Biology 'wants' genetic survival. The mother's reproductive potential must be balanced against that of her children. If she is young and healthy, she can have more children. If the children are very young, many things might happen before they could reproduce.

Note

1 It is interesting to speculate on what information we would have if the police officer had been trained to ask open-ended questions and to probe each of the memory systems in a systematic and ordered way. Instead we see an efficient, Type A approach to getting factual information for a profession that is organized around facts and consequences.

Part 3

An Integrative Approach to Treatment

Chapter 14

Why do we need a new theory of treatment?

There is already a plethora of theories about treatment of distressed people and ways to change deviant or maladaptive behavior. Why do we need another?

Indeed, why do we need a theory at all? Why not just collect the best practices or the evidence-based treatments and use them? Empirically, I could argue that our evidence base is woefully inadequate, but that sidesteps the question. Why theory? Because, without it, one can't organize one's thinking. By organizing thinking about treatment, I mean having an understanding of what is to be treated, why it needs treatment, what successful treatment would look like, and how one might get from distress and danger to comfort and safety.

Not having such a theory is a bit like having a therapist using an A8, externally assembled, strategy. It would seem inconsistent for a therapist to work toward coherence within the patient or client while lacking coherence about the process. Theory gives therapists a road map on which the point of departure and desired destination are defined, and, with the tools to be described in the coming chapters on assessment, functional formulation, and memory systems, a route can be mapped. Of course, there might be more than one possible route. Theories are not straitjackets. Theory, in fact, should clarify one's choices, not impose them upon the therapist. Moreover, to push the map metaphor a bit further, one might discover that one had mistaken the departure point or preferred a new destination. With a good theory, one can adjust the path. Without a theory, one risks wandering off track and wasting effort or arriving at an intermediate way station that feels good or shows competence gained, and mistakenly decide that the job is done. Theory points the way and defines the work to be accomplished.

Moreover, there are three primary reasons for needing a *comprehensive* theory of treatment, both for psychological treatment in general and specifically for treatment of inadequate parenting:

1 *Paradigm change*. The paradigms used to conceptualize maladaptive behavior have changed, with substantial implications for how society

treats troubled people, including parents who are deemed to raise their children in harmful or dangerous ways.

2 *Effectiveness*. All current treatment approaches are less effective than we would like to admit and, in some cases, they may be harmful.

3 *Breadth*. All current theories appear to omit some important characteristic of a sound and comprehensive theory, and thus none offers a complete theoretical guide to treatment.

Changes in paradigm

If we look back to earlier approaches to deviant or dangerous behavior, we see that each reflects, for its time, the state of knowledge regarding what causes disorder and what heals it. Successful treatment of *physical* illness required an understanding of what caused the disease. Unfortunately, mental health treatment is almost where medicine was at the end of the nineteenth century; i.e., we lack an equivalent to the medical theories of infectious disease, autoimmune disorder, genetic anomalies, etc. That is, we have no psychological equivalent to medical pathology (diagnosis), etiology (cause), and pathogenesis (process). Instead, we operate on the basis of cultural belief systems. To the extent that these are accurate or effective, we want to include them in a comprehensive theory. In addition, however, we can find in them the roots of some of the conflicts among, inconsistencies within, and limitations of our current approaches. Below, I introduce three major historical traditions for thinking about psychological disorder, each of which has implications for current practice.

Moral/religious tradition

The moral/religious tradition reflected the belief that 'craziness' was tied to good and evil. Depending upon one's beliefs, this suggested that evil and goodness were innate and immutable, that the affected one had in some way offended the gods or spirits, who required propitiation, or that judicious use of moral instruction or punishment would change unacceptable behavior. In this tradition, individuals were held responsible for their behavior, even if it was believed to be innate and immutable. Three points are worth noting:

1 Under this tradition, moral and religious figures, e.g., priests, shamans, healers, had authority over psychological disorder.

2 When the disorders could not be changed quickly and were dangerous to the individual or the community, the individual with the disorder was removed and protected or removed and punished. The point is that safety (or perceived safety) was a central issue in determining what to do.

3 Treatment consisted of a set of specifiable components:

a *Changing arousal,* either by lowering it, as in placing individuals in asylums to reduce stress, or heightening it, as through exorcisms, dances, etc. In the DMM, we would call this affect-based treatment.

b *Rituals,* i.e., carrying out protective routines, such as absolutions and chants. In the DMM, we would call this treatment based on cognitive procedures.

c *Personal and social connection,* i.e., the healer formed a unique and personal relationship with the troubled individual, one in which the latter was able to trust the healer enough to unburden or reveal him- or herself and to undertake change. Sometimes this occurred in the context of active community support. In the DMM, we could consider the healer a transitional attachment figure, i.e., someone wise and strong with a personal interest in the troubled individual's welfare who could function to protect and comfort the individual when the threats were great and guide the person through a change process to reduce the number of threats that cannot be managed.

The medical/psychiatric tradition

More recent thinking treats 'craziness' as a disease, i.e., mental illness. However, unlike physical disease, maladaptive or unacceptable behavior neither has a known cause that can be corrected nor responds well to medical treatment. Moreover, it is currently impossible to predict from specific symptoms which disorder is likely to develop. Unlike the moral approach, in theory the medicalization of maladaptive behavior holds no one responsible; one is simply ill and in need of treatment. Practice, however, is a bit different. Disorders that involve self-harm, e.g., depression and suicide, borderline personality disorder, and self-cutting, are generally treated within the mental health treatment system, whereas those that harm others, e.g., child abuse and neglect, criminal behavior, are diverted to the legal system, i.e., the secularization of the moral authority. Either way, when there is danger, removal from society to protect someone becomes a crucial component of society's response.

The medical tradition emphasizes factors that cause conditions or cause them to change. Because the causes of mental illness are largely unknown, the focus of the medical approach has been on what causes change. This, in turn, has drawn attention to symptoms and away from the relationships with either the psychotherapist or the family and community.

Most current theories of treatment address symptom reduction. Those that do not, e.g., psychoanalytic theory, have even more difficulty in specifying what should change, how it can be changed, and whether it has changed after treatment. In large part, the recent empirical science of treatment, i.e., evidence-based treatment, is dependent upon the behavioral specificity of symptoms and, as a consequence, tends to favor theories in the behavioral tradition. But as the next section will show, the evidence that behavioral treatments are effective in treating disorder is uncomfortably slim.

On the other hand, pharmacological treatments have effectively reduced the display of symptoms, together with the distress and suffering associated with mental illness, but they, too, rarely cure the dysfunction and do not prevent its occurrence once the drug is discontinued. Ironically, many patients prefer not to continue to take the drugs that are deemed effective by professionals. Among seriously disturbed bipolar and psychotic patients, 30–40 per cent of patients do not adhere to their prescribed medication (Ascher-Svanum *et al.* 2006; Sajatovic *et al.* 2006; Valenstein *et al.* 2006). This is similar to patient compliance with medical regimens for both migraine (50 per cent compliance at one year; Aubé 2002) and major challenges to physical health such as transplant surgery and acute asthma attacks (Cochrane *et al.* 2000; Corden *et al.* 1997; Haynes *et al.* 2000).

An important new contribution within the medical tradition is in the area of genetic and neurological contributions to disorder (cf. Tsankova *et al.* 2007). These, together with experiential factors (Rutter 2007), will be crucial to charting the epigenetic process that yields maladaptive behavior, including harmful parental behavior. Nevertheless, fully understanding the complex interactions of genes and developmental experience that influence psychological dysfunction is still in the future. Knowing how to apply this information to distressed individuals is more distant yet.

Crucial aspects of treatment in the medical approach are as follows:

1 The psychotherapist is more nearly a technician with a scientific basis than a healer (with a basis in faith).
2 The means of change are more clearly specified and change itself is more accurately assessed.
3 The individual seeking or needing help is more isolated from the family and support network than in religious/moral approaches, partly because the disorder is defined as an intrapersonal disorder and partly as a result of issues of confidentiality.
4 Removal from society, either for respite or punishment, is reduced, and drug treatment is correspondingly increased.

Educational approach

The newest 'tradition' is to think of behavior as being learned. When current behavior is maladaptive, so this line of thinking goes, people generally lack information or skills (Kazdin 2005). These, of course, can be taught. Using this approach, assessment identifies the missing skills or erroneous knowledge, and treatment supplies what is needed as directly and efficiently as possible under the notion that if people had the right information and skills, they would do the right things. This approach undergirds current social work practice and primary prevention. Not surprisingly, this approach has not been applied widely to serious psychological disorder (although it is a part of an arsenal of approaches applied to the personality disorders; cf. Bateman and Fonagy 2001; Karterud and Urnes 2004; Karterud and Wilberg 2007). Instead, it tends to be used primarily for prevention of parenting problems (i.e., parent education) as well as correction of them in children with conduct disorders and when parents come to child protection attention.

Other approaches

Although these are the three primary approaches to psychopathology and rehabilitation, there have been and are other approaches. Indeed, the majority of nonpsychiatrist therapists (as well as many psychiatrists) would not subscribe to any of the traditions listed above, much as they might feel pushed to accept either a medical or educational approach. For example, family systems theory does not medicalize the diagnostic process (Bateson 1972/1987). Similarly, 'holistic' approaches try to move away from a medical approach (Cassileth 1998). Psychoanalytic analysts and therapists follow yet another approach with echoes of both the personal guide in the religious/moral tradition and, in its origins if not its current status, a tie to the medical world of neurology. Nevertheless, none of the alternatives has (a) unified psychotherapists, (b) explained from a scientific basis the development of dysfunction, (c) generated a systematic way of thinking about or assessing maladaptation, or (d) explicated treatment in a compelling way, i.e., a way that compelled the field to follow that tradition. Consequently, none fits the notion of a paradigm at this point.

Strikingly, none of these theories is developmental. If conditions experienced in childhood affect the probability and nature of psychological disorder, we may need to consider carefully the contribution of children's development and parents' development to children's adaptation in order to successfully prevent and treat disorder. Viewed in terms of Tinbergen's four levels of explanation, this is the second (Tinbergen 1951). Nor, however, do any of the theories reflect Tinbergen's other questions:

1 Why is the behavior shown now?
2 How did we develop to react that way?
3 What is the general function of the behavior?
4 What is the phylogenetic history of the behavior?

Compared with these questions, it appears that current thinking pays insufficient attention to the development of human behavior either in an evolved sense or in terms of personal development. Indeed, there is even less concern with proximal *causes* than with proximal *means* to inhibit or change the behavior. The difference is between not needing the behavior (removing the proximal causes) and getting rid of the behavior. The question is whether the latter is sufficient.

Good therapists come from all the traditions, and, over time, many of the best therapists, regardless of their training, tend to become eclectic – borrowing ideas from any line of thinking that can help a distressed person. Indeed, as the array of named treatments enlarges, the unifying characteristic is that many therapies combine two or more forms of treatment, e.g., cognitive analytic (Ryle and Kerr 2002), suggesting the implicit understanding of a need for an integrative approach. One of the goals of Part 3 of this volume is to gather and integrate these ideas into the beginnings of a coherent, developmental, and systemic theory of treatment.

Treatment efficacy

The data

In spite of these traditions and a century of scientific work on maladaptive behavior, the empirical findings indicate that we do not know how to treat psychological and interpersonal problems predictably and effectively. One-third of cases of psychological disorder do not respond to any known treatment (in general: Bradley *et al.* 2005, Eysenck 1952; Glick *et al.* 2006; Matthias 2005; parenting treatment: Kazdin and Wassell 1998; Luthar *et al.* 2007), and in almost half of successfully treated cases, symptoms reappear within one year (in general: Fonagy *et al.* 2002; Roberts and Everly 2006; Watanabe *et al.* 2007; Young *et al.* 2003). For parenting treatment, Kazdin (2005) points out that follow-up is unusual, and periods longer than six months are even more unusual; i.e., we don't know. Moreover, 30–40 per cent of parents (Kazdin and Wassel 1998) and 70 per cent of offenders (Thomas-Peter 2006) withdraw from offered treatment because they find it unsuitable to their problems or ways of working. On the other hand, 50 per cent of cases spontaneously improve (Rutter and Rutter 1993), leaving approximately 15 per cent that respond well to treatment in the short term.

That means treatment makes a 15 per cent difference over nontreatment – in the short term (Hubble *et al.* 1999). Moreover, studies indicate that no treatment or theory of treatment is more effective than any other (cognitive-behavioral therapy: Weersing and Weisz 2002; treatment of criminal offenders: Crighton and Towl 2007; parenting treatment: Chambers *et al.* 2004) and most treatments outside cognitive-behavioral treatment eschew the data-based rigor needed to provide evidence and replicable evidence (Fonagy *et al.* 2005). That is, in spite of there being more than 550 published treatments for children alone (Kazdin 2000) and three decades of efficacy research covering more than 1,500 studies (Weersing and Weisz 2002), we don't have evidence that treatment works, that short-term effects are maintained, that effects are replicable, that treatment works under real-life conditions and with samples of real-life children and families, or that positive effects are clinically relevant outside the treatment setting. However, it is clear that treatment has positive effects, but for which individuals and under what conditions is not known.

To the contrary, recently emerging findings suggest that treatment can be detrimental (Lohr *et al.* 2006; Stroebe *et al.* 2005), with rates of 10–20 per cent of patients being in worse condition after treatment (Davidson 2004; Lambert and Ogles 2004; Lilienfeld 2007). If ancillary effects, such as divorce, were considered, the rate of harmful outcomes might be even higher. Occasionally, however, as many as 40 per cent of those treated experienced negative consequences. In the studies published, these were for preventive treatments in which the individuals who received preventive treatment displayed higher rates of disorder than individuals not having the 'advantage' of the prevention treatment (e.g., grief counseling: Fortner 2000; PTSD: Kenardy 2000).

It is puzzling that very few studies of treatment efficacy assess detrimental effects. When drug therapies are used, assessment and reporting of such effects are mandatory, but can lead to the studies not being published if they have been supported by the manufacturing drug company. Given that negative effects sometimes exist and that some therapies (and some therapists) are patently dangerous to some people (Lilienfeld 2007), it seems ethically imperative that we follow the dictum of physical medicine: *primum non nocere* ('first, do no harm'). That means assessing negative outcomes in all our treatment studies.

Viewed together, it appears that the beneficial and harmful effects of treatment are potentially about the same. We must be doing something wrong.

Either our methods don't work or we use them poorly:

1 delivering them to the wrong people; i.e., our diagnostic groupings may cluster dissimilar individuals with different needs;
2 delivering them at inopportune times; i.e., times like the school years when the probability of effective change is low compared with other periods;
3 delivering an inappropriate 'dose'; i.e., either too much or too little.

Psychotherapy

More alarming is the state of psychotherapy. There are four major problems:

1 the need for replicability and its effect on psychotherapists, therapies, and people who enter therapy;
2 a general lack of gatekeeping regarding who may become a psychotherapist;
3 the increasing 'branding' of treatment;
4 the impatience of funding sources.

Although each of these is addressed separately, in fact they reflect different facets of the same problem. That is, in the absence of substantiating efficacy data, the search for effective 'evidence-based treatments' has intensified. The effect of adapting treatment to good scientific designs has had some potentially deleterious effects on treatment, psychotherapists, and individuals receiving treatment.

First, to the extent that psychotherapy is an interpersonal process, therapists, as people who have chosen to help other people, have been overlooked. As the focus on techniques and replicable measurement of change has increased, the opportunity for therapists to form unique personal relationships with the people they help has decreased. Instead, many treatments are structured so that any properly trained therapist can deliver the treatment to any group of patients in a manner that is almost undifferentiable from one therapist to another. That is, the therapist becomes a bit like a mental-health technician.

For patients, the 'manualization' of treatment to achieve empirical replicability probably perpetuates what brought them to treatment in the first place: the inability of important people to perceive and respond sensitively to their unique characteristics. Instead, such treatment may augment the tendency of some patients to feel shaped and defined by the viewpoints of others (both parents in the past and professionals now). Seeing oneself as an object within a technical process would seem to be the opposite of the usual goals of treatment, which almost always include some form of 'self-actualization' (Goldstein 1934/1995; Maslow 1954/1987, 1969, 1943/2006). Put another way, manualized treatment could feel like a Procrustean bed to parents who had to squeeze or stretch themselves to fit the topics and pacing of the manual. Cast in the light of traditions, current evidenced-based psychotherapy may be at risk of losing the quality that made treatment in the moral/religious tradition successful: the human connection between a wise and caring person and a suffering person.

Second, there is no adequate gatekeeping process to ensure that those who will offer psychotherapy have personal characteristics that will promote their being helpful (and reduce the probability of their being harmful). Instead, there seems to be an assumption that a trainee therapist who demonstrates knowledge of a particular theoretical model and competence in applying the techniques suggested by that model will be an effective practitioner, and, with a specified period of supervised psychotherapy, is ready to be licenced to provide psychotherapy.

There may, however, be personal characteristics that affect one's suitability as a psychotherapist (Shaunburg *et al.* 2005). It is, of course, more difficult to assess this than to pass courses, but if it is important to the well-being of those who need therapy, it should be addressed. Given the high rate of trauma and disorder among therapists (Elliott and Guy 1993; Pope and Feldman-Summer 1992; Pope and Tabachnick 1994; Radeke 1998), therapists' history and personal characteristics may not be irrelevant to treatment success (Black *et al.* 2005; Ronnestad and Skovholt 2003). Participating in one's own process of change has traditionally been a part of the selection of healers; the 'calling' of ministers, pastors, and priests; and the personal analysis of psychoanalysts. It is rarely a part of the training of nonanalytic psychotherapists now, particularly not for those whose work is the most empirical, e.g., those using the behavioral and cognitive/behavioral models. For treatment around parenting, it might even be relevant for the therapist to have experience as a parent. Instead, increasing numbers of therapists, including those dealing with parenting issues, have neither a partner, spouse, nor children (Bae *et al.* 2003), suggesting, ironically, a return to the religious/moral tradition of the guide being outside the system (Miller 1987).

Third, psychotherapists are trained in particular disciplines and 'brands' of therapy and apply their brand to all their patients. Instead, we may need to understand how each treatment affects a range of patients, and either have therapists with broad training or use precise assessments that can match particular patients to specialized therapists.

Fourth, mental-health treatment changes in a fad-like manner as one set of ideas fails and new ones are generated, usually by charismatic figures and usually accompanied by a new set of buzzwords. Often this is the result of the politicization of the funding of services such that when treatment fails to achieve the short-term goals of an administration, it is trashed and replaced by another short-term, highly publicized 'fix'. Moreover, thinking about mental-health treatment is often strongly influenced by advocacy groups, such that a political agenda regarding 'victims' of particular disorders or conditions often influences where research monies are funneled and what hypotheses can be studied (that is, political correctness is often dominant over scientific accuracy or public need as defined by prevalence and severity.)

Emerging approaches

The most useful growing edge of treatment-applicable knowledge is the cognitive neurosciences. We are beginning to understand how brain functioning is tied to behavior. To the extent that emerging theory, assessment, and practice build on the cognitive neurosciences, there is both a theoretical basis for treatment and a basis for scientific tests of treatment efficacy for particular subgroups of people. That is, as we gain understanding of differences in brain functioning between troubled people and better adapted people, we begin to have a basis for asking:

1 how that difference came to be (genes(G)? experiences(E)? some interaction of these, i.e., G × E?);
2 what actions in the present can change that (medication? if so, which? – psychotherapy? if so, which?);
3 which effective treatments maintain the change in the long-term (medication? Or must it be taken continually to maintain the effect? – psychotherapy? or must the individual re-enter therapy periodically?).

Whatever the answers, the crucial advance is our ability to tie both early conditions and treatment to differences in neurological functioning.

A risk, however, in our current approaches to neurobiology and genetics is that we may overlook universal processes that have been refined epigenetically across our experience as a species. Instead of focusing on these as they interact with each person's life experience, more attention is being paid to finding the exceptions. For example, we are more interested in seeking chemical imbalance and the gene that accounts for it than in understanding how the human genome and the biochemistry that it generates interact with the near infinite variety of human experience to produce an infinite number of unique humans. The effects of universal processes on unique developmental pathways deserve more attention than the hunt for many needles in the haystack.

Uncertainties, puzzles, and inconsistencies

There are many points of inconsistency or conflict among theories of treatment that could be discussed. Three seem most relevant to demonstrating that a new approach to a theory of treatment is needed.

First, our current medical and symptom-based diagnoses (i.e., DSM-IV (1994); ICD-10 (1993)) neither fit individuals well, nor suggest treatments. That is, many patients have multiple, often overlapping, diagnoses (Kendell and Jablensky 2003). Others have different diagnoses at different times or when assessed by different professionals. Still others, whose behavior clearly indicates maladaptation and risk of harm, fit no diagnosis; e.g., most maltreating parents and criminals. Even when a clear diagnosis can be assigned, it is unclear how the therapist should respond. In this way, psychiatric diagnoses are generally different from medical diagnoses, which function to exclude certain treatments such that a narrow range of treatment options remains. Although some diagnoses suggest a bioneurological treatment, the majority of diagnoses cannot be differentiated on more than a roughly mild to severe scale.

Second, it is not always clear whether our interventions are intended to protect, heal, or punish. For example, foster care is explicitly meant to protect children, but (a) it is often implicitly used as a threat to parents (as punishment would be used), and (b) it is known to harm children (Bearup and Palusci 1999; Craig 1995; Leonard 2003). Similarly, it is unclear whether the prison system is meant to protect the public, punish the criminal, or rehabilitate the criminal (UK Home Office 2001; Rafter and Stanley 1999). Lack of clarity about intentions and inconsistency between intentions and actions makes it highly unlikely that the results will be beneficial.

Finally, pharmacological treatments (which are the clearest advance offered by the medicalization of 'mental illness') are disliked to the point of disuse by many patients. On the surface, it seems inexplicable that someone who suffers would refuse the ameliorative treatment. This happens less with physical ailments and, when it occurs, it can be attributed to side effects. It might be important to ask what important 'side effects' there might be with drug therapies that we have overlooked.

What's wrong?

We must be doing something fundamentally wrong. Possibly, the mental-health treatment system does not need tweaking, adjusting, or greasing; possibly, it needs fundamental changes in how its role is conceptualized, how professionals are trained and work, who receives which sorts of services and at which time during the life span, and how treatment is funded.[1] The changes cannot be limited solely to the mental health treatment system, but must reflect a wide range of systemic influences on personal adjustment and family functioning from (a) the cultural and political levels[2] to (b) neighborhoods and schools, (c) services to families, and (d) service providers themselves. Only a broad array of integrative changes can promote improved treatment of depression, anxiety, violence, substance abuse, etc.

What do we need?

In order to address the social, familial, and personal problems resulting from mental-health issues, we need an integrated theory of psychological dysfunction that can provide:

1 a definition of dysfunction that is tied to its cause and course of development;
2 assessments that enable us to discern the crucial aspects of dysfunction;
3 a theoretically meaningful basis upon which to select treatments, together with empirical tests of the efficacy of the treatments;
4 a receptive service system, in terms of both organizational structure and funding and also appropriately prepared staff.

The purpose of Part 3 is not to reinvent the wheel, but rather to sketch a design for a new cart built from tried and true old parts.

DMM comprehensive theory

Viewed functionally, the moral/religious, medical, and educational traditions each have something to offer to current practice. The moral/religious tradition emphasized the importance of both safety and a guide, a person who assists another to change. The medical tradition emphasizes the specifiability of both the symptoms of the disorder and the means of reducing them. The emphasis on learning could become relevant to mental-health treatment if the focus were shifted from content to learning how to use one's developing brain to generate more accurate knowledge and more adaptive DRs.

The DMM of attachment and adaptation (Crittenden 2006) reflects a fourth, more recent, notion: that maladaptive behavior is the result of earlier attempts to protect oneself and one's progeny. This notion has roots going back at least to the 1960s (e.g., Szasz 1960, 1961) and is reflected today in both evolutionary and transactional psychology (Sameroff 2000). It is not meant to indicate a unitary model of mental illness. Rather, if we think in terms of necessary, sufficient, and contributing contributions to maladaptive behavior, protection of self and progeny (together with producing the progeny) is proposed to be necessary but not sufficient. The model of disorder has been described in Part 1. Part 3 presents a framework for organizing these and other ideas about psychological treatment. Below, a few ideas about the nature of a successful theory of treatment are offered.

Theories must 'want' to grow. No person or group of people or people at one time period *can* know it all. A theory, therefore, should be structured to imply, even require, change. This means differentiating between the theory – as a map – and the content, the information that the theory explains at any given moment.

Lenses and levels

Seeing reality is like looking through many lenses, each highlighting some aspect of what is there, but at the expense of distorting or omitting other aspects of reality. The lenses can be thought of as different levels of analysis, each highlighting some aspect of the process of survival, adaptation, and reproduction. These levels span genetic, biochemical, and neurological processes as well as dyadic, familial, community, and cultural/governmental processes, theory functioning both to place them within the array of important factors and to suggest how they might be connected. For example, theory should point to the processes that might explain how maternal neglect leads to changes in phosphorylation in cell proteins and how this might affect proteins around genes and change gene expression. Or, to take another example, helping to relieve the suffering of children writhing with dystonia might require considering processes from basal ganglia (that make the children writhe so that they become emaciated), to dyadic and family processes that soothe or further distress the children, to government policies and administrative regulations that make some treatments possible and others not. Rather than asking one person to hold multiple models in mind at one time and to guess how they fit together, theory should move toward increasingly clear explication of these relations. (What is 'reality'? The sum of what can be seen and understood by a viewer at a given point in time?) Theory should transcend that to encompass all the potential realities – and that implies change.

The biological and social sciences must come together. All people have bodies and the state of their bodies affect how they feel, what they think, and how they behave. These bodies behave, but the behavior is represented in organs, mental functioning, biochemistry, and the genes that shape that chemistry (Hoffmeyer 1995). Nevertheless, feeling, thinking, and behaving are equally affected by the families, communities, and governments that define the range of people's daily lives. Theory should envision how such disparate influences affect a single, unified person – and all other such persons.

The theory need not tell the content of all of that; that is what specialists do. The theory should, however, propose how these bodies of expert knowledge can go together. Theory, in other words, points to the interactive process. It has a place for important information and for changes in the information.

I choose to place attachment in the center of the DMM for two very basic reasons. No human can survive alone (as Winnicott 1957 so obviously said, but became famous for saying it, as did Stern 1985), and the continuation of our species depends upon two humans having sex together. Attachment, it seems to me, is at the center of our being. Without it, we cease to be, both as individuals and as a species. I begin the story of adaptation with sex and the birth of the baby.

Notes

1 When diagnosis-related groups determine funding allocations depending on what the diagnosis is expected to cost, patients who are expected to take longer will be avoided; e.g., a drug addict with a broken leg, elderly patients who forget that their role is getting better, and take longer to discharge to a safe-enough setting.

2 This cuts both ways, however. Politicizing medicine can lead to fad-like rushes to the new 'treatment of the year', followed by dumping the program (after all its costs in training, administration, and products), often before its benefits and deficits can be adequately assessed, when a new administration comes to power. The result can be disruption in service, displacement of personnel, and lost opportunity to use information to improve service.

Chapter 15

Ideas that underlie the dynamic-maturational model as a comprehensive theory of treatment

This chapter offers an overview of the ideas, brought from many theories of treatment, that are consolidated in the DMM. In that spirit, the limitations of the theories are not addressed. In many cases, an idea is so central to psychotherapy that it is found in many theories and reflects a point of convergence among the theories. For the sake of parsimony, each idea will be included only once, usually where it had its first, most elegant, or most complete formulation. Consequently, omission of an idea from a particular theory should not be construed as its absence from the theory. Put another way, the focus here is on gathering a full list of ideas, rather than reviewing each theory fully. The crucial issue is the idea, not its source. We begin with ideas brought from attachment theory.

Ideas that shaped the DMM

Attachment theory

The DMM is an expansion of the Bowlby–Ainsworth theory of attachment. As such, it emphasizes the importance of (1) attachment figures when children or adults feel themselves (2) threatened, especially when the threat is tied to separation from or loss of an attachment figure (Bowlby 1973, 1980). Following Bowlby, it proposes that, when attachment figures regularly do not help to resolve serious threats, there is a risk of psychopathology and criminality (Bowlby 1944a, 1944b, 1973, 1980). Further, Bowlby lays the groundwork for thinking that the manner of the child's (3) adaptation to threat can be both beneficial in an immediate sense and detrimental for the long-term adaptation of the individual. Bowlby describes clinically, and Ainsworth provides empirical evidence, that there are individual differences in how individuals organize psychologically and behaviorally to resolve threats (Ainsworth *et al.* 1978). These individual difference are described as the (4) ABC patterns referred to in Parts 1 and 2 of this volume. Bowlby also emphasized the importance of (5) systemic thinking about relationships (Bowlby 1949, 1979).

In my expansion of attachment theory, I have emphasized the importance of (6) danger in general (Crittenden 1999c) and of a (7) wider array of strategies than Ainsworth found in infancy (Crittenden 1995). I have also highlighted (8) the strategic function of the behavioral patterns of attachment (Crittenden 1985, 1992b), (9) their adaptive utility in dangerous contexts (e.g., compulsive compliance; Crittenden and DiLalla 1988), (10) their association with mental processing of information (Crittenden 1997), especially (11) transformations of cognitive and affective information, and (12) an array of types of representation that become possible only as a function of (13) maturation. In addition, I have included (14) context as important to understanding an individual's perception of danger (Crittenden and Claussen 2000), thus opening attachment theory to other systemic influences on adaptation. Finally, the DMM returns to the understandings of other theorists in finding most behavior meaningful, albeit, not necessarily transparent; in the case of parents who put their children at risk, maladaptive behavior is seen primarily as the result of earlier attempts to protect oneself and one's progeny (Crittenden 2002).

Within these 14 points, there are many that tie to other theories. It is these points of convergence that have transformed the DMM from a variant of the Bowlby–Ainsworth theory into a comprehensive theory that includes, but is not limited to, attachment theory. We turn to the contributions of various theories of treatment to the DMM.

The DMM and psychoanalytic theory

Both Bowlby and Ainsworth were trained in psychoanalytic theory, Bowlby having undergone training as a psychoanalyst. It is therefore appropriate to address its contribution first. Of course, being a major theory, it has several important variants, some of which use psychoanalysis (for an overview, see Anthony 2002; Bateman and Holmes 1995; Budd and Rushbridger 2005) and others psychodynamically informed treatment; e.g., Kleinian theory (Bronstein 2001), self psychology (Kohut 1971, 1976), object-relations theory (Fairbairn 1944, 1952; Mahler *et al.* 1975; Segal 1964, Winnicott 1956), and ego psychology (Kernberg 1972; Yeomans *et al.* 2002). These cannot be treated separately here, but each has a different emphasis, some being more closely related to attachment theory than others. Crucial ideas that the DMM draws from the work of Freud and his followers are as follows:

1 the notion of an inner psychic life;
2 the idea of defense mechanisms, reframed in the DMM as psychological self-protective strategies;
3 dynamic unconscious processes, treated in the DMM (to fit current neurological understanding) as preconscious processes;
4 transformations of information;
5 the importance of affect;
6 the use of the therapeutic relationship to enact and facilitate change in the individual's psychological organization;

249

7 the conceptualization of treatment as involving a substantive process of psychological and behavioral reorganization (as opposed to symptom reduction).

The DMM and learning theory

Learning theory has been the basis of series treatment approaches, including behavioral, cognitive, and cognitive-analytic. These, in turn, have spawned other treatment approaches: rational-emotive treatment (Ellis 1974), reciprocal inhibition (Wolpe 1948, 1958), cognitive-behavioral treatment (Kazdin 2005; Sudak 2006), dialectical behavioral treatment (Linehan 1993; Linehan and Dimeff 2001), constructivist theory (Bruner 1984; Kelly 1955; Maturana and Varela 1980), post-rationalist constructivist theory (Guidano 1991; Guidano and Liotti 1983; Neimeyer and Mahoney 1995), schema therapy (Young *et al.* 2003), etc. At the core of all of them are the basic principles of learning theory regarding (1) the effect of contingencies on behavior (Skinner 1938, 1950, 1953) and, more broadly, (2) the conceptualization of psychological change as a process of learning involving (3) changes in perception, attribution of meaning, and response. Viewed from the perspective of memory systems, these derivatives of learning theory address changing (4) procedural and semantic memory (Beck 1976), as well as procedurally desensitizing individuals to arousing images.

The DMM and family-systems theory (FST)

Like psychoanalytic and learning theory, FST has led to many approaches to treatment, such as structural (Minuchin 1974), strategic (Haley 1973; Weakland *et al.* 1974), transgenerational (Bowen 1994), solution focused (Berg and Miller 1992; Walter and Peller 1992), and narrative therapy (White and Epson 1990). Their cumulative contribution to the DMM is discussed here. Possibly the most crucial contribution, the one that sets FST apart from psychoanalytic and learning theory, is (1) conceptualizing psychological problems as based in interpersonal processes. Tied to that are the notions that (2) the strategies used by family members are interdependent and the identified patient is (3) not the only person within the family who needs to change and also that (4) the most effective and efficient route to change may be through someone other than the identified patient. These point to (5) the inherent interdependency of change processes among people in close relationships with the notion that (6) whenever one troubled person is found, family members are likely also to manifest dysfunction (Jean-Gilles and Crittenden 1990). FST theorists have described differences in family functioning in ways that closely resemble the attachment ABC patterns, but have carried these further clinically by (7) identifying specific patterns with especially unfortunate implications for psychopathology – for example, triangulation (Haley 1976b) and the double bind (Bateson 1972). In addition, FST has taken the notion of patterning quite seriously from short-term patterns enacted over minutes to long-term patterns repeated across generations (Breunlin and Schwartz 1986). Finally, FST has offered (8) systemic formulations of problems (Dallos and Draper 2005), as opposed to psychiatric diagnoses.

The DMM and transactional analysis (TA) psychology

Eric Berne's work provides another starting point for the DMM emphasis on self-protective strategies. Berne's 1964 volume outlining (1) (strategic) games people employ in their interactions with one another (Berne 1964) lacked the evolutionary basis of attachment theory and the DMM, but the notion of strategies was quite clear, long before it was used by Bowlby. The notions of (2) change requiring safety, including interpersonal safety with the therapist, and (3) respectful equality between patient and therapist were also introduced by Berne. From the DMM perspective, a limitation of TA is the reliance on contracts; contracts imply equality and joint understanding of what is being agreed to. Because people coming to therapy are suffering and do not see the path forward with accuracy, they are not in a position to contract in an informed way about it. Indeed, in practice and if the therapy takes off, it is also unlikely that the therapist could fully foresee the process upon which they were embarking together.

From a somewhat different position, transactional psychology has emphasized (4) the blurring of the boundaries between mental illness and mental health. Instead, transactional developmental psychology emphasizes the need to attend to (5) patterns of adaptation and (6) the influence of the social world on individual development rather than on personality traits. That is, current developmental thinking places deviancy in dynamic relation between individuals and their contexts (Sameroff 2000).

The DMM and Eriksonian theory

Although Erikson's work (Erikson 1950) has not led directly to a school of psychotherapy, it has had direct influence on how psychopathology and treatment have been discussed. The crucial issue is the developmental approach taken by Erikson. Unlike any of the approaches discussed above, Erikson considered (1) development from a normative perspective and viewed it (2) from birth moving forwards. None of the theories of treatment does that, preferring instead generally to ignore developmental processes and focus on problems from adults' perspectives and competencies (learning theory and FST) or to speculate on atypical development from the experience of troubled adults (psychoanalytic theory). Erikson identified (3) a series of age/stage-salient issues (around danger, protection and comfort) that need to be resolved at each age or development in the next stage risks going awry. Like FST, Erikson's approach (4) placed the growing child in a social context, but in this case, it included more than the family, thus, anticipating social ecology (see next paragraph). Finally, Erickson pointed to the (5) crucial importance for serious disorder of the 'transition to adulthood' (16–25 years). In sum, Erickson contributed the notions that something different can go wrong at each stage of development and placed the growing child in a social context.

The DMM and social ecology/Vygotskian theory

General systems theory (Davidson 1983; von Bertalanffy 1968) was 'in the air' in the middle of the twentieth century, and it influenced many thinkers, from Bowlby to Bateson and Vygotsky and, through Vygotsky, Bronfenbrenner (1979a, 1979b). Three crucial contributions have affected the DMM, primarily through Vygotsky. One is (1) the notion of development occurring in the ZPD (Rieber and Carlton 1987). For the DMM, this defines the changing role of attachment figures – in the zone of emerging skills of the attached person. Another contribution, this time highlighted by Bronfenbrenner (1979a, 1979b), is (2) the importance of danger in any of the contexts that are important to an individual. Finally, Bronfenbrenner's social ecology theory clarifies Vygotsky's systemic approach to development by defining (3) several interlocking systems from those that directly include the individual (the microsystem, e.g., dyadic and family relationships) to those that do not include the individual but affect him or her indirectly (the exosystem, as in parents and professionals meeting to discuss the child) and the mesosystem that connects various exosystems to those that affect whole classes of people (the macrosystem, as in political structures, culture). In the DMM, these are elaborated to reflect multilayered systemic influences, including (from micro- to macroinfluences) genes/neurology/biochemistry, individual (health, thought, behavior), family (both nuclear and extended; biological and functional), neighborhood (peer group), culture (ethnicity, religion, and government), and, in the case of those seeking treatment, the professional treatment system (gatekeeper, labels, preferred services, quantity of services).

The DMM and Gestalt theory

Gestalt theory (Perls 1961; Perls *et al.* 1951) focuses attention on the effect of one's perspective. Things looked at from a close, but narrow, perspective seem different from the same things viewed from a greater distance and within a context. This idea, that (1) alternative perspectives give different information (Wertheimer 1938, 1959), is central to the way that cognition and affect and the various memory systems are used in the DMM. Gestalt theory makes clear that (2) no single perspective is fully accurate (McDougall 1936) and that (3) the best approximation of truth comes from integrating detailed and holistic perspectives (Lehar 2003). These notions fit the DMM in two ways. First, when assessing humans, a holistic view tends to distort positively (because the generalities are accepted without confirming or disconfirming evidence), whereas a discrete behavioral view tends to distort negatively (because, without a larger, comparative perspective normal human error is magnified and transformed by the viewer into apparent pathology). Second, in terms of treatment itself, work with individuals on specific issues (the narrow, discrete view) can result in unexpected, even unwanted, outcomes at the more general level (marriage, family). Moreover, as any coder of DMM assessments of attachment knows, (4) the sum of the individual bits of information really is, at the level of patterning, different from its components.

The DMM and pharmacological treatment

Since the 1950s, medications have been used to change aspects of brain functioning, particularly arousal. Psychopharmacology has contributed to (1) our understanding of the biochemistry of disorder and (2) one way to regulate or modify it. Concurrently, the difficulties in finding precise chemical substances that help individuals without either overregulating functioning (thus producing too little or too much sensitivity to stimulation and amplitude of response) or generating unwanted side effects have brought attention to (3) the interconnectedness of aspects of functioning (i.e., a systemic idea on a microscale) and (4) the adaptive value of the processes being changed by the drug therapy (e.g., the function of variability in arousal as an adaptation to changes in context becomes clearer when it is chemically regulated to reduce fluctuation).

Although drug treatment might seem in conflict with psychotherapy, in fact, it is merely an alternative means of accomplishing some of the same outcomes. In particular, pharmacological treatment affects (5) regulatory processes that are essential to other aspects of change: if arousal is too high or too low, psychotherapy cannot be effective because the individual cannot maintain attention adequately. Moreover, it is particularly useful in illuminating (6) the universal chemical processes that link genetic potential with behavior. Drug treatment makes very clear the importance of understanding (7) the systemic and interactive quality of both information processing and (8) the essential interconnection of body and mind. Finally, drug treatment raises questions regarding whether it is possible to change brain functioning in an enduring way without maintaining the drug and, if it is, how best to accomplish that. If or when it is not, the issue of integrating drug treatment with psychotherapy becomes crucial.

Conclusions

The ideas in this chapter suggest that the pathways to dangerous psychopathology involve an accumulation of risks, occurring in both independent and interdependent ways, across development. The risks are shaped by both the biological context of maturation and the social context of increasingly inclusive systems, from the family to ethnic, national, religious, and cultural groupings. The connection among these is each individual's information processing to generate self-protective and reproductive strategies.

An important observation to be drawn from this list of ideas from various theories of treatment is that, within each treatment model, fragmentation is taking place as users of the theory seek more effective approaches. The changes often involve borrowing ideas from other models. This could be taken as evidence of existing integrative processes within psychotherapy traditions. After a century of taking apart the grand theories of the turn of the twentieth century, possibly it is time to again seek a unified view of psychopathology. If so, the 'new' theory should account for the contributions of previous theories as well as the evidence generated by the clinicians who used them and the researchers who tested them. My proposal is that we need an integrated theory of psychological dysfunction that can provide:

1 A definition of dysfunction that is tied to its cause and course of development. The role of danger as a proximal cause of dysfunction is crucial, as is a series of age-salient dangers for serious and pervasive dysfunction. Opportunity for comfort and protection, whether from parental attachment figures or auxiliary attachment figures, such as teachers and therapists, is also important in reducing the impact of exposure to danger.

2 Assessments that enable us to discern the crucial aspects of dysfunction. The assessments should assess (a) psychological processes including, in particular, biases toward using affect or cognition to regulate behavior, transformations of information, and the extent to which psychological processing around exposure to danger is conscious and reflective, and (b) behavioral self-protective strategies.

3 A theoretically meaningful basis upon which to select treatments, together with empirical tests of the efficacy of the treatments. This depends upon item 1 and, especially, item 2. Without sound assessment, selecting appropriate treatments to address problems is simply impossible. It is worth noting that the goal of evidence-based treatment is desirable, but not easily attainable in the current research context. The problems include lack of agreement regarding the desirable outcomes of treatment, our limited ability to assess many of these goals, failure to assess negative outcomes, and failure of researchers to submit, and journals to publish, studies of null and negative effects.

4. A receptive service system, in terms of both organizational structure and funding and appropriately prepared staff. Crucial changes that could improve treatment efficacy are reunification of child, adolescent, and adult services and training.

Chapter 16

The dynamic-maturational model as a comprehensive theory of treatment

A new theory of treatment is needed. Why? Because no existing theory is adequate, because none has shown itself to be better than the others, and because each has important gaps that limit its effectiveness. On the other hand, in practice, the approaches often become less discrete than they appear to be. This suggests that there are some basic 'truths' that many theories discover. Further, each theory has something valuable to offer, often something that is seen uniquely or understood most fully through that theory. The task becomes collecting, comparing and synthesizing the strengths of each theory while identifying and, as much as possible, reducing the limitations of the theories. That is, we don't need another theory. We need a comprehensive theory.

Comprehensive theories

Comprehensive theories incorporate and integrate other theories. They seek convergence among theories and identify discrepancies that need focused thought and research. As shown in Part 1 of this book, the DMM is a comprehensive theory regarding developmental differences in adaptation. This chapter develops the notion that the DMM can become a comprehensive theory of treatment within which the many discrete theories of treatment can be integrated.

Up to now, treatment has been guided by therapists' belief structures. Each future therapist chooses a theory of treatment in which to be trained, receives that training, and goes forth to offer what he or she has been taught to the clients or patients who come seeking help. In most cases, this is done without consideration of whether the therapist's preferred theory offers the best solution to the patient's problem. In some ways, it is as if a physician had a set of favored cures and simply proposed to apply them to all patients without regard to differences among the patients and their illnesses. With a comprehensive theory, one would be in a better position to select treatments that fit each patient's need as well as the psychotherapist's skills.

This chapter offers an overview of the ideas brought from many theories that are consolidated in the DMM. However, trying to write this exposes immediately the difference between DMM ideas and more static and definable approaches to treatment. The DMM ideas about process and bidirectional interaction can't be forced into a static written shape without losing a good portion of their meaning. It's a bit like trying to specify what makes a human by dissecting one, spreading the organs out on a table for all to see, then labeling the parts, with directions on how they fit together. The thing on the table was a human, but it isn't now. It's naked, but no longer sexy. The life has disappeared from the whole and the directions are insufficient to recreate it. Gestalt practitioners would know what this means! Writing forces a linear logic and discrete form on a living process. Affect and the unpredictability that lies at the base of affect risk being squeezed out by the specification of principles and processes. Affect, told cognitively, loses its essence. Nevertheless, something must be said if anything is to change. Therefore, limitations in hand, a short overview is offered, together with examples from the cases in this volume. It should be said clearly that the proposed causal connections are hypothesized and lack evidence suitable to attributing causation. That is, a set of hypotheses is being proposed, not validated, in the examples.

The crucial elements of the DMM regarding treatment of dysfunction

In this age of evidence-based treatment, it seems essential that we consider the basis for a good theory of treatment. The criteria should be both relevant and inclusive; that is, they should not have a self-serving function of defining only one approach as adequate.

Criteria for a good theory

Five criteria are proposed as essential to any theory of treatment, with a sixth as desirable.

1 The theory must be *scientific*; that is, it must honor the existing knowledge base and continue to change as the knowledge base changes.
2 The theory must be *empirical* in the sense that its propositions and hypotheses are testable.
3 It must be *developmental* in outlining the process by which a neonate becomes a well or poorly adapted adult.
4 The theory must be *interpersonal and transactional*; that is, it must treat humans as developing in the context of other humans and as both being influenced by and influencing their context.
5 The theory must be *systemic* such that it reflects the dynamic complexity of a nested hierarchy of systems, from genes to individuals to the

contexts in which individuals live, that communicate both vertically and laterally.

6 As much as possible, the theory should be *parsimonious*; that is, it should offer the least complex explanation that meets criteria 1–5.

The problem to be addressed by treatment

Because they are the focus of this book, I refer primarily to parents and their problems, but the ideas are not limited to parents.

Definition

The starting point is defining what needs treatment. The DMM comprehensive theory focuses on *dysfunction*, as opposed to disease or disorder. Disease requires a pathogen – and we have none. Disorders are based on symptoms, but these are often interchangeable within an individual and used to fulfill different functions by different individuals. Consequently, symptoms are too imprecise to guide treatment (Wilkinson 2003).

Instead, dysfunction is the crucial point: treatment is needed when parents' behavior does not function adequately to protect or comfort themselves and their children, or to support the development of the children. Of course, everyone's behavior is dysfunctional to some degree some of the time. Dysfunction needs treatment when it causes danger or intense and debilitating discomfort for the individual or others, or threatens the survival or adaptation of children. Of the cases in this book, Nick and his parents reflect very minor dysfunction in the context of substantial competence. John reflects quite obvious dysfunction in visible domains (physical abuse) combined with potentially more debilitating dysfunction in hidden areas (masculinity and sexuality). The Brightman daughters reflect very great dysfunction, even fatal dysfunction in one case, that went unnoticed because of high competence in highly visible domains.

Conditions leading to dysfunction

Dysfunction is framed as an interaction among (a) exposure to danger, (b) lack of protection or comfort during and after the exposure, and (c) maturation. Phrased this way, danger interacts with both individuals' maturation and their protective relationships. It is proposed that the single most crucial threat to development is the absence of an attachment figure whose tie to the individual is binding (Bowlby 1958). For children, these are parental figures; for adults, they are committed partners. One difference between John and Susan Smith is that John had a committed, albeit violent, father whereas Susan's father killed himself violently, thus both abandoning her and doing so in a maximally distressing manner. The DMM would suggest that this could have implications that we might see in John's voluntarily seeking treatment and Susan's making suicide threats and attempts, and then killing her children.

Three points are crucial:

1 There is threat at some point in every human's development, but danger alone is insufficient to yield dysfunction.

2 Humans differ in many ways, both genetic and acquired, but this alone does not lead to psychological dysfunction. That is, in an appropriately protective and comforting environment where attachment figures adapt to the child's ZPD, genetic anomaly would not lead to psychological dysfunction (Rutter *et al.* 2006).

3 Dysfunction is inherently an interpersonal process, one that marks a lack of protective synchrony between vulnerable persons and their attachment figures. That is, every person who has been unseen or seen in a distorted way by his or her attachment figure during development is suffering and in need of amelioration. For John, the problem appears to have been being unseen by his mother and seen in a distorted way by his father, whereas, for Susan Smith, the problem was more nearly being unseen by both parents.

The nature of danger

Threat can take many forms, from the presence of something dangerous (e.g., abuse, witnessing domestic violence) to the absence of protection or comfort (e.g., parental depression, neglect). The threat can be danger that was experienced or danger that was only expected and not clearly avoided, such that the basis of the misexpectation was not clarified and corrected. For example, superstitious compulsions (such as hanging a jacket on a hanger) can develop and be carried forward when that behavior has preceded an unexpected danger (e.g., failing a test); if the child thinks that crooked hanging of the jacket augured the failure, then the child may rehang jackets until perfection is achieved whenever he or she expects a test. Indeed, the procedure might come into general use for all kinds of anxiety-eliciting situations. Finally, danger that is clearly visible distorts psychological processes less than danger that is obscure or ambiguous. For example, the danger could be hidden marital conflict or past trauma to the parent that is unmentioned. Monia (as a mother) and Sophie (as a child) are examples in this volume of hidden danger that endangers the child; Rosie is an example that has been published (Kozlowska *et al.* 2006). 'Unspeakable' dangers are generally more disruptive of development than the same problems talked about. That is, the danger you can't see is more dangerous than the danger that you can see (Fonagy 1999).

Maturation

Whether an event or condition poses a threat to a particular person is tied to the person's maturity. Some conditions that are threatening to infants (for example, being without a protective adult for a short time) can be managed by preschool-aged children and are not even noticed as threats by older children. That is, 'danger' is not an absolute condition, but rather is determined in part by the ability of individuals to protect themselves from the threat. Dysfunction becomes a possibility when children are exposed to dangers for which they (a) do not have the biological maturity to organize a protective response, and (b) lack the assistance of a protective and comforting attachment figure. Loss of an attachment figure is a good example. Children cannot successfully manage such losses alone and the remaining parent (if there is one) may be too distraught to be helpful. Donnie is an example, with her oldest child being both neglected and also taking a caregiving role; Susan Smith shows a more complex response, possibly both because of her father's violent form of suicide and because of her mother's affair and remarriage. Jackson demonstrates similar problems around abandonment by his mother and rejection by his father.

Dynamic protective relationships

In most cases, children are protected from danger by their parents. When cared for adequately, they are left to fend for themselves only when they can competently do so. Between these two conditions (being unable and being fully able to protect oneself) is the child's ZPD. In the ZPD, individuals have the *maturity* to care for themselves, but not yet the *experience* and *skills*. It is here, where skills need to be learned, that attachment figures function to facilitate that process, sometimes guiding, at other times demonstrating, and, when mastery is acquired, sharing approval and satisfaction with the child. Luke and his father are an example of a mismatch in a particular ZPD (toddlerhood) that caused difficulties not experienced earlier and unlikely to be experienced later, given the particular issues that activate his father's past trauma. Framing attachment relationships as operating in the child's ZPD enables adaptation and treatment of maladaptation to encompass biological anomalies or limitations by construing the protector's role as adapting to the unique characteristics and readiness of the child. This perspective does assume, however, that troublesome or anomalous behavior varies in concert with changes in other people or the context; i.e., there are contingencies between the behavior and its context.

Further, this perspective implies that parents, too, have ZPDs. Luke's father worked productively with his therapist to reveal his history, his emotions about it, and his behavior when it was activated by his son. His ZPD work involved making thought and feeling conscious, reflecting on the meaning of his childhood experience for his parenting behavior, and generating alternate solutions to use with Luke. More important, however, than these 'solution-focused' processes, Luke's father was learning to use a discrepancy (how could he have hurt his beloved child?) to initiate a process of making information conscious and reflecting on its meaning to generate alternative responses he could use in the future in similar circumstance. Luke's arm will not be broken again, so that event is no longer critical. The important thing for his father is learning to use his mind in new ways. Put in the framework of this book, both his father's parents and Luke himself

259

are 'raising' his father to become a parent, specifically, the parent that Luke needs.

Dysfunction

It is important to recognize that no life is free of danger and that sometimes the most effective way to learn to recognize danger and protect oneself from it is to face it. Of course, the 'dose' must be suited to the person's readiness to perceive the threat, attribute reasonable meanings to it, and organize an adaptive response to it. Framed that way, danger is not inherently negative. To the contrary, the 'bad' dangers are (a) danger that is too great for the individual's development *and* not protected by an attachment figure, and (b) danger that can be managed by the individual *but* the attachment figure acts protectively nevertheless. Put another way, when the attachment figure does not function in the individual's ZPD, the result can be dysfunction. In both cases, the means by which the under- or over-protection at one age becomes dysfunction at another age is information processing. Nancy and her parents are an example of parents who both over- and under-protected their child; although the dangers were not great (compared with other cases offered here), the mismatch between parental responses and Nancy's ZPD probably was tied to Nancy's dysfunction, which did become substantial.

Information processing and dysfunction

Information processing (including past synaptic changes that constitute memory) is the means by which experience at one time influences behavior at a later time. To the extent that individuals (1) misperceive or misattribute meaning to perceptions, (2) fail to generate protective procedures, or (3) fail to regulate their arousal so as to both appraise situations (moderate arousal) and implement solutions (sometimes needing high arousal), their behavior may not fit their circumstances. That is, their behavior is not likely to function adaptively. Essentially, every case in this book is illustrative of parents misperceiving their child's behavior or making misattributions about it. Kate and Andrea Yates provide more poignant examples of being unable to regulate arousal safely.

A particularly important issue is the developmental period in which misinformation was generated. If it was before speech, implicit memory systems will have undue influence over later behavior – and this will not be easily discerned by the individual because the information is neither verbal nor known consciously. Thus, the older the individual was when misinformation was generated, the more easily the mind will find it and have the possibility of correcting it. Consequently, major dysfunction would be expected to have roots in the first years of life, before there was language or consciousness. Albert (who had psychotic breaks) and his mother Maryia are an example of very early adaptation to a mother's needs possibly leading to very dysfunctional behavior two decades later, long after the early distortions had been absorbed preconsciously into Albert's behavior.

Misinformation and behavior

Misinformation generated in past instances of coping with danger is expected to yield comprehensible changes in behavior, albeit maladaptive changes. That is, if (or when) we understand the nature of the misinformation, i.e., the nontrue transformations of affect or cognition, then the individual's behavior will appear meaningful. The default assumption in the DMM is that behavior is interpersonally meaningful unless there is evidence of both neurological anomaly and lack of interpersonal contingency. Kate is an especially apt example of how early self-cutting might have reappeared later in life when both the original and additional functions were fulfilled by cutting.

Faulty information processing and risk of future danger

Every developmental period presents new challenges. If handled poorly, these can become dangers for the individual. For example, going to school presents the challenge of aggressive peers. Essentially, all children face this threat, but children whose behavior is less adaptive, i.e., those with problems from before the school years, are more likely to elicit bullying or become bullies. In addition, because such children distort incoming information, they are more likely to respond ineffectively once bullying occurs. The outcome is that, when children who were at risk at an earlier developmental period experience a new danger for which they must generate a new response, their dysfunction may increase. They may begin a downward spiral where each danger experienced and not managed effectively increases the probability both of exposure to danger in the future and failure to manage the new danger effectively. Candace (who sexualized her son) and Maggie Drucker (who was depressed and violent) are examples of poor beginnings leading to augmenting risk the downward spiral. Albert and the Brightman girls are examples of behavior that functions adaptively in one developmental period (compulsiveness during the school years) but reduces the probability of adequately managing the challenges of a later period (leaving home for Albert and establishing intimate relationships for both Albert and the Brightman girls).

Resilience and nonlinear developmental pathways

It should be noted clearly that, although there are self-maintaining processes at work, this is not a linear, predetermined process (Rutter 2006b, 2006c). Both maturation and luck play a role in opening the developmental process to change. Maturation plays a protective role by permitting the mind to discover discrepancies and organize solutions in ways that were not possible earlier. Unforeseen conditions that bear no causal relation to the self, i.e., luck, affect development as well. For example, when current conditions become safer than earlier conditions were (e.g., a single mother marries a caring man), early risk is less likely to become dysfunctional. Alternately, at some point after the danger, attachment figures may become more able to talk openly and comfortingly about issues that they could not, for their own reasons, address earlier. Benjamin's mother (who disagreed with the drug treatment of her son's ADHD, proposing instead that her marital difficulties caused his problems) became able to consider her own contribution to her son's difficulties only after divorce (Crittenden and Kulbotten 2007). Similarly, an alternate attachment figure, for example, a teacher, may become available even when family circumstances do not change. For Kate, an example might well have been Nick, whose attention might have prevented the often devastating effects of institutionalization from obstructing her opportunity to form intimate marital relationships and, thus, have children.[1] Put another way, dysfunction itself is not an absolute in that what seems dysfunction from one perspective may sometimes be seen as adaptive from another.

Nevertheless, in too many cases, early risks accumulate, dysfunction occurs and is maintained or even augmented, and individuals find themselves unable to solve crucial problems in their lives. There are many possible responses to dysfunction – for example, ignoring it, shaping one's life around its limitations, and using newly maturing potentials to resolve it oneself. The one we focus on is treatment *with* a professional.[2]

Basic principles of treatment

The DMM approach to treatment is guided by several general principles. These are grouped here as goals, the helping relationship, initiating contact and assessment, and treatment, but in practice, these are neither linear nor discrete processes. Instead, treatment often has an irregular circuitous, sidetracking, and recursive quality (as does life), but, when successful, even the backtrackings are temporary, and eventually a forward motion is recovered. Moreover, often something important is gained in the diversion that shifts the direction of the forward progress a bit. All of this is to say that what follows is a bit contrived by the nature of written discourse imposing too logical a structure on the process being described.

Because this is a book about parents who harm or endanger their children, it is important to point out that parents are people. That is, they have a developmental past. Further, their present life presents them with problems and satisfactions. And their future contains their hope for both themselves and their children. Put more clearly, parents are persons first and parents in addition. If they are treated as existing solely for their children, the treatment may be ineffective – both because it will be too narrow and because the individual will feel unseen or seen inaccurately by the therapist. A balance must be found between parents' existence as individuals and their function as parents.

The goals of treatment

Treatment should change information processing in ways that promote adaptive and functional behavior, both in the current context and in contexts not yet experienced or even envisioned. For parents, this includes promoting the survival and development of their children.

Treatment should be a freeing process, one that frees the mind from its unique developmental history, giving each human the possibility to experience human life at its fullest: safely, comfortably, and with a foot in the future through one's children or one's contribution to others' development. Crucial to this process are (a) self-awareness (i.e., uncovering implicit psychological processes), (b) attention to discrepancy, (c) reflective integration, and (d) empathy with others.[3]

Professionals should also work to affect the larger systems in which individuals and families live in ways that promote the safety and comfort of everyone and the children-rearing capacity of adults. Put another way, treatment should not be restricted to or isolated in the therapist's office. Therapists should attend to how families live outside the therapy as well as the extent to which the culture supports or impedes adaptive family functioning.

The helping relationship

Psychological treatment involves two or more people engaged around the process of change. I have used the all-purpose term 'treatment' to cover everything (a) from educational parenting interventions to long-term psychotherapy (b) for individuals, parent–child dyads, couples and groups. In order to discuss the relationship between those who seek treatment and those who offer it, I need to be more precise about the type of treatment under consideration because this affects the relationship greatly.

How does the therapist function in the treatment relationship?

As a general notion, the more individuals seeking help are able to manage reflective integration, the less they will need the professional to function as a transitional attachment figure. That is, individuals who can reflect productively are presumed to have had or found reasonably adequate attachment figures who protected and comforted them well enough.[4] The result is that they developed no major distortions of information processing that preclude their gaining access to most of the information, identifying and correcting at least some discrepancies, and constructing reasonably integrated representations. Because these psychological processes do not develop prior to adolescence, it is presumed (hypothesized, because this can be tested) that these parents were cared for well enough in an attachment relationship during childhood. When they need help with parenting, such individuals need access to semantic information and procedural skills rather than needing to learn how to use information appropriately. For them, the relationship with the professional is less important than the professional's ability to provide the needed information and skills.

At the other extreme, the more individuals were left early in life to manage serious threats beyond their capacity and without assistance from an attachment figure, the more it is expected that they will have substantial distortions in the preconscious memory systems. This could affect their needs in treatment in several ways:

1 Having been left unprotected and uncomforted, they may either hesitate to form close, helping relationships in which they would feel vulnerable or, conversely, throw themselves precipitously into new relationships, expecting the relationships to provide more than can be provided.

2 They may have seriously inaccurate transformations of information that function out of their awareness, thereby making it very difficult for them to discover errors themselves.

3 Their preconscious knowledge may forbid conscious awareness and articulation of such discrepancies.

4 They may lack both episodic recall and experience with integrative processing.

These conditions suggest both a very great need for their therapists to assume the role of a transitional and corrective attachment figure, and distortions of how that role would be conceived and managed by the parents. The relationship with the therapist will need to be unique, personal, and established slowly. It is likely to begin superficially and change over time, as increasingly threatening topics can be opened to exploration. Moreover, the progress of the relationship will itself be both the process and a goal of the treatment. Because the therapist functions as a transitional attachment figure, the relationship will necessarily be intimate. As such, it cannot be duplicated; that is, no other therapist can replace the original one without an experience of loss. Such a relationship is, therefore, at the opposite end of the spectrum from that of a professional who functions primarily to make information available or to teach skills.

How is the professional-parent relationship organized?
Again, using the extreme poles of being able to integrate reflectively and having only slightly transformed information, as compared to being unable to integrate and having highly distorted, omitted, erroneous, and false information, the personal characteristics of the professional carrying out an educational intervention are of negligible importance. As long as the professional is reliable and knowledgeable and has access to the needed information, personal characteristics (even if not liked by the parent) are relatively unimportant. Moreover, if needed, someone else with similar training could take over the function without substantial disruption to the parent or the intervention. That is, the personal connection is quite superficial, not going beyond that of a social contact.

At the other extreme, people whose past history of being endangered and uncomforted has resulted in substantial distortions of information processing and close relationships are likely to need to form personal relationships with their therapists. These relationships will have many of the characteristics of naturally occurring attachment relationships, especially in that no one else can fulfill the same role and that both the professional and the parent will be changed by their experience together (Crittenden 2000c). That is, the healing relationship will be asymmetrical (in power and authority) and reciprocal (by involving a mutual change process). In sum, the professional can function like a teacher/guide (behavioral and cognitive-behavioral model), an attachment figure (working in the parent's ZPD), as part of a transference–counter-transference dyad (psychodynamic model), or as an interested equal, working outside the system (family systems model).

Between these extremes, there is a range of relationships between parent and professional that vary in intimacy, specificity, and assumption of an attachment function. In practice, the term 'client' tends to be used for less personal relationships with less hurt and more competent help-seekers, and the term 'patient' is usually reserved for relationships in which the person seeking help suffers, lacks integrative skills and processes, and needs far more than information or new skills. In cases of minor dysfunction or only risk of future dysfunction, the term 'client' fits better than 'patient'. In fact, the more the individual can take charge of the process or even choose to discontinue it altogether without risk of serious dysfunction, the more the term 'client' is appropriate.

One way to think about the distinction between 'clients' and 'patients' is that clients may be uncomfortable, but, compared with patients, they do not suffer. That is, clients' affective state and management of their feelings is not a central issue. Instead, the cognitive issues of knowing what to do or how to decide what to do are more often central. In addition, clients are sufficiently well organized that it is not essential that the therapist comes to know them uniquely or even personally. Clients can manage to extract what they need from group interventions[5] that are not adapted to fit them uniquely, e.g., manualized interventions. Further, 'client' implies that the parent knows what he or she is contracting to purchase. Moreover, as is implied by being able to make an informed decision, clients already work verbally, consciously and, often, reflectively.

On the other hand, patients often just want relief from suffering and have no idea what that entails nor what the therapist is able to offer. Except hope. Suffering and hope are the crucial issues. Suffering brings patients to treatment and hope enables them to sustain the process. The process? It will take more patience than they could possibly imagine at the outset. It is particularly in cases of hope for relief from suffering that the relationship with the therapist has itself a healing function.

Initiating the relationship and assessment

The next chapter is devoted to a lengthy discussion of assessment. Here it seems most important to indicate that assessment is a constant process, beginning with the first voice tones on the telephone when the appointment is made, continuing through the first look and handshake, and progressing through the formal assessment in the early sessions and remaining a subscript of ongoing reassessment throughout the treatment. Like all else, however, assessment is a two-way street in which the parent who has come for treatment is assessing whether this therapist can be useful. Gaining access to parents' understanding of what is helpful to them is not, however, easy or direct. Even when asked explicitly, many parents will feel uncomfortable admitting to evaluating the therapist or to announcing their evaluation. It may be necessary for the therapist to watch for and respond in an inquisitive way to subtle indicators.

Because the helping relationship is crucial to the parent's being able to change and because parents who endanger their children are often in managed forms of treatment, it is crucial that their preferences be discovered and honored. If one or two of the professionals assigned to a parent seem unable to work with the parent, or if the parent expresses negative views regarding them, other professionals should be offered. The kind of change that is needed is unlikely to occur when the client/patient feels uncomfortable with the helping professional. Our pride or sense of authority should not stand in the way of parents being given the best opportunity for change.

Treatment

Treatment is the process of engendering change. As with all development, change reflects learning, i.e., changed perception, attribution, selection of a behavioral response, and implementation of the response. Moreover, what is learned must be retained, i.e., stored in the brain in a retrievable manner.

To some therapists, this might sound foreign and as if treatment were being framed exclusively as didactic learning; their theories and goals would be intensely opposed to managing treatment as 'education'. For others, especially those from a learning theory perspective, this statement would appear to fit their practices quite well. What I mean falls between these two perspectives; that is, the learning I refer to is not primarily educational or didactic, but it can be organized developmentally and does result in both changed knowledge and changed information processing.

In the DMM, learning refers to new ways in which information is processed to yield new perceptions, attributions, solutions, and ways to implement solutions. Didactic learning is a very small part of this and generally is only appropriate for those parents who can already reflect and decide what is suitable for them and their children. That is, didactic learning is not a primary aspect of treatment for parents who endanger their children. For endangering parents, learning is both less direct and more typical of the learning that constitutes children's development. It is *experiential* learning that is processed through many neurological pathways (which we have referred to as memory systems). It is retained as neural networks with increased probabilities of being activated under particular temporal or associative conditions. Creating these networks, generating the eliciting associations, and regulating both of these, i.e., deactivating some networks, and reducing some associative processes while generating other networks and associations, is what is 'learned' in psychotherapy. One function of therapists is to present opportunities for relevant learning experiences that are in the parent's ZPD.

The conditions that promote experiential learning vary. Some parents will need pharmacological treatment to initiate or maintain change; others will need strong and pervasive contextual support, e.g., an inpatient experience or daily visits from professionals or removal of their children; and others will manage on 50 minutes a week or a two-hour group meeting or some variation thereof.

Conclusions

To conclude, treatment of parents who endanger their children should focus on the dangers the parents have experienced and the psychological and behavioral strategies they developed to cope with them. When their strategies are framed as accomplishments achieved under difficult circumstances, the nullifying effects of accusations of inadequacy can be diminished and possibly even replaced with pride and awareness of having some control over important aspects of their own lives. Keeping in mind that people whose behavior is maladaptive have had to shape themselves around others' limitations can give legitimacy to parents' need to be seen accurately and adapted to sensitively. Working in their ZPD is the most pragmatic way to promote change, but more than that, doing so can become satisfying to both parents and their therapists when the parents' developmental experience is appreciated. Understanding this experience requires that therapists listen carefully to what is said and even more to what is meant. Finally, compassion for parents' suffering, both as children who suffered and now as adults who have failed to accomplish their own dreams, and recognition of their intent and effort can make empathy and compassion possible. When these are founded on shared knowledge, they may enable therapists to assist parents to bridge the gap between perception of danger and the possibility of safety and comfort.

Notes

1 This is a good example of complexity. Nick's behavior met criteria for sexual abuse, i.e., morally offensive and criminal behavior. Nevertheless, he maintained a personal and intimate relationship with Kate for seven years while she lived in an institution without any family contact. Kate thought he was the best thing in her life – and, functionally in those circumstances, he might have been.

2 The usual preposition would be 'by' a professional. The choice of 'with' emphasizes the transactional quality of treatment.
3 The usual preposition is 'for', but that implies a separateness and superiority that I prefer to avoid.
4 Of course, after successful treatment, formerly endangered people also function integratively.
5 It is not presumed that all group work lacks individual adaptation, but when it does, it may not be suited to patients.

Chapter 17

Assessment relevant to differential treatment

Good assessment is crucial to good treatment. It is the link between the problem and its solution. Without it, it becomes difficult to designate which treatments are appropriate and which contraindicated. This is true even when the treatment is brief and delivered in a group setting. For example, even prevention services and parent education require some assessment to ensure that the intervention is appropriate and will not be misapplied, possibly even causing harm. Put another way, good assessment enables us to deliver services appropriately, with maximum benefit to the recipients and minimal risk of waste or harm.

The primary focus of this chapter is on assessment of attachment and the skills needed to deliver the assessment procedures and interpret their meaning. In addition, a few brief assessments are offered that can help to suggest when a full assessment of attachment might be needed.

What sort of assessment is needed?

Assessment can be expensive and time-consuming. When families' problems are pressing, it can be tempting to do a cursory assessment and get on, as quickly as possible, to treatment. This might not only be 'penny wise and pound foolish'; but also dangerous to some families and one reason why our services are so ineffective. If we deliver services that are unsuited to parents' needs and skills, we waste the services and risk making the families appear incompetent, resistant, or uncaring – or all of these.

Strangely, it is in the cases in which the most momentous decisions are being made that I most frequently hear that a quicker, less extensive assessment is needed. Specifically, professionals doing court evaluations regarding child custody (in cases of child protection and divorce) often require an assessment of attachment, but do not feel they have the time to deliver a formal assessment and almost always decide that having it interpreted by a reliable coder is unnecessary. Because nothing is more crucial to a child's future than where and with whom he or she will grow up, I cannot understand not wanting the most valid assessment possible. Of course, at present, we lack any assessments that are known to predict satisfactory placement success in an empirically valid sense (after all, we cannot run a double-blind experiment). Nevertheless, when attachment is understood properly as being *self-protective strategies and the information processing that underpins them* (as opposed to the secure/insecure issue), then properly delivered assessments of attachment can be very useful to decision-making and, over time, can build a body of clinical data that can inform future decision-making. Our current random use of 'attachment' in court settings cannot either inform individual cases or build a body of validating information. Forgoing formal assessment that is coded by trained, reliable professionals who are naive to the specific case may, I think, be the sort of shortcut that can generate long-term damage.

Current assessment of parenting adequacy

At present, most evaluation of parental adequacy is carried out by licensed PhD psychologists or MD psychiatrists and social workers (with a wide range of training). Nowhere, however, does this training necessarily include the study of attachment or training in delivering assessments of attachment. Instead, the usual assessment begins with consideration of the family history and evidence of harm to the children. Psychological evaluation usually adds formal, standardized assessments, carried out in an office, that are used to determine (a) whether a disorder is present; (b) if so, which DSM-IV or ICD-10 diagnosis fits best; and (c) the intellectual functioning of the individual. Social work evaluation more often consists of direct observation, usually in the family home, of (a) the parents, (b) children, and (c) home environment. Both sorts of evaluation sometimes also address attachment by noting whether parents and children appear attached and, if so, whether the relationship appears secure. Frequently, however, professionals untrained in attachment misconstrue clinging to the parent as 'strong' attachment and, therefore, assume that it is secure attachment. In Ainsworth's empirical work and in the DMM, such attachment behavior is more often indicative of Type C (ambivalent, coercive) and carries risks. This suggests the risks incurred when professionals without formal training in attachment theory and standardized assessments of attachment render informally derived evaluations. Because they lack formal methods and empirical validity, such evaluations often lead to disagreement among 'experts' with no evidence with which to resolve the disagreement.

Neither psychological nor social work evaluation directly addresses (a) the information processing leading to dysfunction; (b) the reasons the parents behave as they do, i.e., their self-protective attachment strategy and its historic roots; or (c) the relative appropriateness of different types of intervention or treatment. That is, lacking a coherent theory of parental dysfunction, it has been difficult to use current assessment practices to link the basis of dysfunction to differential selection of treatment. Instead families with more problems tend to be offered more treatments. Moreover, the treatments are whatever the community has available delivered in whatever theoretical framework the clinicians have been trained.

It is proposed here that *self-protective strategy* and *the information processing* underlying it, i.e., 'attachment', are the crucial variables for indicating which sorts of treatment are likely to be beneficial, have no effect, or be contraindicated because they might do harm. It is further proposed that assessing attachment is a specialized task, which, like other forms of psychological assessment, requires appropriate training and authorization and, when carried out properly, can provide a basis for others to evaluate the expert's conclusions.

What we need to know before beginning treatment when parents have endangered their children

Assessment can be a time-consuming and expensive process. Nevertheless, without sound assessment, treatment decisions can lead to wasted effort or, worse, harmful interventions that could make conditions worse for both parents and children. In this section, a hierarchical set of questions are posed, each with a suggestion regarding a brief evaluation. The common denominator, of course, is danger, its presence, proximity in time and space, probability of occurrence, and severity of effects.

1 *Are the adults aware of the need for change?* Discrepancy identifies the need for psychological treatment, in this case, the discrepancy between what the parent intended and what happened or between how the parent sees the situation and how others do. Only when some discrepancy is stated openly, either by a person recognizing the problem him- or herself, or by someone else defining the behavior as a problem, can there be an impetus to undertake a process of change. Ironically, change itself is threatening such that the degree of discrepancy needs to be managed well. Mild discrepancies rarely result in seeking treatment. Moderate discrepancies produce sufficient discomfort that treatment may be sought, even though the bias in processing that produced the discrepancy is rarely apparent to the parent. Severe discrepancies often result in treatment being imposed on the parent, such as child protection, psychiatric hospitalization, or imprisonment. Put another way, recognition of discrepancy and perception of danger are linked in complex ways. The issue is whether the parents understand the risks of their behavior and recognize the need to protect their children differently. For professionals, the question is whether they can modulate the risk that they pose so as to engender a productive response without eliciting unproductive self-protection from the parent.

2. *What level of service does the family need?* A simple scale, the Level of Family Functioning Scale (Crittenden 1992d), can help professionals make some quick decisions about how to direct the family to appropriate

271

services. Families at levels 3–5 (Box 17.1) will need full evaluation and careful provision of services. It is important to note, however, that community resources often determine whether a family is 'supportable' or 'inadequate'. The consequences of that difference are immense – for children, parents and the community at large. If the children are removed (i.e., placed in 'care'), a series of negative consequences is likely to ensue. These may be balanced by benefits, but removal is never a cost-free, safe solution.

Box 17.1 Level of family functioning

I. Independent and adequate
Families in this category are able to meet the needs of their children by combining their own skills, help from friends and relatives, and services which they seek and use. Such families, like all families, face problems and crises. It is their competence at resolving these problems which makes them adequate.

II. Vulnerable to crisis
Families in this category need temporary, i.e., 6 months to 1 year, help in resolving unusual problems; otherwise, the family functions independently and adequately. Examples of common precipitating crises include birth of a handicapped child, divorce, loss of employment, death of a family member, entry of a handicapped child into school, and sexual abuse in day care of a child. Because each of these crises could result in chronic problems, it is the nature of the family's response, not the nature of the crisis, which results in the *vulnerable* classification.

III. Restorable
Families in this category are multiproblem families who need several types of training in specific skills or therapy around specific issues. Following intervention, it is expected that the family will function independently and adequately. The period of intervention can be expected to last 1–4 years and require active case management to organize the sequence of service delivery and to integrate the services.

IV. Supportable
There are no rehabilitative services which can be expected to enable these families to become independent and adequate. With specific ongoing services, the family can meet the basic physical, intellectual, emotional and economic needs of their children. Services, and management of those services, will be needed until all the children are grown. Examples of supportable families include those with a mentally retarded mother, a depressed mother, or a parent who abuses alcohol or drugs chronically.

V. Inadequate
There are no services sufficient to enable these families to meet the basic needs of their children, now or in the future. Permanent removal of the children should be sought.

---

3 *What sort of services can the parents use effectively?* Various services require different skills and readiness to be used effectively. If applied to parents who are not ready for them, the service might be wasted or, worse, do harm. The gradient of interventions (Box 17.2) (Crittenden 2005a) suggests which parents might benefit from which services. It is worth noting that the most frequently assigned intervention, parent education or parent training, is unlikely to be helpful and may be harmful to parents who endanger their children. This is because the intervention requires that parents be able to function reflectively by engaging in problem solving and applying their solutions to child-rearing at home (Kazdin and Wassell 2005; Webster-Stratton and Hammond 1990), whereas many, or even most, such parents are likely to be stressed or psychiatrically disturbed (Kazdin and Wassell 2005). This resource is better reserved for parents at Level of Family Functioning 2.

4 *Do the parents have psychiatric problems?* If they do, further evaluation of the family is needed, even if the immediate danger is not great. Parental psychiatric disorder is among the most powerful indicators of risk of child disorder, including both acting-out sorts of problems and role-reversing care of the troubled parent, i.e., A3 compulsive caregiving (Falcov 1996; Fombonne *et al.* 2001; Howard 2000). Depending upon the study, 60–80 per cent of mothers with psychiatric disorder ultimately lose custody of their children (Göpfert *et al.* 2004). Moreover, when the child has symptoms, the mother's psychiatric state is related to poorer outcomes in both child treatment and parenting treatment (Kazdin and Wassel 2005). Although that might be explained by genetic contribution,

Box 17.2 Gradient of interventions

- **Parent education**
  Parent can integrate, but needs new information

- **Short-term counseling**
  Parent can integrate and has information, but needs another perspective and dialogue around the perspective to promote problem-solving

- **Parent–child intervention**
  Parent can use explicit information to describe problems, including their own contribution, but cannot integrate discrepant information

- **Adult psychotherapy**
  Parent's behavior is generated implicitly, i.e., not consciously, and is maladaptive, sometimes dangerously so

  Parents need understanding of implicit 'triggers', verbalization, recognition of discrepancy, integration, and the experience of being understood empathically before they can understand others (for example, their children) empathically

---

the data suggest otherwise (Barnes and Stein 2000; Murray and Cooper 2003). For example, parents with psychiatric disorder are more likely to show maladaptive parenting than those without, and this, in turn, is related to children's disorder, but when maladaptive parenting behavior was not shown, the relation between parental and child disorder did not hold (Johnson *et al.* 2001). Finally, the evidence indicates that psychiatric personnel rarely consider the effect of their patients' condition on their children even though more that 50 per cent of psychiatrically distressed women are mothers (Göpfert *et al.* 2004). This in spite of the fact that professionals were alerted to this problem four decades ago and frequently thereafter (Hawes and Cottrell 1999; Rutter 1966).

The importance of assessing attachment

Attachment has become an important aspect of most child protection and custody cases and is increasingly seen as relevant to prevention and treatment of psychological dysfunction. Its assessment, however, has been treated informally, as something any observant professional can evaluate. One aim of this chapter is to change that notion by arguing that attachment is a complex construct and its assessment requires skill and active maintenance of the skill. It is proposed that attachment should be assessed only by trained and authorized professionals.

Because the DMM is both a comprehensive theory of the development of dysfunction and a comprehensive theory of treatment and, in addition, has a set of age-appropriate assessments, it has the potential to link history, diagnosis, and treatment in meaningful ways that could increase treatment success, reduce treatment failure, and lower costs by reducing inappropriate or harmful treatment.

What is assessment?

Before addressing the assessment of attachment, a few concepts regarding assessment in general are relevant.

Sampling behavior

Assessment *samples* behavior to generate a *working hypothesis*. This hypothesis is not definitive. It is very important to keep this in mind. Assessments do not tell how a person is, but rather how they *most probably* are. This is because assessments elicit a subset of behavior and use that bit to estimate the nature of the whole of the person's behavior. But if the person is having a bad day, or feels sick, or is irritated by the professional, the assessment may elicit behavior that is not typical, and the results of the assessment may be skewed. Moreover, no assessment is perfect even under ideal conditions.

The outcome of the assessment is a *working hypothesis* of how the person, in this case a parent, functions. For example, if the assessment is a few screening questions to ensure that the parent fits criteria for a prevention service, it generates hypotheses of no risk (and, therefore, no eligibility for the service), mild risk (and therefore eligibility and suitability for the service), or high risk/known dysfunction (and, hopefully, exclusion from the prevention service and referral to a more intensive service). However, those families accepted for a service continue to be observed, and a few will be observed to have more or less risk than was initially thought. If the prevention program is functioning properly, these families will be terminated from an unnecessary service or referred to a more appropriate service. The point is that decisions are taken on the basis of the initial assessment, but that assessment only samples behavior and cannot be assumed to be absolutely accurate. It functions as a working hypothesis until new information permits its refinement.

Formal assessments, measures, and clinical judgment

Assessment can be carried out with either formal tools (e.g., tests and procedures) or in some unspecified way that yields a clinical judgment or expert opinion. The focus here is on the use of formal tools because the consequences of judgments regarding parents' adequacy or inadequacy can have such a profound impact on both parents and children that unverifiable information seems inappropriate.

Formal assessment tools assess some construct (e.g., heath, intelligence, attachment) and have a research literature regarding their validity. That is, simply writing an assessment and giving it a construct name is insufficient to verify its validity for the construct. Assessment of parenting should be limited to formal assessments with validating data that are relevant to the population from which the parent comes. This, of course, can mean revalidating the existing tools for new populations, such as immigrants, or handicapped adults or children.

Measures are a special type of assessment; they literally measure *how much* of the construct is present. Weight, income and intelligence are all measured. Attachment is not. One does not have more or less attachment or a strong or weak attachment. *Attachment is a pattern of behavior that serves a self-protective function.* Many behaviors can do that, but counting them does not reveal their patterning (Ainsworth *et al.* 1978).

Qualitative assessments yield a categorical outcome (as opposed to a continuous measure). Assessments of attachment are complex qualitative assessments in that they yield, for any given person, a number of categorical outcomes, e.g., the subclassification, designation of unresolved traumas and losses (or not), and modifiers (or not). Moreover, assessments of attachment are not 'tests',[1] in that there are no correct answers and one cannot fail. An important point to note is that qualitative assessments are formal assessments with specified and replicable data collection and data-reduction procedures.

Clinical judgment and expert opinion, on the other hand, are informal assessments because they lack a standardized procedure and specified method of deducing the outcome. They are very concerning when applied to attachment. The best assessments, particularly for court use, follow a *standard protocol*, and have a *physical product*, and *formal method of analysis* that other experts can examine. For example, radiographs of bone fractures constitute evidence of child abuse. Their power lies in the fact that any number of qualified experts can look at the films and render an opinion, together with the evidence in the film and in the published literature, supporting that opinion. Similarly, a psychologist's statement regarding a parent's IQ is based on a formal measure of intelligence (e.g., Stanford–Binet), together with the protocol of the parent's responses and the published normative data.

Far too often, clinical opinion regarding attachment is relied upon, even in court cases where custody and placement in care are issues. Clinical opinion regarding attachment is concerning for three reasons:

1 Most of the 'experts' rendering the opinion have no formal training in attachment.

2 The basis for their opinion cannot be examined by anyone else. That is, there is no physical evidence underlying their opinion and no evidence of validity for whatever they did to derive the opinion.

3 The crucial features of attachment are not always readily apparent in live observation. That is, relationships can appear one way and be another. Without physical evidence that others can view and validating studies in the published literature, one opinion is a bad as another. In court settings, conflicting opinions regarding attachment are usual – with no one having appropriate evidence.

Assessing attachment and information processing

Attachment has become an important topic in assessment and, at the same time, is managed very imprecisely. In this section, a brief guide to assessing attachment and information processing is offered.

Knowing which model is used

There are two major models of attachment, the DMM and the ABCD model. The DMM and ABCD coding methods and classificatory systems can, in most cases, be applied to the same observational procedures.

The crucial point for practitioners is that the models often yield very different outcomes when applied to the same procedures (Crittenden *et al.* 2007). Further, mixing the models introduces dissonance into outcome. How can one structure an intervention around a mixture of self-report taken at face value, observed 'disorganization', and the complex organization drawn from the DMM assessments? They lead in different directions. Put another way, they generate incompatible DRs that dispose the clinical individual to different responses. At some point a decision must be made regarding which sort of DR to use to guide intervention. It might be most economical to make that decision before assessing, use a coherent set of assessments, and then use them to focus the treatment.

In general, the DMM methods:

1 yield more differentiation within clinical samples (as opposed to labeling most clinical cases 'disorganized' or 'cannot classify');
2 are focused on the effects of danger on information processing and self-protective strategy (as opposed to the presence of security);
3 treat unresolved trauma and loss with more complexity than other models (as opposed to finding only preoccupying lack of resolution);
4 identify various forms of 'broken' strategies (i.e., depressed, disoriented, and with intrusions of forbidden negative affect, each of which appears to have different clinical correlates and implications).

As a consequence, these assessments have greater clinical utility and are more directly tied to implications for differential treatment than the ABCD methods. Finally, the DMM model has a telescoping set of developmentally expanding assessments that cover the life span. Thus, a single individual can be tracked over time or an entire family can be assessed at one time with the same model. On the other hand, the ABCD methods, having been developed earlier, have more published validity data.

Essential aspects of assessing attachment

There are several crucial elements to a good assessment of attachment. If they are missing, the assessment is unlikely to yield a valid conclusion.

1 Because assessments of attachment attempt to predict an individual's response to threat, it is crucial to *observe how the individual responds to threat*.

2 The procedure should permit the threat to be *regulated*. Without threat, everyone looks fine. With extreme threat, everyone panics or freezes. Moderate threat best displays the strategy.

3 Threat should be introduced in such a way that it can be *compared with the absence of threat and the presence of opportunity for comfort*. That is, the behavior of interest is a pattern of behavior, not an instance or a specific behavior.

4 The basis for the assessment should be *recorded* in such a way that it can be reviewed later to derive the pattern of attachment.

5 The assessment should tap more than one memory system, including in all cases procedural and imaged memory (the implicit memory systems

that are less easily controlled and that more often organize dangerous parental behavior).

6 It is very important that *the assessment be standardized* so that protocols are comparable across individuals.

7 The procedure should be *validated* by published research findings. Especially if one is making judgments about adequacy of parenting, one needs to be able to compare the focal parent with known competent and incompetent parents.

When assessment is being made under threatening conditions, i.e., for child protection or court applications, the coder should be alert to the reasonable quality of the parent's perception of threat and not necessarily attribute it to excessive vigilance for threat. The strategic response is still of interest, but parents who are very vigilant or cautious may be behaving reasonably, given the possible consequences of the investigation.

What formal assessments of attachment are there?

The array of DMM assessments is not finite and can be expected to increase in the coming years. Right now the assessments that I have developed are as follows:

1 The *CARE-Index for Infants* (birth–15 months; Crittenden 1981, 1988c, 1979–2005) is a three-minute, videotaped, play interaction included in many published studies; it assesses procedural and imaged memory (of both infant and adult).

2 The *CARE-Index for Toddlers* (16 months–3 years; Crittenden 1992a; Crittenden *et al.* 2007) is a three-minute, videotaped, play interaction that is included in some infant studies, but no separate studies as yet; it assesses procedural and imaged memory (of both toddler and adult).

3 The *Infant Strange Situation (SSP)* (11–15 months) is the classic Ainsworth procedure involving 20 minutes with and without the mother in a structured context. There are many published studies.

4 The *Preschool Assessment of Attachment (PAA)* (2–5 years; Crittenden 1992c, 1988–94, Crittenden *et al.* 2007) is a 'Strange Situation' adapted for 2–5-year-old children; it has many published studies and assesses preschoolers' procedural and imaged memory as well as very limited aspects of verbal representation (sometimes even including episodes).

5 The *School-aged Assessment of Attachment (SAA)* (6–13 years) (Crittenden 1997–2005; Crittenden and Landini 1999) is a seven-card, story-eliciting procedural that is transcribed verbatim and coded; there are conference presentations and studies under review; it assesses all memory systems, although integration is in concrete (episode-specific) terms only.

6 The *Transition to Adulthood Attachment Interview (TAAI)* (16–25 years; Crittenden 2005d) is structured on the Adult Attachment Interview (AAI), i.e., with probes of each memory system, but focused on late adolescence; there are clinical data, but no studies to date; it assesses all memory systems, although integration is in current and abstract terms only (i.e., generalized across episodes, but only in the present, not from early childhood).

7 The (modified) *Adult Attachment Interview (AAI)* (Crittenden 1999a; George *et al.* 1986/1996) is a semistructured, hour-long interview about early-life experiences that is transcribed verbatim and coded by DMM discourse analysis. There are many studies on the secure/anxious distinction, several conference presentations on the DMM patterns, seven theses and dissertations, and three published studies; it assesses all memory systems with full integration being possible.

8 The *Parents' Interview (PI)* (Crittenden 1982; Crittenden *et al.* 1991, 2000) is an hour-long interview for parents about their childhood, marriage, and child-rearing; it is transcribed verbatim and coded by the same discourse analysis as the TAAI and AAI. There are two published studies. It assesses all memory systems around parenting behavior.

The DMM assessments are ahead of the database. Some have reasonable empirical support (the CARE-Index, the SSP, and the PAA), but only the PAA has comparative DMM/ABCD data. Others are tied to well-known assessments for which there are data regarding clinical validity (AAI and TAAI); in these two cases the data are based on Main and Goldwin's classifications of AAIs and, although they differentiate normative from clinical cases, they are less precise than we might want and also lack differentiation within clinical cases. That is, from a DMM perspective, these data do not invalidate the AAI (coded by Main and Goldwyn's method), but they also fall short of being clinically useful. The purpose of the DMM method is to improve the clinical utility of the 'Strange Situation' and the AAI by (a) producing a more differentiated set of outcomes that are (b) tied to the presenting problem and (c) suggest directions for treatment. Three sorts of studies are needed at this point: (a) comparative DMM/ABCD studies, (b) studies that seek differential patterning among clinical groups, and (c) studies of the utility of these for improving treatment.

What is assessed when one assesses 'attachment'?

Assessments of attachment at different ages yield different information.

1 infancy (birth–18 months):
   a CARE-Index: adult sensitivity, control, and unresponsiveness and infant cooperation, compulsiveness, difficulty and passivity;

b The 'Strange Situation': the basic strategy, plus modifiers of depression or intrusions can be discerned;

2 preschool years (2–5): the strategy, modifiers of depression and intrusions and, occasionally, unresolved trauma (tied specifically to separation) can be identified;

3 school years (6–13): the strategy, modifiers of depression, disorientation, and intrusions and unresolved trauma can be discerned regarding several common threats that school-age children experience (i.e., moving, rejection by peers, bullying, father leaving, running away, and mother going to hospital);

4 adolescence and adulthood:
  a an attachment *strategy* or state of mind, i.e., the way speakers use information to organize their behavior when they feel endangered or believe their children to be endangered;
  b a possible set of *unresolved traumatic experiences* that distort people behavior without their being aware of it;
  c an *overriding distortion* of the strategy such as depression;
  d an *interpreted developmental history* of the speaker, combining information provided directly by the speaker with information derived from the pattern of errors (i.e., dysfluence) in the transcribed discourse;
  e the speaker's *level of awareness* and '*level of parental reasoning*'.

The information in the SAA, TAAI, and AAI is obtained by evaluating (a) what speakers say, (b) what they don't say that they should have said, (c) the dysfluence with which they speak, and (d) how they interact with the interviewer. The last two are especially important because dysfluence shows when there is conflict in the speaker's mind and how it is resolved whereas the interaction with the interviewer shows the speaker's strategy in use.

Information processing

The information processing data that can be derived from the assessments listed above are tied to the maturation of the individual. All of the assessments yield information about the individual's bias toward affect or cognition, and all display the types of transformations of information (true, distorted, omitted, erroneous, and false prediction) used by the child or parent.

The infant and preschool assessments provide assessment of preconscious, implicit functioning (procedural and imaged memory). The SAA provides, in addition, semantic memory and connotative language and episodes, but only as applied to concrete instances. The TAAI and AAI permit the full range of types of information, including abstract forms of explicit information, as well as unresolved traumas and losses of many types and modifiers of the basic strategy. The Parents' Interview permits assessment of (a) the same constructs as the AAI, albeit with less detail, and, in addition, (b) aspects of the couple relationship and each parent's level of parental reasoning. The last is especially useful in determining what sort of intervention or treatment is appropriate.

Training: Procedures, coding and classification

Carrying out the observation procedures requires training. This is true whether it is the 'Strange Situation', a story-eliciting procedure, or an attachment interview. All require skills that can be taught, but in the absence of the skill, the procedure can be rendered unclassifiable without the (untrained) clinician being aware of this. Professionals who have been trained to administer the DMM procedures have certificates that indicate authorization.

More importantly, the coders who will classify the procedures must be carefully trained to reliability before coding the assessments and must maintain their reliability. Coders who are qualified to code assessments of attachment have certificates of reliability authorizing this work. These certificates have a closing date (beyond which the certificate is not valid) and indicate what applications the coder is reliable for (a) screening, (b) clinical application in one's own cases, (c) anonymous research data, or (d) person-specific data that may be included in case records. Coders whose findings will contribute to making life-changing decisions (e.g., out-of-home placement, adoption, fostering) must be reliable at the highest level, and their reliability must be current.

All coders of attachment assessments should be blind to everything about the case, including especially the risk status of the case, i.e., the reason for the classification, the diagnosis of the individual, and any other personal information (except age and gender).

Of course, one might respond that this just isn't possible! It requires too much training, and few people are prepared to undertake that training and then to maintain the skill. Surely the amount of effort is substantial. The question is whether we can do with less without risking doing harm in a substantial number of cases.

Two observations are relevant. First, in the decade or so after Klaus and Kennel's monumental discovery of 'maternal bonding' (Klaus *et al.* 1972; Klaus and Kennel 1976, 1982) not only were hospital birth procedures changed to allow fathers to be present and babies to stay with their mothers, but also nurses and social workers began making judgments of whether mothers had 'bonded' or not. In court settings, these unfounded, observational judgments sometimes contributed to infants being removed from parental custody. At a distance of some decades, we know that every parent who takes the baby home and feeds it (i.e., the infant lives and wasn't abandoned) has 'bonded' in some way. The changes in hospital procedure have been retained because they are humane and appreciated by families, but the quick and uninformed judgments of bonding have disappeared almost completely. A good idea can be misapplied and do harm. Second, it is my experience that, when a proper assessment of attachment follows either a long treatment process or a series of court actions, suddenly the whole picture changes. The patient in treatment or the parent in a child-maltreatment proceeding suddenly is seen to be acting from a new set of motivations and with a coherent, if misplaced, strategy and that this strategy calls for a different professional response than has been given to date.

These points are based on personal observation and are used, as they should be, to question current practice. The answer to the question, however, should be empirical. If the observations are confirmed by others' observations and if the issue is deemed important (i.e., is it important how we direct psychotherapy? Is it important what we conclude about attachment in child-protection proceedings?), then we have the basis for addressing it in a controlled research framework asking whether informal and formal assessments of attachment, carried out completely independently, reach similar or different conclusions, and which produces better outcomes for children and families.

In the meantime, lacking the answers to these questions, should we be using informal judgments of attachment in decision-making situation? If we have case evidence that we can do harm by making informal judgments about a complex and not obvious construct and we do not have access to appropriately trained and skilled professionals, then possibly that construct should be left as an unknown, rather than having information of unknown validity used to make life-changing decisions. Bad information is not necessarily better than no information.

Deducing a classification

Except for the CARE-Index, the classification consists of a subpattern, plus possibly one or more Us, plus possibly a modifier. This information is derived from the videotape or written transcript in a recursive, meaning generating, manner. That is, the procedure is viewed or read in its entirety. Then it is reviewed or reread to identify the crucial information. For the 'Strange Situation', this is an episode-by-episode running narrative of parent and child behavior. For the transcripts, it is annotation of specific sorts of discourse. The bits of observation, which are fully verifiable by other viewers/readers, are then accumulated into constructs (for discourse, this is memory systems). These are then reduced to a possible subpattern, unresolved traumas or losses and modifiers (within the range possible for the specific assessment).

This provisional classification is then reconsidered in terms of possible disconfirming evidence and its fit with the content of the procedure *as understood through DMM theory and empirical studies*. The italicized phrase means that the content is not expected to state directly the strategy; indeed, if it did, there would be no need for this lengthy process – we would simply ask people to self-report their strategy. Instead, on the basis of theory and research, certain types of experience are expected to result in certain sorts of behavior. For example, adults who were in care in childhood are expected to laugh more, to use more positive statements about their various attachment figures, to downplay the impact on themselves of problems, and to take more personal responsibility for problems than people raised at home by adequate parents. The content, in other words, sounds like a secure and balanced B whereas the telegraphic, self-omitting discourse tells a different story. Theory and research findings are used to find the consistency between content and coded discourse.

If there is disconfirming evidence or a misfit of content to classification, the process is repeated until all the data can be subsumed into a single best-fitting classification. The point is that the coder is searching through layers of patterning which, when they have been brought to light, reflect recognizable and adaptive patterns in the person's developmental context.

Who should be assessed

When the well-being of children is the primary issue, it is the parents who need most to be assessed; specifically, their self-protective strategies and information processing should be assessed. This is true whether the case is in the child-protection, mental-health, or adoption system. Moreover, assessing both parents' attachment is important, as is assessing their relationship to each other. The child's attachment to each parent will yield additional information, but is overall of less importance than understanding the parents' psychological organization. This is because changing the parents' behavior will have fairly rapid and strong effects on the child's behavior (especially with younger children), whereas changing the child's behavior will make parents more comfortable and less threatened, but have relatively little effect on their processing of information or self- and progeny-protective strategy. When threat recurs, they will use the old strategy, just as they did before the child was treated.

The best solution, especially in serious cases, is to assess each family member, siblings included, and the family's functioning as a whole. This is expensive, but family problems are rarely limited to one person and are hardly ever resolved by 'fixing' one person.

Integrity of assessments

All of the assessments of attachment depend upon (a) surprising the mind by introducing something unexpected, (b) regulating the threatening elements of the procedures, and (c) a careful, ordered accretion of information. If aspects of the procedures are taken out and used separately or combined with other procedures or questions, the attachment assessments will eventually become useless (as if one had practiced the answers to an IQ test in school). In addition, the extracted parts are unlikely to yield valid results in their new context because the structure of the process is the 'active ingredient', not the specific questions. Put another way, these assessments have a carefully organized internal structure that is essential to displaying the strategy. When naive professionals use them out of context, they both weaken the original procedure and fail to gain the value they sought in the new context. It is very important, therefore, that these procedures ('Strange Situation', picture cards, and interview questions) remain intact and be used sparingly.

What assessments of attachment can't do

There are two major limitations to assessing attachment. First, assessment of attachment cannot identify abuse or neglect. This must be done with the usual evidentiary methods. In fact, even the history revealed by instruments like the AAI is factually uncertain. Because information is biased and because it is always reshaped to fit the self in the present, the facts cannot be known for sure from recall of any kind, including attachment-based recall.

Second, attachment cannot be assessed quickly and easily, or be assessed by a professional who is not carefully trained in *assessing attachment*. This is because attachment assessments seek to identify a complex psychological and behavioral process, one that has *implicit* and *biased* aspects. Therefore, the assessment cannot be explicit, e.g., self-report or casual observation. These are 'heavy-duty' diagnostic procedures that can only be used by properly trained personnel – as is the case with other psychological assessments.

How much effort should be put into assessment?

Good assessment is crucial to delivering appropriate treatment to individuals and families. It is also essential to conserving precious resources by not delivering treatment in wasteful ways. However, the appropriate amount of effort and cost depends upon its ultimate use. If the goal is prevention, some screening questions about risk conditions (e.g., danger in the past or currently) should be sufficient to decide whether a fuller assessment is needed. For psychotherapy, a proper assessment of attachment for all relevant individuals is called for, both to begin the treatment efficiently (it can take many weeks to reach the same understanding without formal assessment) and to avoid misdirecting the treatment. When life-changing decisions will be based in part on the outcomes of the assessment of attachment, fully qualified and authorized professionals should code, classify and write up the results of the assessment, it being certain that they are not the same individuals who carried out any of the assessments. Such conditions include removing children from their parents' care, divorce-related custody decisions, and selection of foster and adoptive parents.

Contraindications: Avoiding the wrong treatment

DMM thinking suggests that it is not true that some treatment, any treatment, is better than no treatment. To the contrary, the wrong treatment may be worse than no treatment. For example, giving abusive parents a parent education or parent-training intervention is likely to increase their array of techniques for managing child behavior (e.g., 'time out'), but not change the way they process information or resolve lingering childhood traumas. This creates risk that the parent will misuse the new tools – for example, using time out too frequently, threatening it but not following through, or, worst, using it for excessively long periods.

Another issue is screening for exclusion from service, as opposed to inclusion. That is, many services have inclusion criteria, e.g., certain symptoms or diagnoses, but lack exclusion criteria even when the inclusion criteria have been met. Usually, such criteria would have to do with multiple diagnoses or conditions where the additional problem rendered the service inappropriate. For example, one might have criteria for inclusion in a cognitive-behavioral therapy program for reducing anxiety. But if one did not screen out those anxious individuals who were also suicidal, one might risk both overlooking a serious and imminent threat and also augmenting it by appearing to offer hope and not fulfilling that hope.

In addition, lacking valid information on a person's self-protective strategy and style of information processing can mislead a psychotherapist into misdirecting the treatment. That is, having a symptom-based diagnosis does not indicate the Type A and Type C distinction. If the parent's violent acts, as well as the diagnosis, lead the therapist to assume an aggressively coercive pattern when, in fact, the parent uses a compulsively compliant strategy in a context of unresolved childhood trauma, depression, and sudden and unexpected intrusions of forbidden negative affect [ina]s, then anger management could become part of the treatment. This, unfortunately, would reinforce the compulsive compliant strategy, thus possibly making the individual *more* likely to have violent intrusions.

Depending upon the specific assessment and the number of assessments used, the cost can range from quite low (the CARE-Index) to fairly high (the TAAI and AAI). If this is viewed in the light of the human and financial cost of misdirecting psychotherapy or a poor choice regarding child placement, the upfront cost of good assessment is quite minimal.

Ongoing assessment following formal assessment

Although I have argued strongly against informal, clinical opinions about attachment as a basis for making decisions, it should be made very clear that any assessment (of anything, including attachment) is only a sample of behavior leading to a probabilistic hypothesis about the assessed individual's status. Therefore, it is highly appropriate that personnel working with the parent or family should continue to assess attachment, through informal observation as an ongoing part of service, after the formal assessment and functional formulation are complete.

Note

1 The usage 'strange situation test' is a misnomer; Strange Situation Procedure (SSP) is correct.

Chapter 18

Functional formulation and the plan for treatment

DMM formulations are the bridge between the problem and its potential solutions. They are the therapist's DR of the relation between the parent and the therapist.

Functional formulation

Defining functional formulations

DMM formulations are built on the ideas of systemic formulation, but contain a few differences. The most significant, the focus on the functions of protection and reproduction, leads to the use of the term 'functional formulation'. This highlights that it is the function of the behavior that is the central interest in understanding problematic or dangerous behavior. This *focuses* the process of examining information and generating explanations for behavior.

In addition, the DMM *structures* the process of gathering and organizing information in order to arrive at a functional formulation. Particular attention is paid to the sources of information and the possible biases that each source might have. This means that, for a user of the DMM, not only will the source person be noted with care, but also the form of the information (in terms of memory systems and possible transformations of information) will be treated as important information. Indeed, form is conceptualized as being at least as important as content. The notion is that the functional meaning will be contained in the form of the information in essentially *all* cases and that the form will match the content *only* in cases with high levels of both intrapersonal and interpersonal coherence. Because such cases rarely come to professional attention, form is treated as crucial information. Because form is much harder to discern in action, video can be crucial, especially for supervision of the therapist where what is recalled may differ substantially from all that occurred, particularly in the nonverbal form of the dialogue. When therapists report only verbally to their supervisor, the supervisor cannot be an independent source of information; he or she is constrained by the perception and biases of the therapist.

In order to keep sources of information clear and discrete, attachment theorists have constructed formal assessments to be applied and coded by people who do not know the history or presenting problem. Formal assessment and blind coding/classification permit (a) multiple DRs to be generated and compared, and (b) each DR to be evaluated in terms of its probable validity without contamination from other information. That is important because if, for example, the coder already knows that there is a charge of child sexual abuse or a diagnosis of schizophrenia, it will almost certainly bias the coder's attribution of meaning.

Although clinicians reading this might think, 'Oh, that's about research; it doesn't apply to me', this does apply to clinicians. If clinicians want to know more about their patients, they need a fresh mind that does not know the story. 'John' from Chapter 12 is an example. His therapist was working on the assumption that John's aggression indicated that he was using a Type C5, 7 strategy. If the therapist had coded the AAI, he might have found the aggressive *fuckin*'s and have been confirmed in his expectation. But I classified John as A4, 7. That not only presented the therapist with a discrepancy, but it also opened a new perspective, eventually changing the treatment in ways that engaged John more fully and, possibly, avoided the potential harm of guiding John to reinhibit his anger (as one might do if he used a Type C strategy).

A major point of agreement between systemic and functional formulations is the emphasis on including all family members in the assessment and the preference for obtaining their perspectives directly from each person, i.e., the source issue again. That is, it is explicitly presumed that each family member will have biased representations of both themselves and other family members and that this will be especially true in cases that come to professional attention. Having multiple sources of information, including each person's representations, other family members' representations, and the clinician's representation from direct interaction with each person, can facilitate generating a reasonably accurate picture. Of what? Of family members' strategies for self-protection and reproduction and the ways in which these fit together or clash. Having multiple perspectives on the same behavior clarifies where there are points of disagreement and conflict. These discrepancies are important because they are thought to mark places where not enough is known and this can suggest an opening for the intervention.

Further, a DMM functional formulation takes a strengths approach, assuming that people organize their behavior to solve problems as best they can (Lewontin 2001), given their maturity and conditions as they were perceived when the behavior was first organized. It is the 'conditions' (actual danger, important people, resources, etc.) and 'perceptions' (psychological processes) that are most obviously the focus of change. Developmental change is among the most important conditions because it continually changes the family by creating new psychological, behavioral, and strategic possibilities. When development leads to less adaptive strategies, one should consider how perceptions and attributions, both currently and, for adults, across the course of their childhood, may be biased. Reducing biases can become a goal for treatment.

Finally, functional formulations are systemic and holistic in assuming that the various aspects of functioning are interdependent such that changing any one affects all family members. An image that might elucidate this idea is that of a mobile composed of connected and suspended parts. Each part can move separately, but, when it does so, each affects all the others. This image makes clear how improbable stability in a family system is. Although one can't expect homeostasis in mobiles or families, it would be helpful if the process of change could be gentle, avoiding harmful disruptions or misunderstandings. With a good functional formulation, the therapist can predict, monitor and guide an evolving process of change.

To summarize, 'functional formulation' gathers all available information about past and current functioning (as well as foreseeing the next developmental steps) in order to state a concise hypothesis about how things are, how they came to be so, and what maintains them as they are, and, on the basis of all of that, to suggest what might promote change. That is, if good assessment connects past and present, good functional formulation addresses the adaptive quality of that relation and then points a way into the future. It is like a signpost at an intersection of family members' developmental pathways.

The components of a functional formulation

Assessment of attachment makes a crucial contribution to the functional formulation of individuals' adaptation, i.e., to their search for personal effectiveness (Bandura 1998). Nevertheless, it is insufficient to yield an adequate understanding of a person's behavior. In addition, one needs to assess at least the following:

The individual

1 biological adaptation (general health; acute and chronic pain; too much or too little sleep, food, exercise, etc.; genetic influences, biochemical imbalances that require change before other functions can change, etc.);

2 developmental history (the parents' childhood history, particularly exposure to danger, i.e., abuse, neglect, deception, separation, severe or excessive illnesses, bullying, triangulation, domestic conflict, etc.);

3 current context (again, danger is the issue: inadequate income, poor housing, limited access to or use of medical care, domestic violence, dangerous neighborhood, etc.);

4 current adaptation (i.e., the ways in which the various aspects of the parent's life function: marriage or other adult partnership, employment,

social life, extended family relationships, and, of course, the parent–child relationships for *all* the children in the family);

5 attachment in all important relationships (e.g., to parents, spouses/partners, and children) because it addresses, directly and with complexity and detail, information processing, self-protective strategy, and impediments to adaptation. This is crucial to how the parents organize their behavior with the child and defines what the treatment needs to address.

The therapist

6 the attachment history, strategy, and information processing of the therapist, defined in the same terms that are applied to patients or clients. As the guide to the therapeutic relationship, therapists should know themselves and what they have to offer;

7 the skills/training of the therapist, including limitations that might affect the treatment of the specific individual in question;

8 the parent–therapist relationship (to the extent that the parent does not feel the professional to be empathic, available, and competent, the parent may not be able to benefit from the service).

The context

9 the availability of ameliorative services (dysfunction will be greater when helpful services are not available).

Inclusion of supportive services, both in the parents' childhood and now, is important. Talisha reminds us that, without services to her mother when Talisha was a child being punished harshly, she has, of course, repeated the process. Why are we surprised?, she implies. These words of John put the point even more bluntly:

> *I just want the anger to stop ... and the voices to fuckin' stop and the ... thinking to stop. I just want some sort of medication to help me to stop ... just a quick fix if you like ... and I feel as though I'm not getting the help ... I don't think I'm getting the fuckin' help. I've been fuckin' ... been asking for help for years ... Jail doesn't work from me ... Jail does not work for fuckin' me! I am trying to do it differently, but the anger is still there, the resentments are still there, fuckin the hate.. and the hurt are still there. It spills up from childhood. I'm a 41-year-old fuckin' man now, for Christ sake, why am I still feeling things like this? Why do I still feel that I need to hurt people as well?*

When the services aren't appropriate and the danger is great, great suffering for both the parent and his children can ensue, leaving the parent to find his own solution. In John's case, he'd like treatment, but will accept drugs, and if we can provide neither, his choices might be reduced to getting his own drugs in his own way or risking continued harm to his children. Treatment that answers his question of why he feels and acts as he does and uses the answer to free him of the anger that he wishes to free himself from depends upon both a sound functional formulation of the problem and the resources to address it.

Putting it together

The process of putting the components of a functional formulation together is complex, demanding intelligence, experience and maturity from professionals. The complexity comes from the number of perspectives that need to be accounted for at one time and the challenge of understanding how they fit each person's developmental pathway up to now.

Inability to keep all components in mind at once will distort the professional's understanding and may result in skewed treatment that may not be helpful and could be harmful (just as biases and omissions distort parents' understanding of their children, resulting in inadequate parental behavior). If the professionals see only society's perspective, they will not be able to engage the parent (for example, Talisha). If they see only the parent's perspective, there will be no basis for change. To be maximally effective, professionals need to find a balance among all the perspectives that promotes safety and comfort. That is, Talisha's daughter needs us to protect both her body from her mother's blows and her opportunity to be raised lovingly by her mother. To enable that, we need to reach her mother, enabling her to feel safe enough with her therapist to explore the DRs (often memories from her own childhood) that motivate her excessively harsh punishment. It is almost impossible to hold both sets of needs in mind unless we truly understand that Talisha (and John ... and Kate and Andrea and ...) loves her children and means to protect them. If that knowledge enters the therapist's DR as compassion for all family members, then the probability of finding a pathway toward the shared goal of raising one's child in safety and comfort is increased. Without the varied tugs on our compass needle, we risk being pulled off course – in which case both parent and child will suffer.

Compassion is an elusive quality. It is not sympathy for a particular person or family. Sympathy can make it difficult to see conflicting needs or to impose unwanted change on a dangerous or endangered person or family. Compassion depends upon full awareness of both the experiences of each individual and their potential for growth and change. With compassion one can, like a good parent, hold all the needs and perspectives in mind, weigh them, and make the difficult choices that will ultimately benefit the whole family.

The roles of professionals

The DMM conceptualizes the role of professionals a bit differently than current family-systems therapy where the role is one of equality and nonknowing. In this 'nonknowing' role (Selvini-Palazolli *et al.* 1980), the family-systems therapists' contribution is being neutral and curious observers, from outside the family system, who can report on their observations to the family.

Being a transitional attachment figure, in DMM terms, the therapist is looked to as someone stronger and wiser, to use Bowlby's terms. That is, therapists are expected to be experts, but specifically experts on *how to do things*, as opposed to how the family members are. Consequently, family members retain their expertise regarding who they each are, what the problem is, and how they can work together. The therapist/transitional attachment figure 'earns' the right to join in the process by bringing expertise in knowing what information to seek, how to go about gathering it, alternate ways to express it, and how to frame the information in ways that clarify meanings rather than antagonizing others. In troubled families, these skills are very unusual and, therefore, very valued when the therapist demonstrates them by using them.

This leads to another aspect of the therapist's role. Therapists observe important aspects of individual and family functioning, but unlike teachers, they do not simply pass this knowledge to the family. Instead, their role is to enable the family members to discover it. They do this by creating situations that highlight the opportunity to notice and, as needed, pointing in the significant direction. The trick is for the therapist to stay in the individual's ZPD, i.e., to point where the individual is just ready to see. If the therapist stays attuned to the parent, there will be no need to tell. This is important because what is told might be forgotten, might be mistaken, and can never give the parent the delight and satisfaction that comes from discovery. If parents are ever to carry on reflecting on themselves, they must find this delight more powerful than their dismay at what they might observe or understand. Once this long-term goal is seen, short-term, 'right-answer' or instructional treatments can be seen to defeat long-term purposes.

When troubled individuals choose not to look or to distort what they see, they are indicating that what they expect to see will dismay them. Again, the role of the therapist as a transitional attachment figure is highlighted. In this role, the therapist has the compassion to foresee this, to soften the blow by laying a groundwork of human fallibility, to understand that both the Type A self-denigration and Type C self-aggrandizement leave space for the therapist to help the individual to find the laudatory aspects of him- or herself, and demonstrates an acceptance of that which hasn't quite been said yet, but is lying half-seen between them. That is, compassion for 'everything' is too general to be helpful. Compassion for what is already said is fine, but it doesn't affect the process of saying it. (Its absence might stifle the future process, however.) It is anticipatory compassion that is specific enough to be real and imprecise enough for the parent to give it precision that is most helpful in guiding the parent forward. This is the role of attachment figure as comforter.

Finally, the therapist/transitional attachment figure functions like a parent in helping each person to address a problem from which they can learn without being overwhelmed by the complexity of the entire problem.

In terms of functional formulation, the professional works with the family around the formulation, but may not reveal everything that seems important at one time. Instead, the professionals' formulation may exceed what one or another family member can manage and yet still be an important, or even essential, part of the overall formulation.

For example, John, from Chapter 12, had serious problems with violence and sexuality. His concern about violence brought him voluntarily to treatment. The AAI and, later, the functional formulation indicated that masculinity and sexuality were possibly greater and more basic issues. When these were suggested gently, John refuted them strongly. If the many issues around sexual abuse were true (which could not be known for certain), John was not ready to address them. Keeping them as questions in the therapist's mind, however, enabled him to work on building the necessary reflective skills while actively creating a therapeutic environment of sexual openness and curiosity (as opposed to morality and censure – which is what John had brought to therapy). The point is that the therapist functioned helpfully by finding the 'growing point' between knowing better than the client and knowing less than the client. He took an expert role, functioning in John's ZPD to assist John to examine his experience and functioning, but only John could know what had actually happened and how it might have mattered to him.

Adding meaning

A functional formulation, like an attachment classification, adds meaning to the set of information. The process of adding meaning requires that professionals attempt to understand reality from each family member's perspective, taking their developmental experience into account. Doing this in cases of parental inadequacy can be very difficult because understanding one person's perspective can feel like devaluing another's. That is, if one understands the abusive mother's experience and intentions, it can feel like overlooking the harm done to her children. For example, having empathy for Vanessa can feel like disregarding what she did to her twins. It takes very mature and compassionate professionals to be able to hold multiple, conflicting perspectives in mind at one time without implicitly valuing one person over another. This is especially true if each of the perspectives involves suffering and is yet more difficult if the legitimate needs of the individuals are in conflict. These features, suffering and conflicting legitimate needs, typify troubled families.

Donnie (from Chapter 11) is a case in point. She was in deep depression, having been seriously neglected as a child, then losing a child to death, followed by being left by her husband. All of this went unnoticed until the two younger children were identified as being neglected and placed in foster care, thus creating two more losses for Donnie. When child protection entered, they focused on the children's needs, not really thinking of Donnie as a woman with needs of her own. Protecting Donnie's children, by placing them in a foster home, increased Donnie's depression, thus making her less able to care adequately for her children. The problem was to reconcile the apparently conflicting needs of a parent and her children. Once the attachment assessments, carried out without knowledge of the case history, revealed Donnie's history and depression, it became possible to see the unifying aspects of the family situation. Donnie desperately needed her children, but was too depressed to care adequately for them. Her children needed their mother and a permanent home. Donnie, more than many people, was compulsive and obedient. Given specific safety advice, she would do as she was told. But she could not show affect or take chances if watched. Readjusting the treatment plan to meet Donnie's needs provided a way to meet her children's needs.

Compassion for children (of any age!) rarely harms others, whereas sympathy for one without having the perspective of the other in mind can harm everyone. My rule of thumb is that if there seems to be a 'bad guy', then we don't really understand the situation yet. For example, the aunt in the Blackstock case (Chapter 12) was clearly the 'bad guy', and the two boys were glorified for forgiving her. I would argue both that their forgiveness was premature (and within their old compulsive compliant strategy) and also not reflective of a mature understanding of their aunt's behavior. When the boys understood their own suffering and hers, both currently and growing up, then compassion would become possible. The change in understanding, in these two cases, began with believing that everyone wants to be safe, that all parents want their children and want them to be safe, and that all parents have strengths – if one knows how to tap them.

What maintains the inadequate behavior?

Once one understands how the family members function now and, historically, why the parents learned to behave as they do, it becomes important to understand what maintains the behavior in the current setting where it is harming the children. There are three likely causes of the inadequate parental behavior. One is that the current context is threatening and the parent's strategy is an adaptation to the threat. If this is the case, the threat needs to be identified and reduced or the parents need help in finding an effective alternate strategy to protect themselves and their children. Among the cases described in this book, at least the following were living in immediate danger: Candace, Maryia, Donnie, Monia, Albert's mother, Susan Smith (being left without a partner), Denise (spousal abuse), the aunt of the two caged boys (being beaten by her husband), Andrea Yates (being trapped with her children, having no control over her own reproduction), and Kate (losing her child, having no partner). It should be kept in mind that the services often pose a threat to families, and part of what professionals observe may be a reaction to the threat that they bring.

Another possible cause of parents continuing a childhood strategy in parenthood even when it becomes inappropriate and maladaptive for the children is biased information processing. Because the old strategy is biased in how the person perceives information, with 90 per cent of perception being memory (Gregory 1998), that bias may affect what the parent perceives now. If misperception, leading to outdated attributions of meaning, is motivating inappropriate behavior, then treatment needs to address information processing and strategy. Simply addressing strategy may not change behavior, because misperception will trigger the old one and not engage the new strategy. Among such cases in this book are the following: Luke's father, Nancy's parents, Vanessa, and John (intrusions tied to childhood trauma); Talisha and Nick's parents (beliefs about good parenting); David (use of a parenting reversal strategy); Denise, Maggie, Donnie, and Andrea Yates (depression, i.e., the belief they could do nothing to change things).

Third, maladaptive behavior may be maintained by other family members' behavior. Indeed, if the parent does change, family members may not perceive it. In that case, a dyadic or family level plan of intervention will be needed. Cases that fit this explanation, among those described in this volume, are the fewest: Gerd (disorientation and autism); Mary Brightman (family compulsiveness); Sophie, Kari, and Susan Smith (triangulation, cited only).

Given these conditions that maintain the inadequate parental behavior (and the conditions that caused it in the beginning), the issue becomes how one can efficiently change the situation. Addressing all of the parent's childhood problems will be slow, laborious, expensive and, possibly, ineffective. Dealing with each current problem may overwhelm the already stressed family.

Attachment and critical causes and case planning

Mary Ainsworth and I proposed that 'critical' causes were more important for intervention and treatment than discovering and addressing all the multiplicity of causes that affect behavior of family members (Crittenden and Ainsworth 1989). By 'critical cause', we meant the thing which, if changed, would initiate a cascade of changes that would ultimately resolve the most serious threats to family functioning. We suggested that 'attachment' was a critical cause of change. Today I would refine that by saying that distorted information processing (around danger and reproductive opportunity) is the critical cause of dysfunction. Correspondingly, opening information processing to awareness, balance of input information, reflection and integration can initiate a life process of improving adaptation.

If this is true, then there is no need for treatment to address or correct every problem, nor will it be beneficial to attempt that. Too many goals and too many professionals working toward the goals are likely to distract parents' attention, generate anxiety about performance and change, and obscure the critical aspects of the treatment. Especially when parents' family relationships are troubled, adding numerous professional relationships could be counterproductive. Similarly, when parents cannot already reflect and integrate, offering numerous interventions leaves parents with the not-yet-possible task of integrating what the professionals failed to integrate (see Crittenden 1992d). That is, the DMM idea is that instead of addressing multiple problems with multiple solutions and professionals, only essential issues should be addressed. Surely, current danger must be one of them, as must achieving a state of arousal that enables thought. When these are minimally achieved, the focus on the critical cause, information processing that yields explicitness, reflection, and integration, becomes possible.

Put another way, the hypothesis regarding the process of future change should be economical and organized around 'critical causes' (Crittenden and Ainsworth 1989). Learning to use one's mind more effectively, i.e., learning to (a) make the implicit explicit, (b) access both affect and cognition, and (c) reflect on and integrate all the information, has the power to change the individual's future long after the treatment is completed. Indeed, learning to use one's mind effectively can permit the treatment to be ended before the changes that were initially sought are fully achieved.

Chapter 19

Psychological treatment and information processing

In the DMM, treatment is the final step in an overlapping and recursive sequence of activities. Treatment follows referral, assessment and formulation and, at the same time, is part of them. If the central goal of treatment is to foster an adaptive process by changing the way information is processed, then the focus of treatment should be the nervous system particularly brain functions.

The brain is where biology, history, and the current context come together to shape behavior. The psychological operations that shape behavior are collectively called 'information processing'. Information processing enables individuals to behave in ways that increase the probability of their survival and that of their progeny or, alternatively, increase the risk of distress, injury or death. When behavior repeatedly increases risk or jeopardizes survival of oneself or one's progeny, the process is maladaptive and needs to change. If the individual cannot both discern this and also begin to make the necessary personal changes, then professional assistance may be needed or, in some cases, mandated.

Genes, neurological structures, environment and psychological disorder

The scientific cutting edge in the study of psychopathology is genetics and the cognitive neurosciences. Moreover, the most exciting and informative work is going on at the most basic levels of understanding. What is being found has the potential to change greatly how we think about and treat distressed humans, including those who become a danger to others.

Many people expect the new discoveries to be in the form of anomalous genes that *cause* particular disorders, especially the most serious and intractable disorders. Moreover, depending upon one's perspective, this expectation leads to feelings of doom or relief. The sense of doom is based on the belief that, if one has a gene that causes some particular disorder, one may be doomed to that disorder. The feeling of relief is tied to the notion that, if this is the case, then psychotherapists cannot be expected to cure what, up to now, they have not successfully cured. That is, if psychological disorder is genetically determined, psychotherapists can't be held responsible for changing it. On the other hand, this mistaken belief in genetic causation can have the unfortunate outcome of enabling families to think that children who are diagnosed with troublesome disorders have a genetic defect; i.e., the child is the source of the family's distress. Further, if the presumed cause is genetic, then each parent can accuse the other of responsibility for passing on that 'bad' gene. Family harmony and the child's relationship problems are not improved by these misapplications of genetics.

The search for pathology-producing genes has not, in general, fulfilled these expectations. Few genes have been discovered that differentiate samples with and without specific diagnoses, and, when such genes are found, the amount of variance accounted for is very small, with most people diagnosed with the disorder not having the gene in question. Moreover, to date, few if any of these genes have been shown to *cause* disorder. More generally, the scientific literature does not uniformly support the notion of genetic determinacy. For example, even in such a clear and classic case as phenylketonuria (PKU), the anomalous gene is necessary for the disorder, but so is the environmental contribution of phenylalanine in the diet. That is, the gene alone does not *cause* the disorder. In fact, genes simply encode directions for producing proteins. When that is accomplished and how the proteins function depend upon the environment.

This does not mean, however, that the study of genetics and neurology is irrelevant to treatment of individuals with psychological and behavior problems. Instead, I think it means that we should seek a different sort of contribution from these disciplines. Rather than seeking anomalies, we should be looking for a basic understanding of our universal human potential, asking what advantages there are to (a) various aspects of the human genome, (b) the biochemical processes that it generates, and (c) the neurological structures and psychological processes that mature across the first two to three decades of life. In addition, we should ask how these processes might have been adaptive during our evolution and under what conditions they might be adaptive now. This will highlight the psychological requirements for surviving an array of dangerous circumstances, both across our evolution as a species and across the vicissitudes of individual lives. When psychological processes are considered with reference to dangerous contexts, universal processes that enhance survival might be seen to produce both safe and dangerous affects on both psychological well-being and distress. Further, the central advantage of humans, compared with other species, might be our psychological and behavioral flexibility in the face of changing circumstances.

Genes, context and adaptation

We can't change the genetic complement of a person. If some of an individual's genes increase the probability of maladaptation or even cause a specific disorder, we must work within the context of those genes. Nevertheless, genes are much less determined in their function than they are often thought to be (Edelman 1989; Rutter 2006a; Rutter *et al.* 2006). Gene expression is affected by the context of other genes as well as by maturation and a hierarchy of environments from cellular to cultural (Lipton 2005). Moreover, work by a number of investigators in nonhuman species shows that the effect of genes on development and behavior is regulated by aspects of the environment, specifically those related to danger and reproductive opportunity (Diorio and Meany 2007). Moreover, these changes in the promoter regions of genes (that affect when genes are turned on and off and what effects genes have on the organism and its behavior) are both passed to future generations (without changing the genetic code itself) and can be reversed when the environment changes (Weaver *et al.* 2006). It is unlikely that such processes that permit a better fit of organism to context would exist solely in nonhuman species. For example, emerging data on suicide suggest the presence of similar markers in humans (Meaney 2008).

In our search for the genetic contributions to disorder (Ogren and Lombroso 2008), we have more often focused on anomalous than universal aspects of the human genome, although more sophisticated thinking is shifting toward gene–experience interactions (Rutter *et al.* 2006). One contribution of the DMM is to identify *universal* human processes that, in interaction with varied experience, can explain some maladapted or disordered behavior. That is, maladapted behavior could be associated with anomalous genes, anomalous genes interacting with specific everyday environments, or normative genes interacting with particular sorts of dangerous environments. The DMM focuses particularly on the latter two conditions, because psychological treatment can modify the environmental component.

Neurological structures

The human brain and its activity are probably more plastic than those of any other species. Both neurological structure (synapses) and neurological activity (neurotransmissions) are highly plastic; for example, synapses can come and go within the course of a day and neurotransmitter levels fluctuate in milliseconds. That does not imply infinite plasticity, but it does suggest that one advantage of a long period of maturation is that the effects of early experience can be modified.

Abuse, the intrusion of something dangerous, and neglect, the absence of something protective, are the two opposite forms of danger (Crittenden 1981). One effect of abuse in the early years is that the experience-expectant mechanisms of the overproduction of synapses followed by pruning of excess synapses that occurs in the second year of life could mold brain structure in ways that markedly reduce brain connectedness (Glaser 2000). Subsequent experience-dependent mechanisms may refine the area of applicability of the circuits. For example, repeated separation may change neural structures and accompanying neurotransmitters such that experience that would elicit neural activity in most individuals could lead to states of inactivity (i.e., neural depression) in formerly separated individuals (Post *et al.* 1998). As a consequence, integrative functioning would be reduced; this may be reflected in the DMM Type A compulsive patterns. An important question is the extent to which later maturing brain structures can compensate for this limitation. For example, could reflective functioning at the cortical level connect that which should have been connected at earlier processing levels with experience-dependent mechanisms?

In cases of neglect, many of the initial overabundance of synapses do not receive the input necessary for their continued existence; they wither away, leaving a paucity of neuronal networks. This may be reflected in those DMM depressed Type A patterns that lack an underlying compulsive organization. Rectification of the effects of neglect will depend on production of new synapses and their organization into neural networks. What we do not yet know is the extent to which the brain can readapt later and what conditions facilitate this readaptation (Perry *et al.* 1991).

Plasticity and change

Even though early brain organization is probably less flexible and open to change than later brain organization, the process leading to behavior can be modified. That is, peripheral/somatic, procedural and imaged networks can be expected to change slowly and slightly compared with semantic, verbal and episodic networks. Further, reflective and integrative processes both mature last and also are the most plastic. The crucial points are that:

1 The brain is always (re)organizing itself.
2 The process of organization is dependent upon communication both laterally within each system and vertically among systems.
3 Early organizations, especially those that have persisted in an unchanging context for a long time, can be expected to change less than later organizations, i.e., those that are verbal and integrative or developed in a more recent context (Schore 2000).

Because implicit processing operates more quickly than verbal and integrative processing, under conditions of threat we should expect a bias toward repeating responses that were first organized during childhood exposure to danger. Such effects are often labeled 'trauma responses'.

I'd like to suggest an alternative perspective. Adapting to danger early in life before the brain is fully mature magnifies the impact of early experience on brain development and functioning (Post and Weiss 1997). This is adaptive because it attunes the individual *to the dangers in that context*.

However, the costs of such early specialization can be (a) less sophisticated responses than could be organized after maturation had progressed further, and (b) reduced flexibility if the context changes. That is, there may be a trade-off between short-term adaptation, in the form of specialization of brain functioning around specific sorts of danger, and long-term adaptation around varied responses and the full range of possible contexts. Of course, if one does not survive in the short term, one need not worry about long-term adaptability. The unfortunate irony is that, for some people, this could mean that successful early adaptation to severe threat will interfere with long-term adaptation, including the survival of their children.

Adaptation and maladaptation

The point to be made is that what we call 'psychological disorder' may often result from specialized and protective information processing that is applied to an unsuitable context (Sameroff 2000) or used when more nuanced responses would have been more effective. If so, unless the individual's processing of information is expanded, behavior will continue to be maladaptive.

This framing of psychopathology moves away from (1) the reductionist perspective of psychological disorder, in which something (genes, chemicals, structure) is wrong, unhealthy or malfunctioning; (2) the ethical-legal perspective, in which the parent is choosing to behave immorally and harming the child for some unspecified reason that punishment must curtail; and (3) the newer educational perspective, in which the parent lacks knowledge or skills that can be taught in a didactic manner. It also highlights the importance of prevention and of differential treatment that reflects differing neurological processes.

Treatment

When I give talks, the information in this chapter is what most people want. In fact, I've been told, 'Don't tell us about disorders or development. We know all about that already. Just tell us what to do.' Quite clearly, I see treatment differently. I think framing the problem and its potential solutions is crucial to the success of the treatment. Moreover, the things one can do need to be done in a way that the parent can accept. That is, it's less the technique itself than the way it is used with respect to the parent(s) and the therapist. Still, without a judicious selection of techniques, the therapy may not be successful.

Treatment

I have left the term 'treatment' undefined intentionally so as to include all the processes that are used to relieve distress and change behavior. That includes, at a minimum, everything from spiritual and religious practices to psychoeducational treatment, counseling, short-term psychotherapies, long-term psychotherapies, psychoanalysis, and pharmacological treatments, both brief and ongoing. In every case, however, *the goal of treatment would be to change information processing in ways that promote adaptive and functional behavior, both in the current context and in contexts not yet experienced or even envisioned.*

If therapists had:

1 a clear understanding of the presenting situation;
2 an adequate assessment of information processing and strategic behavior (of both the therapist and patient/client);
3 a relationship in which the therapist functioned as a transitional attachment figure to the client/patient;
4 knowledge of the effects of various treatments on information processing and behavior,

then they should be in a position to chart a provisional plan for the treatment. If the plan was implemented in ways that provided feedback, i.e., continuous reassessment, then one might be able to make reasonably efficacious decisions about treatment and to modify them in a recursive process of multiple iterations. That is, every time something new was discovered or learned in treatment, the situation would be reviewed and a better-fitting plan developed. This might be termed a transactional or *dynamic* model of treatment.

Treatment planning

Why is it necessary to plan at all? Many psychotherapists to whom I have spoken believe that planning is undesirable because one cannot predict at the outset where a therapy will go. Moreover, they say, one should not even try, because having a plan risks constraining the therapy and losing potentially important opportunities. Finally, almost everyone says they just don't have time for this.

They don't have time to make judicious treatment decisions? They prefer to plow ahead with whatever treatment, assuming that something, anything, is better than nothing? I hope my dentist doesn't start drilling without a plan, and, for sure, I want him to think about the plan, have a back-up plan, and be ready to change the plan when new information makes the original plan a poor choice. I want my dentist to *think* before he drills, even knowing that doing so takes time.

I include planning for mental-health treatment because I think it is necessary to strike a balance between all encompassing, nondirected or free-wheeling therapy and predefined, narrowly construed or solution-constrained therapy. Moreover, I think attention to discrepancy is crucial to solving problems. Because plans that are reviewed highlight discrepancies, they promote wise selection of treatments.

Knowing where one is going is crucial to getting there. Without a plan, one risks either wandering through topics and processes that are not necessary or overlooking crucial issues. Put another way, one risks being sidetracked or never finding the track at all. It's like the joke about the drunk searching in the gutter under a streetlight. A passerby asks what he is doing. The drunk answers that he's looking for his car keys. 'Did you lose them here?' 'No, but this is where the light is.' Without a plan, we may focus on (a) what parents are prepared to talk about, never noticing that they lost their way around the unspeakable topics, or (b) what the therapist is prepared to offer, never noticing that it throws no light on the parent's problem.

Even if the therapist isn't so easily misled, without a plan one hasn't any way of judging one's progress in the treatment or even of saying when the goals of treatment have been met. For example, treatment might be discontinued when the 12 lessons of the program have been completed. Or when the parents report that they are feeling better. Or when the money/approval for service runs out. But these events do not necessarily indicate that the job is complete. Alternatively, the treatment might continue much longer than is needed.

A plan keeps the focus on the goal clear. Again, the DMM aims for balance: Neither too precise/concrete a goal (e.g., getting rid of a specific symptom) nor too general/indefinite a goal (e.g., sound mental health). The DMM keeps the goal (i.e., of information processing that promotes increased safety and successful reproduction) in clear view. A plan permits parent and therapist to evaluate whether they are making progress toward the goal.

Basic principles of treatment planning

Once one has experienced the initial relationship between parent and therapist, performed an adequate assessment, and derived a functional formulation, one can address how to structure the treatment. As said before, safety is the first issue. If danger is imminent, it must be addressed even before the assessment is complete. Beyond that, the extent of danger, particularly danger that is generated by the parent, will affect how extensive a treatment will be envisioned. This leads directly to the issue of information processing. Distortions of information processing can occur at many levels from peripheral/somatic to cortical integration. Knowing which levels were disrupted might be helpful in focusing the treatment in terms of order, duration, techniques, and individualization. Beginning with the least extensive implications and going toward the greatest, these are lack of or distortions of

1 reflective and integrative processes;
2 explicit processes (semantic, connotative and episodic memory);
3 implicit processes (procedural and imaged memory);

4 peripheral processes (both sensory input to the brain about the state of the body and organic/muscular responses of the body to the state of the mind).

In addition, bias toward cognition or affect in each of these processes is relevant to which treatment strategies might be useful. Finally, when strategies are nonstrategic (i.e., unresolved trauma or loss, depression, intrusions, disorientation and reorganization), this should be addressed in the plan.

Treatment planning is carried out *during* the treatment and, like assessment, is ongoing. It uses incoming information in an integrative way to generate reorientations of the treatment toward its goal;[1] it is the therapist's integrative process of successive approximation. I can almost hear a chorus of family systems and psychoanalytic therapists calling out, 'But we do that!' My response would be, is it articulated verbally? Written down? Consulted some weeks later to see how the treatment is going and whether the direction taken matches the direction charted? Are discrepancies highlighted and used to consider whether to continue as is or to shift direction a bit? If the answers are 'yes', then, indeed, you do that and we agree on the importance of doing it.

On the other hand, the planning that I am suggesting is different from stating a hypothesis and testing it without redirection during the testing process. This is what randomized controlled tests (RCTs) do. RCTs are behind most of the 'evidence base' of treatment efficacy. But as many people have noted, this is not 'real-world' treatment. Nor should it be – if therapists are less than all-knowing gods who can predict the future, if the people seeking treatment are uniquely variable, or if successful treatment increases individuals' sense of agency in their own lives. If real-world conditions pertain and personal agency is a goal, then treatment planning really needs to become a *process* that fits the formulation to the treatment in a series of successive readjustments based on feedback from action taken.

Changing information processing

Knowing how to modify information processing to increase flexibility and adaptability depends upon knowing the effects of various therapeutic techniques on brain functioning. Some of the needed information exists now, particularly for drug therapies. Some of the rest can be hypothesized with relative confidence. Some is simply unknown at present and will need a systematic program of research to clarify how various treatments affect the processing of information. Consequently, the discussion of information processing and maladaptation (Parts 1 and 2) is on firmer empirical ground (albeit far from definitive) than that of selecting appropriate treatments.

The ideas that follow go beyond the database of empirical evidence as it exists today. In many ways, this chapter is better construed as a proposal for a program of research, together with a few examples of hypotheses. The program is built around the notion that changing information processing in an interpersonal context requires (1) a working relationship between the persons and (2) tools for changing DRs.

The therapist as a secure base

It has become common to think of therapists as being a secure base for their patients. The DMM perspective is more complex. When the therapist functions as a transitional attachment figure, both the therapist and the patient contribute to their relationship. The patient's motivation for initiating the relationship is usually tied to reducing something painful. The therapist's motivation is less clear and probably differs from one therapist to another. Nevertheless, the nonverbal subscript of their communication will communicate each person's understanding of the relationship. The question is whether and how these can be made compatible.

The central issue to the patient is safety. To the patient, therapy is like uncovering a gravel-filled wound and allowing someone else to assist in digging the gravel out. Even if one knows that it is necessary, one cannot feel safe or comfortable during the process. Leaving the metaphor aside, I think psychological security in therapy (or any relationship) is impossible until one has come to feel safe and comfortable with knowing oneself. For a child, this is easy if their attachment figure has always treated them as valued and loved; they see and feel what the mirror has shown. For patients, however, this was hardly ever the case. However much their parents actually loved them, patients felt unloved and, at least at times, without value. This makes participating in a reciprocal process of change around revealing negative aspects of self very anxiety eliciting. Put in the opposite form, if the parent could use another person as a secure base, he or she probably would not need psychotherapy. For the therapist, this means (a) being aware that, much as they consider themselves safe and helpful, this is rarely the patient's perspective, and (b) knowing enough about the patient to avoid evoking the patient's self-protective strategies unintentionally. This is especially true if the patient is a parent and if the topics under discussion are tied to the harm the parent inflicted upon their child.

Consequently, a therapist can make him- or herself available as a secure base and can behave as a sensitively responsive attachment figure should, but actually feeling secure is the patient's contribution. Thus, the connection between the therapist and the patient is the therapist's willingness to become a secure base and the patient's desire for one. In other words, becoming a 'secure base' might be a goal in therapy, but it is a distant one in most cases. Instead, therapy is about making that transition.

If that is accurate, the issue becomes whether the therapist can tolerate not being accepted as a secure base. The challenge is to remain available as a possible secure base even while the patient repeatedly fails to reciprocate that understanding of the relationship. Depending upon the therapist's motivation for being a therapist, this may or may not be comfortable or even possible. However, if the therapist fails to acknowledge and accept the patient's wariness, the relationship with the patient must necessarily be misattuned and become even more anxious.

Managing this complex attunement requires sensitive responsiveness on the part of the therapist. For example, in the transitional attachment function, the therapist would need to show genuine feeling, including especially comfort, but display it in a manner that can be corrective for the parent. That is, for parents using a Type A strategy, the therapist might model expressing feeling, especially negative feeling, whereas for parents using a Type C strategy, the therapist might model containing and transforming negative affect to language (in both cases, in the patient's ZPD). When it becomes possible for the therapist to become spontaneous with the patient in the normal way, as opposed to thoughtfully organizing to meet the patient's strategic needs, then one might imagine that the patient is now secure – and the therapist is no longer needed as a transitional attachment figure. Ironically, at the point when the patient's understanding of the relationship matches the therapist's, the relationship may be concluded.

Therapeutic tools

Almost nothing is known, in an empirical sense, about how to change DRs and the information processing that produces them. I propose, however, that *all* our treatments function to change information processing (or they fail). The task at hand is to discover *how* they function and *in what way* they change information processing. If we knew that, we would be able to select treatment strategies and techniques in a more informed manner than we can today.

The point is that, for parents who endanger their children, assessment, formulation and the relationship with the therapist are so crucial that discussion of technique without these other issues risks being more harmful than helpful. Having a set of techniques in the absence of good assessment and formulation and a comfortable relationship with the parent is like handing out weapons and hoping for the best. Too many professionals want to be told what to do, in a talk or a book. Unfortunately, the adviser (person or book) cannot know enough about the specific parent in the therapist's mind to be able to shape the information dynamically to the precise situation. Generalized information applied specifically may backfire by leading the parent to feel that they are not seen or heard as an individual.

What professionals need

My work with professionals suggests that many are as desperate for something that works as are endangering parents. Like such parents, they know that what they offer is often ineffective, and I think that many wonder whether at times they haven't been harmful. The data confirm the accuracy of these concerns. At present, however, we lack the solution.

Nevertheless, even if we had it, it would not be a recipe for treating this disorder or that disorder. Indeed, treating 'disorders' is not the goal. To the contrary, we seek to treat people who suffer from psychological distress and use strategies that no longer fit their circumstances. That is, the DMM does not define people by their disabilities, but rather sees their intentions and imagines their potential for change. Once the goal is stated that way, it becomes obvious that each person, each relationship between person and therapist, and each process of discovery is unique. Nevertheless, knowing how treatment techniques affect information processing would open the process of constructing treatment to shared intellectual inquiry and precise description.

Good assessment, good formulation and good therapeutic relationships are within conceptual reach, but beyond what most health systems can afford. Instead, the field is looking for the silver bullet, the quick, easy and inexpensive tool that will solve mental health problems that have taken years, sometimes generations, to develop. Resolution of the complexities that resulted in dangerous parenting (regardless of whether the danger arises from action, inaction or misdirected action) is unlikely to follow from simple or brief interventions. Nor will the process be the same for everyone (which is why good assessment and formulation are crucial).

In the next chapter, some ideas about how therapeutic techniques might be used in the process of psychological treatment are offered. Because we lack data on the precise effects on brain functioning of our many treatment techniques, therapists must continue to use theory, experience-informed intuition and feedback to guide their selections. DMM theory regarding information processing can suggest the likely effect of the techniques (i.e., a hypothesized effect). Experience-informed intuition draws upon a store of cases (both directly experienced cases and those gleaned from expert sources such as texts, journals, and this book) to compare the current case to exemplars. Feedback permits case-by-case, week-by-week, evaluation of the fit of hypothesis to reality. It permits immediate modification of the plan and the means of implementing the plan to bridge more effectively the gap between the functional formulation and the goals of the treatment. Three cases that differ greatly in the information processing of the client/patient are offered to illustrate this process.

Note

1 This is similar to Bowlby's original concept of 'goal corrected partnerships', as opposed to 'goal directed cooperation'. The goal is continually being adjusted in the parent-therapist partnership (Bowlby 1969/1982, 1973).

Chapter 20

Psychological treatment: Three cases

Three cases are described to illustrate how the principles offered might play out in reality. The cases offer a range of parenting problems:

1 mild parenting difficulties during a period of developmental change (normative parenting; the Shoemaker family);
2 moderate parenting problems (parenting cluster 3; Justin);
3 severe life-threatening problems across the lifespan (parenting cluster 5; Kate).

In reading these cases, it should be kept in mind that the first is offered descriptively, based on the therapist's observations. If the therapist offers an internally coherent story based on inaccurate observations, we will find it difficult to discern the error or to think differently from the therapist.[1] Thus, the first case which lacks transcribed discourse, feels very convincing but denies the reader untransformed evidence such as is provided for the second and third cases.

In cases 2 and 3, actual transcribed discourse is offered, together with my analysis of the discourse (using the DMM method of discourse analysis). This permits readers to evaluate its meaning themselves. The use of discourse analysis highlights the importance of detailed work to identify psychological discrepancy. For example, Justin's content is highly coherent and socially acceptable; it is easy to approve of what he says and, without discourse analysis, we could easily agree with him and think that the treatment had been highly successful. The discourse analysis casts doubt on that.

Discourse analysis also emphasizes the general point in DMM theory that discrepancy which the speaker does not perceive marks cases of serious psychological and behavioral problems in a way that is not seen in mild cases. That is, the first case, the Shoemakers, displays much less discrepancy between the content and form of what is said than the second and third cases (Justin and Kate, respectively). We begin with the Shoemaker family.

Mild and transient dysfunction (normal parenting)

Mr Shoemaker had called the center, saying he needed an appointment for his adolescent daughter who was having problems at school (dropping grades, cutting classes, forging her parents' signatures, and hanging out with undesirable kids) and at home (where she was sullen and withdrawn or, conversely, absent for hours at a time without telling her parents where she was, nor when she would return). Mr Shoemaker seemed both angry and concerned and, most of all, he was urgent: he needed this appointment now and he guaranteed his daughter would be there. An appointment was set for the next week, in the evening so that Mr Shoemaker could attend without lost time at work. The entire family was to attend. Mr Shoemaker objected, especially to bringing his son, who, he said, was doing just fine, and he didn't want him 'getting any notions'. The offer was repeated firmly: to be helpful, we need to see everyone, next week, 7 pm. The Shoemaker family came.

In the initial meeting, Mr Shoemaker took the floor, listing the many complaints he had about Barbara, his 13-year-old daughter. While he explained the situation, his wife looked at him supportively, nodding in rhythm to his speech, and occasionally glancing at their daughter to ascertain whether she had gotten the message. She had. Barbara sat slumped in her seat, shoulders thrown forward and head down; there was a certain belligerence to her position combined with her expectation that there was nothing in this for her. She didn't say a word, but everything about her hissed her rejection of her father's story. Kevin just fidgeted and tried not to look at anyone. By the end of the appointment, Mr Shoemaker had made his and his wife's position clear. Barbara had declined to put her thoughts in words, but her refusal to accept her parents' summation was equally clear. The battle lines were drawn and the basis for Mr Shoemaker's concern about his daughter's activities away from home seemed more than justified. Kevin, at 10 years old, loomed as the next problem.

The therapist first needed to assign the family to a level of family functioning (LFF) (Box 17.1); this determination would affect what sort of assessment was offered. The presenting problem suggested predelinquency, but it had not been preceded by a history of escalating problems. Mr Shoemaker had sought service himself, based on the problems at home and contact from the school about his daughter's truancy. It appeared that Mr Shoemaker was able to use the discrepancy between his image of his family as well functioning and the evidence of problems to initiate a problem-solving process, i.e., LFF scale 1 or 2 ('independent and adequate' or 'vulnerable to crisis'). Further, the family was middle class and financially independent, and, except for their daughter's absence from school and home, everyone was safe. In information-processing terms, Mr Shoemaker spoke in prescriptive semantic statements about what his daughter should do, with episodic evidence to back up his claims. The school's concern supported at least the gist of his concerns, and his daughter did not deny the substance of what he said even though her silence and body language suggested that she might have told the story differently. Finally, Mr Shoemaker spoke connotatively with strong tones, sharp sentence structure (short declarative phrases), and powerful words (the negative descriptors with which he described his daughter's behavior). In addition, however, he compared Barbara's current behavior with the sweet and loving daughter she had been up to about a year ago. In information-processing terms, all the explicit memory systems were functioning, including at least some reflective capacity; however, it came packaged in negative affect which detracted from its effectiveness. Mr Shoemaker appeared to be using a Type C1 strategy. Taken together, this brief assessment suggested on the gradient of interventions (GI) (Box 17.2) that parent education or counseling services would be appropriate and probably sufficient.

And Mrs Shoemaker? She agreed with her husband, as a nice C2 wife would. For Barbara, it was a bit different. She was the image of resentment and seemed to be without words. At 13, she should have been able to articulate her position and to begin to gather an array of similar situations and draw some more general conclusions about herself and the problem. She should even have been ready to consider her parents' perspective. None of that was evident. If this family used a low and normative Type C strategy, Barbara appeared ready to escalate that to something higher. Nor for that matter was it clear that her father could articulate anything about her perspective or even the need for her perspective to be articulated. Kevin didn't care; none of this was his business and being present seemed to make him anxious. Barbara was the sore point; she needed to be able to imagine that the intervention was *for* her and not to fix her. Kevin, on the other hand, needed to see that problems were rarely located in, or resolved by, one person; he also needed to be included in this crucial developmental transition in his family.

The initial functional formulation was of a paternal family structure that had operated well enough while the children were young, but which was failing to meet the daughter's needs at the beginning of adolescence. The groundwork for goal-corrected problem-solving needs to mature along with the family members' aging. The daughter's inability to articulate her perspective combined with her father's maintenance of his 'strong protector of the family' role (that had worked in childhood) had thrown the family out of balance, affecting everyone's functioning. This was a ZPD problem in which failure to communicate in mutually satisfactory terms was creating dyssynchrony and risk, especially for the daughter. The family was temporarily assigned to LFF 2 with probable integrative capacity and, therefore, a readiness for parent education or counseling services (Box 17.1). All of this suggested that a full evaluation was unnecessary. Because there was no imminent danger, if our brief evaluation proved insufficient later, we could administer AAIs and a TAAI then. In the meantime, we would remain observant, ready to modify our practice as events unfolded in a transactional process with the family.

Only one issue was in question and that was the daughter's readiness. She had not spoken in the family context. The therapist chose to meet with Barbara alone for the next meeting. That pleased Mr Shoemaker – he knew where the problem was. Whatever pleased him pleased his wife.

The meeting with Barbara confirmed the initial functional formulation: this was a developmental crisis at the onset of adolescence. Barbara felt overcontrolled: her father had a rule for everything, he poked his nose into her business, only her friends understood her, her parents simply couldn't, there was no point in talking to them – she was always wrong anyway. Her mother? What's the point? She talked gently enough, but, no matter what she said, she went with Barbara's father. Underneath this 'who cares' exterior, displayed only in her slumped position and her sad eyes, was Barbara's need to be cared for, her feeling of loss as she made this transition from sweet little girl to young woman. Did Barbara feel underprotected around the new adolescent issues? The therapist explored that a bit. How was she managing puberty? Did her mother understand and assist her? Her mother had prepared a little package of information and materials and the necessary hygienic supplies were always available, but Barbara thought her mother was too embarrassed to talk about it; the school program on sexuality was clearer.

The third meeting was scheduled for the whole family, to give them feedback. Puberty had required new strategies and they hadn't been found. Nevertheless, it was clear that both parents meant well. They had the competency to make the changes, but hadn't understood what was needed. Barbara hadn't known how to tell them what she needed and no longer needed, and she hadn't understood that, to have her freedom, she needed to reassure her parents that she would behave safely, especially around sexuality. It was the preoperational shift (from infancy to the preschool years) come again, only this time, instead of taking authority, her parents needed to cede authority to their daughter while shifting in their protective role to one of being available for listening and advising around the challenges that Barbara felt. Put another way, Barbara needed to know that her parents were available as a protective resource to her, but also needed to understand that to enlist that protection she had to communicate in language. Framed that way, two things were needed: communication in Barbara and her parents' ZPD (keeping in mind that parents too must grow into their role) and restructuring of the family relationships to give Barbara's mother more authority and a direct woman-to-woman relationship with Barbara.

This third meeting was crucial. In an unusual move, the meeting was scheduled for the family's home. This looked like a very brief treatment process, so the transfer of learning from therapy room to real life needed to begin as quickly as possible. The agenda, from the therapist's perspective, was to enable the family to see themselves in ways that would yield the functional formulation without the therapist having to announce it.

They met in the family's living room, with the therapist taking the offered seat, the parents sitting together on the sofa and Barbara pulling up a dining-room chair because there weren't enough seats with the therapist there. The therapist's seat appeared to be the father's habitual seat, i.e., the best in the house. The therapist began neutrally, 'How has it been ...?' As expected, Mr Shoemaker answered for everyone, and his wife concurred. Kevin fidgeted and Barbara withdrew. The therapist began with Kevin, with a little joke and an assignment: 'Kevin, you seem to be the only one not caught up in this mess! But I bet you see and hear a lot.' Kevin nodded with a covert little grin. Then came the bait: 'I'd like you to be the official family observer. You watch and observe. I want you to keep track of what's going on and to signal, like this, when you think things might be getting too hot.'

This might seem off-center at first, but it functioned to give Kevin a meaningful role, i.e., an evident reason to be part of the sessions, and concurrently, it announced his actual role. He was next in line for adolescence; what he saw with his sister would shape how he approached this change for himself. We might as well get him and his family focused on this thus maximizing the impact of our treatment.

Next came the central issue, Barbara. How could the therapist get the parents (and Kevin) to see that she was isolated and speechless? The therapist chose to focus first on comfort, but if that didn't work, there were other approaches. 'Kevin, you look comfortable now and set up in business. Mr and Mrs Shoemaker, are you comfortable together on the sofa?' ... It was both a question and a long pause that expected an observation on their part. If they noticed that Barbara was isolated and in the uncomfortable chair, we'd move to addressing Barbara's discomfort. If not, possibly the official observer should be asked what he saw. Alternatively, Barbara might be asked directly, and, depending upon the fullness of her answer, the therapist would assist or move directly to the point: 'I'd like to try having someone join you. Kevin is busy. Could one of your parents join you for just a moment to see whether we can understand your perspective a bit better?'

The therapist's intended goal was to get Barbara's mother aligned with her daughter around articulating her daughter's perspective. If this happened, the mother's consultant role could be highlighted as well as the structural shift within the family subsystems. But if her father ended up offering or being invited, the notion of fathers being protective by taking other perspectives and fostering a daughter's femininity could be emphasized. Either way, the goal was to enable the parents to see Barbara's isolation and silence and to find ways to reduce it, i.e., to conceptualize their executive role as using their strength to foster inclusion and communication.

The final goal was using Barbara's communication to set up a process of negotiation around an adolescent's need for freedom and her parents' need to be assured their daughter was safe. Once that was accomplished, it should be a slam-dunk for Barbara to promise to give that assurance in a meaningful way and for her parents to offer the trust she sought – and for each parent to find a way to ally with her around the process of becoming a young woman. Depending upon how it went, maybe an assignment to practice a simple negotiation and report back would be needed. Maybe a little role-play. Or possibly, just the statement of the need and wishing them a good night. Only in the moment, looking at the family members, reading the consistency between their nonverbal and verbal communication (the issue of the *form* of the communication versus the content), and making that on-the-spot, experience-informed intuitive judgment could the selection of one of these possibilities – or another – be made. The process, however, was far from a play-it-by-ear, blindly intuitive one. Communication, realliance among family members, and negotiation skills remained the focus.

As it turned out, there was only one more meeting. It occurred two weeks later. The family was relaxed. Mom and Barbara had the sofa, Kevin had the dining-room chair, Dad held the floor from his own chair, and the therapist had the second best. Dad opened the meeting, summed up what they each had done, and praised Barbara for talking, for her schoolwork, for her 'attitude'. Then he asked her for her perspective! She glanced at her mom, who nodded reassuringly, and she told her story. She got off-track, however, talking about her friends and how much she wanted to go to the party this Friday night.... Her father looked a bit exasperated, then came back with a comment to the therapist that Barbara could hardly keep her mind on school since this invitation had come, but he understood, he remembered. And his voice softened as he remembered. He closed his bit by saying he just wanted to know where she was going and that the friend's parents would be there.... Barbara half-brushed him off, but in fact she looked reassured that he cared and would let her go. They were talking and the therapy was done.

The Shoemaker case highlights important issues. One is the difference between appearance and reality. It certainly looked as though Barbara was the source of the problem and it would be possible to overlook the interpersonal and family issues and focus individual treatment on 'fixing'

Barbara. Another is the importance of keeping an eye on critical issues and not getting distracted by presenting problems. This case could have been construed as predelinquent. Instead, putting it in a developmental framework kept it normal – as it was. The LFF scale and GI focused us on family members' strengths, demonstrating that they were enough to justify omitting a full assessment. In fact, had the therapist focused on dysfunction and offered therapy to Barbara, the situation might have escalated to her actually becoming a problem and the family both concurring and not finding their role in resolving family problems.

That is, too much treatment might not only be a waste of resources, but also harmful. Although I have characterized therapists as functioning in a transitional attachment role, in the Shoemaker family, the parents were functioning attachment figures both to their children and to each other; their functioning could be improved, but they did not need to be replaced, and the therapist was careful to work through them and to strengthen them. Including Kevin was important; it reduced the focus on dysfunction while also reducing the risk that he would face similar problems. It capitalized on observational learning.

Puberty had changed the meaning of safety for both Barbara and her parents, but instead of reconsidering their relationships, they dug in their heels and clung to the strategies that had worked well in the past. In the face of new threats from Barbara's sexual maturing, Mr Shoemaker became more authoritarian. As a consequence, Barbara felt more constrained exactly when she had expected more freedom. However, with the lack of a history of danger and interpersonal failures, very simple focused changes enabled everyone to discover the means to new and satisfying roles. The means? Communication. Open and direct communication of their intentions and feelings. Enhancing clear communication was a simple critical cause of change in the ZPD of Barbara *and* her parents. And, yes, they did live happily ever after.

In this case, as with the others that will be described here, I have used information processing as my primary criterion for deciding what sorts of treatment strategies are appropriate and for suggesting a progressive approach to treatment. Basically, I have suggested that if sensory input and somatic functioning are adequate, one can move to considering preconscious procedures and images. If these are reflected accurately in words, then semantic, connotative and episodic functions can be addressed. If these are represented with reasonable accuracy, then reflective and integrative functioning can be addressed. The members of the Shoemaker family were healthy. Moreover, they could describe their behavior in ways that closely matched what they did procedurally and the imaged information they used. Indeed, their connotative and semantic DRs were congruent and they could supply episodes to support their generalizations. They were ready for reflective and integrative work and, indeed, the parents already knew how to do this. What was needed was clearer communication about the changes that puberty had created. They could have made it with a didactic parenting course that supplied the missing information about puberty from adult and adolescent perspectives. However, by focusing on communication as a 'critical cause', the treatment gave the Shoemakers the tools with which to sort out other changes in the future without having to return to treatment.

Moderately severe dysfunction (cluster 3)

The second case is more serious. It is the case of a released sexual offender who had served his sentence and was understood to be doing well. Justin had had an extremely lonely and isolated childhood, so without affection that, after discovery of his sexual abuse of children, he had said he would *'have loved to be touched like that'*. After charges were placed and before going to trial, Justin had voluntarily sought treatment for the explicitly stated purpose of the therapist's being able to report favorably on Justin's effort to change to the court. In his report, the therapist had indicated that he thought Jason had been making strides in understanding himself, his inner motivations, and his inappropriate, sexualized behavior with children. He also stated that he thought that prison would be detrimental to Justin's psychological state. Following Justin's release, the therapist had occasion to meet with Justin. This followed both the experience of imprisonment and the group-based, recidivism-prevention treatment offered in prison. The dialogue that we have occurred when Justin returned to his therapist after release from prison.

I wouldn't want to repeat going inside, but I also wouldn't want to miss it. At least in prison you know exactly where you stand all the time. If they didn't like something I did, they gave me an immediate reaction so I became more careful in how I spoke to and approached people.

I have to wonder whether Justin used a Type A strategy that prison structure and treatment reinforced. I see the temporal contingencies (if/ then contingencies), the use of feedback, the distancing of self ('you'), the need for vigilance to inhibit 'bad' responses. But where are his negative feelings? Where is his desire for comfort and understanding? Where is his fear of being all alone – the fear that may have driven him to children? I am left wondering whether treatment has helped him or whether it might have increased the very needs that he cannot address.

Later he said:

Because I'd always felt so small, I had no idea until that moment that I actually had any power at all. ... You are literally naked, with strip searches as the outer symbol. Unlike my life at home, in prison nothing was too terrible to speak about and I learnt how to talk about what mattered. This means that now if I ever thought I was about to abuse a child, I'd be able to let someone know and stop myself.

Reading this through DMM discourse analysis and recognizing a history that I now associate with some sexual offending, I wonder whether Justin didn't replace his own feeling of being small with others' perception of his power, thus replacing a true vulnerable self with a borrowed 'bad' self. If so, he would now have less access to his actual motivations than before treatment. I wonder at the image of nakedness, something imposed on 'you'. Then I hear the borrowed mantra of what to do if he was about to 'abuse' a child. Do offenders, at the moment of abuse, think about using their 'power' to 'abuse'? Is this their language or ours? Is this their motivation or is some other desire organizing their behavior? If the actual motivation is different, what is it and how is it known; i.e., which of Justin's various DRs regulates his 'abusive' behavior? In Justin's case, he stated that he thought the work on 'grooming' and 'victim empathy' was unrelated to him, but because he was in prison, he *'played the game'* and tried to pass the 'treatment task' so he would be released. I doubt that Justin was motivated by a feeling of 'power' or a desire to 'abuse'. I think these words, borrowed from his treatment program, have moved us – and him – *further away* from his actual motivations, thus making it *less* likely that we will understand and he will be able to stop himself. Finally, I am concerned that, following treatment in prison, Justin believes that he alone caused his inappropriately sexual behavior. Were there no signals from the children? If there are children who use coy behavior, who lean in too close, or who sit with open legs that display their underwear, then there are signals in the real world of children that some men, men like Justin, might interpret as being sexual signals. Justin seems unaware that his behavior might be instigated by actual perceptions that were followed by misattributions of meaning. I think that Justin cannot be safe until he is consciously aware of the signals and able to change his attributions.

Later he said that, before being in prison, he had felt unloved, but because he had received lots of letters while in prison:

Now I know that [I am loved by my friends] in my heart and this gives me a tremendous motivation to stay on the straight and narrow so as not to put those friendships at risk.

This discourse presents several problems. Turning to friends (actually friends' *letters*) for love is very distancing and holds an A5 quality of turning to distant people for affection without there being a loving relationship between them. Further he is using the perspectives of other people to organize his behavior; this is very Type A and involves (again) a loss of true self.

When others praise him, Justin turns the praise away saying:

I'm awfully sorry but I did ... There were boys who were very much victims and I regret what happened.

The components of apologizing (twice), focusing on the victims' perspective, maintaining a narrative of self-identity that is defined by sexually inappropriate acts, and his overriding failure as a human (such that he believes he must stay away from everyone under 18) are consistent with a Type A strategy. Possibly we have not understood that he was once an uncomforted and shamed child using a Type A strategy. Maybe we have not understood that he relies on powerful people to tell him semantically what he should think and that, when he takes their thoughts and borrows their words, he loses even more of his own perspective and his unspeakable need for comfort increases. If need for comfort, repeated victimization in childhood, and feeling powerless to cope with adult relationships, all organized in a Type A strategy, were part of the motivational state that led to his sexual behavior with children, then our use of prison and manualized treatments that focus on (a) taking responsibility for the acts, (b) focusing on the victims' perspective, and (c) isolating the self from normal people, may have *increased* the probability that this man, and others like him, will reoffend.

Treatment of sexual offenders

If this story points to places where current practice falls short of meeting our goals, what should we have done or what could we do with other, similar men? For sure, an alternate approach would begin with careful assessment of information processing and strategy, e.g., an AAI. If we did that well, we would have managed three things at once:

1 establishing an empathic, listening relationship in which relevant questions were posed, but only the speaker held the answers;
2 gathering the sort of life details that are absent from the usual intake protocol but which generate a bond of shared knowledge between speaker and listener;
3 gathering information processing and strategy information for inclusion in a functional formulation of his situation.

The sections that follow describe a possible approach to treatment of Justin. It is important to keep in mind, however, that not all sexual offenders would be in the same situation and their treatment might better be organized in some other way.

Assessment and functional formulation

In Justin's case, we conclude that his body functions normally (the peripheral nervous system); he perceives sensations as adult men do and he regulates his arousal adequately. On the other hand, he is procedurally constrained and lacks access to images of many of his affect-laden childhood experiences, such that he does not know how these motivate his behavior. That is, implicit DRs motivate him in ways that he cannot articulate and forbidden feeling states (such as desire for comfort and fear) are transformed into sexual arousal and are expressed in sexual ways. Justin needs to discover these feelings, experiencing them as normal and acceptable, and then learn to redirect their display in more appropriate ways, e.g., to an adult who reciprocates his feelings. Verbally, there is substantial incoherence between what Justin says and what he does and feels. Reflectively, he seems unaware of the incoherence, i.e., he does not attend to discrepancy.

From there, we would move to a functional formulation, one that took into account his probability of reoffending and its probable severity if it were to recur. In this case, Justin had hugged and caressed children, including stroking their genitals. These were children whom he knew and liked, and he did not use force or violence. Further, he had not denied his behavior. We would decide that placing him near children would not be safe, but he was unlikely to seek them out or engage in threats or deception. In LFF terms, he fits at level 3: restorable (in 3–5 years of comprehensive work). In terms of information processing, his gaps appear in the implicit memory systems, with a strong bias toward a Type A organization. Finally, on the gradient of services, he needs individualized psychotherapy (keeping in mind that group programs can be individualized). A critical issue will be enabling Justin to find himself, i.e., his own feelings and motivations. This will require communication in which his input is substantial and from which he receives an empathic and personal response.

This suggests that our initial intervention needs to address awareness of procedural and imaged functioning. This choice is corroborated by Justin's previous treatment experience, which had addressed verbal semantic memory and left him thinking about himself and his behavior in 'borrowed' and negative semantic terms. Rather than trying to correct that, it might be more effective to intervene around preverbal information.

After transforming his imaged feelings to language, we can move to semantic generalizations, with special attention to differentiating prescriptive from descriptive generalizations and enabling Justin to deduce his own generalizations. All of this should be fleshed out and familiar to Justin before we press for reflection and integration. Put another way, we want the information that will be integrated to represent Justin's experience accurately.

Danger and protection

This plan will take a long time and Justin will not be safe (for either children or himself) until he is well along in the integrative process.

Because Justin felt comfortable with structure (as most people using a Type A strategy do) and was at little risk of seeking children, our plan might be something like a protected community or day treatment center where he would be kept apart from children until he better understood himself, i.e., his motivations and ways of regulating them. Intimacy and the need for comforting relationships stand out as central to change and, in this protected setting, we would want to provide several professionals for him to get to know, allowing Justin to settle on one with whom he would work closely.

Changing the process or stopping the behavior?

Before starting the treatment, we need to consider whether we wish to work from the beginning, i.e., from Justin's motivations, or from the end, i.e., his inappropriate behavior and its consequences. Practically, this is the difference between (1) letting Justin discover his motivations (using the treatment to facilitate this process and to assist him to find more appropriate ways to meet these motivations) and, conversely, (2) focusing on stopping the unacceptable behavior (using the treatment to interrupt the process leading to sexualized behavior with children while emphasizing the consequences if he failed to stop the behavior). As Justin described it, his actual treatment was based on the latter process, i.e., stopping the inappropriate, sexualized behavior. Indeed, this is a widely accepted practice in sexual offender treatment.

If we choose to work from the beginning, we will want to clarify Justin's motivations (not assuming that all sexual offenders share the same motivations). For example, if Justin has confused desire for comfort (a forbidden affect when he was a boy) with sexual desire (an acceptably adult affect that men are permitted to display openly), then we will want to help him to clarify the difference between these two feelings and to redirect his desire for comfort in appropriate ways for an adult man.

On the other hand, if we wanted to focus on stopping the inappropriate behavior, then we would want to stop sexual fantasies, avoid access to children (how restricted must life become if one is never to be near children!), focus on the rules for what to do when the feelings arise so as not to act on them, and emphasize the negative consequences of acting inappropriately. Such treatment hinges on isolation and maintenance of inhibition; in Justin's case, it requires that he retain and emphasize his Type A strategy. Nevertheless, it leaves the man vulnerable to unexpected contact with children, breaks in his inhibition, and momentary lapses when knowing the consequences is no longer relevant to his behavior. Especially for sexual behavior, consequences have little meaning for anyone once

319

sexual arousal is underway and especially if one's partner is also aroused (even if the partner's arousal is negative, e.g., fear or anger).

I prefer beginning with changing the motivating process because it assumes that each person's motivations are normal, human and worthy of fulfillment, and then helps the person to find an appropriate way to accomplish that. If such treatment is successful, men like Justin will become both safer and happier. Their basic humanity will have been found and returned to them without shame. On the other hand, managing treatment from the endpoint backward seems both risky, in terms of how it might fail in real-life contexts, and inhumane because it leaves the man with his shame intact and his motivations unfulfilled.

Unpack and restack: Treatment focused on implicit DRs

If we work from imaged representations forward, we will want to address imaged representations and bring them to conscious awareness. As part of this process, we might want to explore Justin's sexual fantasies (as evidence from imaged memory), identifying the feelings associated with them and analyzing their function with him (Hochman 2002, 2007). Images are information; they are not inherently good or bad, but instead they are informative. Our goal will be to assist Justin to examine his imaged knowledge, both unpacking it to extract its meaning and restacking it to generate more adaptive meanings.

In Justin's case, his extreme loneliness as a child had led to fantasies of sexual contact from adults and peers. Once these images were put into words (which has the effect of lowering arousal and the probability of acting on the feelings, Lieberman *et al.* 2007), we could help Justin identify the feelings that preceded them (i.e., that elicited them), accompanied them, and followed them. The last of these is likely to include feelings of shame and excessively low arousal, which in turn would create a need for comfort and increased arousal – which sexual fantasies and acts accomplished. Put in information processing terms, the exploration of images could lead to uncovering his procedure of using sexual fantasy and behavior to regulate arousal.

To unpack the images, we might suggest changing the fantasy to identify its crucial elements. Is *sexual* touching needed? Will bodily caressing, with a response from the other, be sufficient? Can Justin feel the response in any way other than sexually, etc.?

In addition, we would explore his feelings when he was with the children (did their coy behavior seem flirtatious to him?) and after the sexualized intimacy with them. Especially if his pleasure was tinged with regret and shame, we would want to focus on how to satisfy his motivations without these negative outcomes. We would also want to explore how he experienced adult relationships with both men and women, with an eye to what misunderstandings might have been carried forward from childhood.

Once his current status was explicit, we might 'restack' the images by modifying the fantasies so as to meet an adult man's needs without harming his partner (i.e., shift the fantasies to comfort with children and sex with adults). That is, having clarified with Justin what he sought (his motivation), changing the images or fantasies could help him to find an acceptable route to it.

Parallel to exploring his images, we might use semantic representation to discuss his normal human need for comfort, the sadness of not having had it as a child, and the possible ways to achieve it as an adult. For this, we might employ the power of connotative language to express affect without needing action.

People sometimes speak of therapy as 'restorying' childhood, parenting the parent, or recapitulating development differently (Byng-Hall 1995). The sequence above might look like that. But this time, we begin with language, albeit constrained or distorted. And we begin with experiences already lived; they can be thought about differently, but they cannot be erased. Finally, we begin with a mature brain – and to be successful in our treatment, we will need all of its adult capacity. Treatment isn't childhood relived, even though selected aspects of childhood may need to be examined and even though the process will move from regulation of arousal to implicit knowledge, explicit knowledge, reflection, and ultimately integration. Instead, treatment enables adults to shape the impact of childhood on their functioning and to imagine a different, more adaptive and satisfying way of living while developing the skills to make it possible.

These sorts of activities would confirm or disconfirm our initial assessment, possibly pointing to some modification of our formulation. An ongoing transactional process would facilitate the gradual progress toward a goal-corrected partnership between Justin and his therapist (Wilkinson 2003), rather than the goal-determined approach that guided his treatment in prison. In doing this work, we want to stay with Justin's perspective, not letting it slip toward an echo of a conformist perspective, our perspective, or the victim's perspective. All of these are known. Justin's perspective is the unknown, and he must find it before he can establish a genuinely empathic relationship with anyone else.

How will we know which techniques to use?

In the section above, I suggested some techniques, but in fact it isn't yet known how each affects information processing. This is the gaping hole in the empirical understanding of treatment. Nevertheless, therapists who are able to assess, formulate, and listen while working with patients can use the patients' responses to tell them how they are doing. If we want our patients to change, we should be ready to do so as well. The treatment seems not to be working? We have a discrepancy. We explore it – with the patient (cf. session-by-session gathering of feedback; Duncan and Miller 2000). We do ourselves what we want our patients to learn to do.

At present, we can guide treatment with some general principles. Start where the patient is.[2] Be a bridge from his reality of suffering and danger to ours of hope and satisfaction. Every case is different; one size does not fit all. If there is danger, start there. (In the case of Justin, we began with a protected therapeutic community.) If implicit information can't be made explicit, address that. If negative affect is inhibited, free it. If contingencies are unknown, reveal them. Listen more than talk. Question more than tell. Remember that maintaining a transactional stance means retaining genuine curiosity with openness to all that the patient presents and hesitating before rushing to rescue or guide. Prepare carefully for the suffering that will be revealed. Don't be dazzled by the speed of semantic communication until implicit DRs are revealed and the process of revealing them is managed well by the patient. Get the episodes, being certain to work concretely before leaping to the great generalizations. Highlight discrepancies (small, safe discrepancies first!) and share the joy of resolving them.

My concern is that, not knowing how sexual offenders' minds are organized, we have made assumptions based on their behavior and words and our feelings of outrage and moral disapproval, and then constructed treatments to correct these. For all our good intentions, we feel so uneasy, even when sexual offenders have been punished and treated, that we isolate them from children and, in many cases, track their whereabouts on sexual offenders' registers – sometimes forever. We could, and do, argue that something about sexual offending is beyond the scope of treatment. I'm not convinced that it is. The developmental approach offered in this volume suggests that we might have misunderstood what sort of treatment was needed and may have inadvertently offered treatments that backfired, possibly even making the initial problems worse.

Retribution and punishment

But what about Justin's violations of children? Is there to be no punishment or retribution? It is not clear to me that Justin, who uses a Type A strategy, will benefit from further negative consequences. Justin already feels shame and regret. Possibly it would be more useful for him to 'pay back' in a meaningful way. To contribute some community service, but not in a menial way, e.g., not picking up highway trash. Instead, why not have the paying back both reduce his debt by doing something beneficial to society and build his pride? Let's use a skill that Justin has to give something valuable to someone who doesn't have it. Why not create something good for all parties where isolation has, in the past, led to shame-filled outcomes?

Conclusions

Review of childhood history is passé in many forms of treatment where the focus is on the here and now, problem solving, and learning new skills. For a man like Justin, too strong a focus on the here and now leaves him only an offender, not someone who was offended against. As a child, he was a victim himself, one who had to distort his development to stay safe at home. This then put him at risk at school and again in adulthood when he found himself unprepared to love and be loved and to begin a family of his own. Instead he 'borrowed' children and they functioned for him as parents (who should have caressed him comfortingly), lovers (who were absent from his adult life), and children (whom he would love and comfort). Framed that way, Justin's intentions are normal; it is his development that has skewed the way he meets his needs. I think we need to let him see that. If we can use our relationship with Justin to illuminate how old patterns have been brought into the present when they are not needed, we might assist Justin to free himself from the invisible grasp of the past (Bowlby 1988).

In prison, Justin found himself to be like other offenders; in treatment, we want him to find himself to be like other humans. How? First, with his therapist. Only as Justin finds and reveals himself, detail by detail, will we be able to say that we know Justin; only then will Justin know that he is really known and appreciated. There are no shortcuts to this. We can't announce it, can't cite the literature, can't wave our AAI and say, 'Here! See! We know.' We must reach our state of knowing *with* Justin. We must discover him together. Our contribution? Pointing in potentially useful directions and not getting sidetracked by the irrelevant topics that are easily talked about. So why do the long, complex and expensive AAI if we can't use it directly with Justin? To increase the probability of getting on the right track. Once on it, Justin can signal how fast and how far we can go.

If we take this long, slow and personalized approach, how will we know when treatment and restitution can be ended? Based on today's technology, we might say that the treatment will be complete when Justin himself finds the discrepancies, when he initiates exploring them, and when that work is productive. We will know he has really freed himself from his past when he arrives at his appointments telling us with satisfaction of the discrepancies he found by himself, the ways he explored them, and the adaptive resolutions he found. Especially if Justin can express this in open, reciprocal and spontaneous dialogue, we will conclude that he has balanced mental processing, is accepting of himself as normally human and of others as compassionate, and experiences security in the relationship with his therapist. If we look to the future and anticipate the as-yet-untried uses of new technologies, such as functional magnetic resonance imaging (fMRI), we may be able go further and say that therapy will be seen to have been successful when Justin's fMRI lights up like a Type B's when he addresses problems.[3]

Severe parenting dysfunction (cluster 5)

Kate was the mother of a 3-year-old boy in foster care who was being considered for adoption by his foster family (Chapter 12). Kate herself had been raised in a children's home, where she had a long-term sexual relationship with a young member of the institutional staff. She later married another resident of the home and together they had a child; then years later, they divorced. Kate remarried and had the son who was now in care, following her husband's death and her own delusions of the need to cleanse the boy in bleach. Kate now experiences dramatic changes in arousal (from depression to mania) with periodic delusions and self-harming in the form of cutting.

Assessment and formulation

Kate's history, symptoms, and situation (living alone as a widow and with a child in care) suggest the possibility of very grave danger. With her son, her LFF is 5: inadequate. Alone, she might manage level 4: supportable, but only if we are prepared to offer stable, ongoing and appropriate support. Whether she can ever reach level 3: restorable, depends greatly on whether she can find a committed and stable attachment figure (e.g., a man, her daughter). Kate's information processing displayed problems at the peripheral level, where she did not respond to sensory stimuli, including pain, with self-protective arousal and action. On the gradient of services, she needs individualized psychotherapy. If that fails, re-institutionalization becomes a possibility.

Somatically, Kate responded both too little and too much, failing almost entirely to find a life-preserving balance between depression and mania and also failing to change state in synchrony with actual change in the dangerousness of her situation. At the preconscious level of awareness (i.e., procedural and imaged memory), Kate has both erroneous information and also self-generated, delusional information that she attributes to sources outside herself. This suggests both problems with source memory (common among children growing up in numerous placements or with numerous caregivers) and conflict between what she thinks prescriptively she should feel or do and her actual feelings and intentions. In fact, Kate's AAI classification includes an A8, in which external authorities define her 'self'. All of this suggests a strong need for Kate to know herself as she is and to find acceptable the person that she is.

Danger and protection

Safety is always the first issue. Because she cuts herself, Kate is not safe. Short-term hospitalization when she does this addresses it briefly, but does little or nothing to prevent recurrences; indeed, it may encourage them. Because Kate lives alone and has a traumatic history of loss, a different living arrangement is needed, such as living near her grown daughter or in a residential community. Parallel to this immediate attention to safety is the issue of basic physiological stabilization and, later, establishment of contingency between her state of arousal and the actual dangerousness of her situation. Stabilization is needed before other forms of psychotherapy can be usefully undertaken.

Accomplishing this may require a committed therapist who can function as a transitional attachment figure over possibly as long as several years. Within this relationship, the focus that DMM theory would suggest is on identifying, expressing, and talking about her feelings, particularly negative feelings and false-positive displays of feelings. Because Kate uses an extreme form of the Type A strategy, this is likely to be a long and sometimes painful process. In addition, however, because institutional living often involves both too little stimulation and aversive stimulation, Kate may have a constrained neurological basis for change processes (i.e., fewer neural networks and connections among networks). It simply isn't known how much this can be changed in midlife, but Kate's experience as a wife and mother suggests a certain degree of either resilience or recovery.

Regulating arousal

Reducing extreme states of arousal that are not tied to actual threat can be accomplished either directly through pharmacological means or indirectly through Kate's use of state-altering techniques, e.g., meditation, exercise, biofeedback, etc. In some cases (and Kate might be among these), regulation will need to be a part of the context, either temporarily (inpatient status) or for the long-term (protective living contexts). The advantage of pharmacological therapy is its speed (although even this can take some weeks before it is maximally effective); its disadvantages include the lack of self-regulatory control by Kate, reduced ties between Kate's state and her context, and any side effects that she might experience. Self-regulating techniques have the benefit of being under Kate's control; therefore, they promote her long-term adjustment. The primary disadvantages are that they require a degree of motivation that Kate might lack, and their effects might accrue too slowly or be insufficiently intense to meet her needs.

A crucial issue, I think, in deciding how to use these treatment possibilities (separately, in combination, or in succession) is the extent to which Kate can understand how they can function for her benefit. That is, if she can understand her need for greater stability and reduced extreme fluctuations, she can participate meaningfully in the choice of technique. Moreover, if she understands that changes in arousal should be tied to changes in environmental conditions, she can begin to think of her feelings and behavior as serving the useful function of connecting her safely to her context. Life should become less frightening when these relations are understood intellectually and, later, experienced physiologically. However, while the body is dangerously extreme in its state, it is probably premature to rely solely on psychological functions, except as these are directed toward somatic regulation. Once that has improved, other psychological issues can become more prominent in the treatment (cf. Levine 1997; Linehan *et al.* 2007; for similar perspectives).

All of this is to say that managing arousal and attention is crucial at the outset of treatment for Kate and that giving her awareness of the process and increasing control over it may eventually enable the process to move into the background – where it is for most of us most of the time.

Treatment from the start point or endpoint

When Kate was discussed earlier (Chapter 12), I wondered whether it might not be better to focus on redirecting the 'start point' of information processing than to try to eliminate the 'endpoint', i.e., the cutting, etc. This is an important distinction because the behavioral and cognitive-behavioral treatments that she (like Justin) had received focused on stopping inappropriate behavior, i.e., the endpoint behavior. Instead, it might be necessary to focus on the sequence that led to perception of danger, i.e., the point at which information processing went awry.

Two effects could be expected from identifying 'start-point' errors. First, once the misperception occurs, it may be nearly impossible to stop the self-protective process. Assuming we clarify Kate's feelings and motivations, making them verbal and conscious, it is entirely possible that hardly anything will need to be done to correct her semantic functioning, beyond correcting the input and assisting her to resist her tendency to rely on others' prescriptions. Put another way, it is not evident that semantic, connotative and episodic processing has been affected beyond the distortions and limitations of the information made available. Second, once we correct the misperception, it is likely that Kate's original (childhood) problem will reappear, now more clearly. Consideration will need to be given to whether that problem is still valid in any way. If it is, Kate will need a better solution than the misconceived one. For example, in Kate's case, the uncovered problem might be how to connect securely with other people so as to be able to regulate arousal better. For Kate, the connections will need to be conceptualized around the possibilities for a middle-aged woman with a young child, an adult son or daughter, and a grandchild. That is, the childhood problem is relevant, but the context of its solution is changed.

Returning to John (who had been abused by his father and imprisoned for physically abusing his own children, and who later confessed to having sexually abused them as well) as a different example, the newly revealed problem from childhood might be how to manage touch, at the peripheral/somatic level where in early life he was exposed to the mixture of love/sex/hate/aggression. Now, in adulthood, the basic problem of using touch both for self-regulation and for intimate communication in an array of family relationships (from children to lovers) will need to be solved in a new manner. That is, it won't be enough to stop the bad touching. Once the origin of the problem is pushed back to the peripheral nervous system, the therapy will need to solve this very basic, very human problem in a satisfactory way – for a 41-year-old man.

In both cases, if we were to get so far, reflective processing would probably need to be shaped. This can be begun early by focusing on resolving discrepancies in perception, but will, in all likelihood, need direct effort toward the end of treatment. For example, the therapist might articulate a variety of possible descriptions of Kate's state, helping her to both match words to feelings and behavior and to differentiate these (cf. Taumoepeau and Ruffman 2006). It would be essential, however, for the therapist assiduously to avoid giving Kate the 'right' words because Kate is only too ready to yield her perspective to someone else's. For John, the problem might be learning not to dichotomize solutions as right or wrong and, instead, seeing how compromises can enable interpersonal conflict to generate win-win solutions that strengthen, rather than destroy, relationships.

Finally, if we explore the issue of 'start-point' or 'endpoint' treatment for the Shoemakers, we note that they have clear and accessible DRs in all memory systems – so we do not need to address the start-point issues further. Instead, having assisted the family members to see and articulate the problem, we can focus very promptly on the reflective process that can yield a new solution. That is, there is no need to go back further than the point at which the individuals' information processing became distorted (with regard to conditions in the present).

Treatment in cases of severe danger

To summarize, for seriously endangered and endangering parents such as Kate (or John, Victoria Climbié's great-aunt, Susan Smith, or Andrea Yates), treatment must begin with safe living conditions, progress to assessment and stabilization of their somatic state, and then pick up at the memory systems (where Justin began) and carry forward to reflective integration (where the Shoemakers began). Moreover, for parents with serious problems that have jeopardized their ability to establish or maintain relationships, learning the basic skills to do so and finding opportunities to meet people with whom they might establish enduring relationships are crucial to maintenance of their recovery. This, in other words, is the newly uncovered problem that was 'solved' in dangerous ways that must now be stopped, but which still needs an age-appropriate solution. Kate could possibly begin to redefine herself as a grandmother to her grown daughter's child. This is a less demanding role than parent, but one that would connect her to her family in many ways. Resolving Kate's overwhelming array of losses is probably counterproductive because therapy can only change thinking and behavior; it cannot replace what is lost, and, for Kate, the losses are beyond imagining. Maybe Kate, like other victims of severe and irreversible trauma (cf. Wajnryb 2001), should use her dismissing strategy to keep this source of pain at bay. Justin will have problems finding suitable companions, with prison being an unfortunate meeting ground. John has children and a partner; we should include them in the treatment in appropriate ways. Indeed, we have already seen that protecting these threatened relationships is the reason John sought treatment. Susan Smith and Andrea Yates will face even greater problems because murder is irreversible. Both women, however, gave signals of their distress, combined with histories associated with serious disorder. Their situations are clear reminders that prevention, that is, timely intervention and appropriate treatment, is the better choice and, sometimes, the only choice.

Conclusions

I chose to offer ideas about treatment through three case studies. Doing so fits the DMM notion that each case is unique and, like life, not completely foreseeable at the beginning. Further, each case was formulated on the assumption that the troublesome behavior developed at a time and in a context that made it the best solution possible in that situation. In almost every case, a part of that context was the absence of an attachment figure who protected and comforted the individual; this lack created the occasion for the strategy and behavior that would become problematic later in life.

The three cases demonstrate the relevance of basic human motivations for adaptation and maladaptation. The Shoemakers were concerned with protecting their daughter at the beginning of her reproductive maturity, Justin had not managed his own reproductive maturity, and Kate faced problems keeping both herself and her child safe. Protection of self, reproduction, and protection of progeny were the organizing issues in these cases and are proposed as central to all or almost all maladaptive behavior. The cases also demonstrate the crucial importance of protective human relationships for adaptation and, when there is maladaptation, for treatment. Finally, the cases ranged in severity from needing (a) brief assistance in applying reflective processes to opening communication during a period of developmental change, (b) substantial protection and assistance at disentangling confusions carried forward from childhood and redirecting basic needs in adaptive ways in adulthood, and (c) protracted protection and assistance with the most basic life-maintaining processes.

In each case, treatment was an attempt to expand and correct information processing and strategies in ways that could more appropriately meet the individual's needs. A crucial notion was the idea of the therapist functioning as a transitional attachment figure engaged reciprocally with the individual in the individual's ZPD. These ideas highlight the contribution of the DMM in cases where the parent is endangering. They enable us to keep the humanity of all the individuals in sight, regardless of behavior that needs to be changed or needs that have been misunderstood. The contrast is especially clear in Justin, the case of child sexual abuse. Indeed, sexual abuse or offending is highlighted throughout the book for this very reason: the DMM analysis of the problem and perspective on its solution differ substantially from treatment as it is most often delivered. When the complexity of each person's relationships is seen in terms of developmental needs, suffering when these go unmet, and the hope that accompanies being understood accurately, treatment has the maximum possibility of generating change.

Notes

1 This limitation is equally applicable to treatment supervision. If audio or video information is not provided to the supervisor, he or she cannot form independent ideas about the patient or the treatment. In that case, the therapist seeking a new and potentially helpful perspective will have limited the supervisor's potential to provide that, instead biasing the process to be confirmatory.
2 This is crucially important because the treatment alliance within the first weeks of treatment is the best predictor of outcome (Hubbel *et al*. 1999).
3 Although it is not yet ready for application to treatment, work on fMRI and DMM attachment patterns suggests this potential application (Strathearn 2008).

Chapter 21

Improving the safety of children and families

The Dynamic-Maturational Model (DMM) of attachment and adaptation represents an attempt to organize ideas from other theories and bodies of knowledge (including clinical expertise) into a coherent developmental model of human adaptation that is inclusive of regulatory processes from genes to cultures. Very little of the DMM is new; in fact, most is drawn from the work of others and is only new in how the work is connected. Even many of the patterns described in the DMM have been described by other people. What is new are the hypotheses regarding the way that they are connected developmentally (as person–experience interactions),[1] functionally (as context-specific, adaptive strategies), and structurally (in terms of underlying information processing). It is hoped that this organization will enable new findings and observations to be related to the existing knowledge base more easily such that their implications will be understood more quickly.

Two notions are central to the DMM organization:

1 Maturation and behavior function to promote safety and reproduction.
2 Cognition and affect are two types of information that concatenate through development to yield a near infinite variety of human organizations that promote survival and reproduction.

It should be stated clearly that the DMM is a *theoretical* understanding leading to hypotheses about prevention and treatment. It is not data-driven, but rather reflects a dynamic interaction between data-production, theory development, and clinical insight. In other words, the DMM is data-informed, but also informed by theory and experience. Theory, of course, cannot be proven, although hypotheses drawn from it can be disproved. DMM theory is thought to be consistent with both the empirical base at this time and with clinical experience. Nevertheless, as with all theory, some of the ideas and hypotheses will stand the test of time and others will be found to be inadequate or misguided. Over time, new studies and clinical experience will add to our factual knowledge base and be used to modify theory and reformulate hypotheses.

In addition, however, the utility of theory is important and that, like theory itself, is not a purely factual matter. Put another way, although it is important that the facts underpinning theory be accurate, it is not possible to say whether or not a theory of treatment is 'true'. Better questions might be the following. Can the theory lead to new thinking and better treatment? Does it open the mind to new perspectives? Does it create new connections between the client/patient and therapist? Can these be used to reduce suffering? Does it generate hope, accompanied by helpful behavior?

The theory offered here is intended to offer professionals new ways to represent the experience of endangered parents and children. It is hoped that this will enable us to protect both children and their parents better. That is, the proper test of these ideas is whether or not their application increases the safety and comfort of children and their parents in the future.

Maladaptation and treatment

A developmental approach to understanding maladaptive behavior reflects the notion of learned variations in behavior that use universal human processes. This suggests that changing learned patterns of information processing is crucial for changing behavior and increasing adaptation. In other words, *treatment should change information processing in ways that promote adaptive and functional behavior, both in the current context and in contexts not yet experienced or even envisioned.*

Framed functionally in terms of safety and reproduction and the development of strategies to promote these, behavior, even maladaptive behavior, can be seen as meaningful. Thus, when behavior is maladaptive, one can ask under what conditions and at what age might the behavior have developed and, given that developmental context, how might the behavior have been adaptive. This reframes maladaptive behavior as a learned strength and focuses attention on (a) differences between then and now (i.e., reflective integration), (b) the ability of the individual to articulate these differences (i.e., explicit verbal information), (c) awareness of what one does and how one feels (i.e., implicit information), and (d) the limitations of the individual in perceiving these differences (i.e., perceptual information known somatically).

Level of awareness and focusing treatment

These four levels of awareness (integrative, explicit, implicit and peripheral/somatic) can provide psychotherapists with a guide to the extent and depth of the needed therapeutic process. For example, if people perceive discrepancy well and can articulate discrepant perceptions verbally, they are ready for integrative, problem-solving types of treatment that depend upon verbal and abstract processes. At the other extreme, if the individual misperceives changes in the context in basic somatic ways and is unaware of the discrepancy, the treatment may need to begin with perceptual and somatic forms of knowing and means of regulating the biological connection of self to context. Such treatment will rely much less on language as a *source* of information and instead focus on discovering the language that can *express* what is experienced. Only much later, after words have come to have meaning independent of immediate somatic and psychological states, will reflective and integrative processes become useful. This is not to say that such people should be treated as if they did not have language or cortical reflective capacity. Instead, I mean that these advanced capacities should first be directed to making the least explicit information clearly evident and that higher-level integrative processes should be reserved until the individual is safer and more comfortable, and has explicit access to much of the needed information from all levels of functioning. That is, integration is best attempted after the person knows him- or herself well and is comfortable in the relationship with the therapist.

Type of information and focusing treatment

A second dimension is the individual's relative reliance on cognition (i.e., temporal contingencies) and affect (i.e., arousal-based feeling states) to organize behavior. Some individuals rely primarily on cognitive information, specifically the invariant temporal sequences of events leading to expected outcomes, whereas others rely more on their feelings, particularly their negative feelings, to predict outcomes. Knowing the bias of a particular individual can permit the therapist to focus the treatment on correcting this bias both by making the meaningfulness of the less-used source of information clearer and by reducing the distortions in the preferred source of information.

A particularly important aspect of framing feelings as information is that negative affect becomes information about possible danger to the self, one's reproductive opportunity, or one's progeny. Information about such threats is obviously important. Moreover, the stronger the feeling, the more important to the self the information is perceived to be. Focusing on the information value of negative affect takes negative feelings out of an evaluative framework in which negative affect is 'bad' and strong negative affect is worse, and reframes it as important information that should be examined. For individuals using a Type A strategy, this implies that important information has been overlooked because, in the past, displaying it led to negative consequences, whereas, in the present, its absence is leading to maladaptive behavior. For individuals using a Type C strategy, this implies examining the accuracy of the affective prediction, using cognitive information as a way to assess that accuracy, and, when feelings are observed to predict with insufficient accuracy, learning ways to regulate feelings or the way that feelings organize behavior.

Recent empirical approaches to treatment have emphasized its 'cognitive' characteristics and their compatibility with a scientific, evidence-based approach. The DMM suggests that affect is equally important and that treating affect in a cognitive manner (e.g., through an emphasis on verbal labeling and semantic regulation of negative affect) may miss the unique advantage of affect. In particular, the state of the client as a distressed person or of the patient as a suffering person may have received too little attention. Treatment of sexual offenders (i.e., individuals who jeopardize their own and others' reproductive potential) is offered as an example of how the DMM would redirect treatment.

Consider the concept of 'choosing' in accredited sexual offender programs in the UK. In such programs, there is an understanding that some schema form very early, before words, and that these have a profound affect on the way one perceives the world and other people. Nevertheless, the programs are not yet good at assessing how information is processed nonverbally and focusing treatment accordingly. Instead, the programs tend to rely on explicit (verbal and conscious) communication. Moreover, they are organized around the notion that inappropriate behavior can be brought under control of reflective integrative processes; i.e., that men consciously choose to offend or not.

The DMM idea is that there are two more basic levels that dispose behavior. These two, peripheral/somatic arousal and implicit procedural-and-imaged knowledge, are neither conscious, nor verbal. A behavioral response is selected, but the process by which this happens could hardly be called 'choosing' because it is neither conscious nor volitional. If that is accurate, then talk therapies that focus primarily on explicit information would be less likely to enable offenders to live fulfilling lives and avoid reoffending than programs that begin with assessment of information processing and attention to implicit information.

To return to the cases presented earlier in this volume, David was probably minimally balanced at the peripheral/somatic level (this could support his idealization of his comforting mother, who accomplished this regulation of his bodily arousal in early infancy), but distorted at the preconscious level of procedures (run away and hide yourself alone) and images (fantasize about being held and loved, etc.). Rather than trying to stop the fantasies, treatment would address the fantasies, helping David to describe them, select his labels for the feelings in them, and assign his meanings to that information (i.e., 'I feel like that because ...' and 'When I feel like that I change my feeling by ...'). Only then, when the description is accurate on David's experience and available verbally to him, can the treatment begin to address, reflectively, (1) what conditions now elicit those feelings/fantasies, (2) how the *conditions* can be changed to reduce the need for the fantasies by increasing the appropriate satisfaction of the man, and (3) what can be done *after the fantasies* (dispositions) occur to address the man's feelings in an appropriate way that won't result in harm to others and shame/disgust for the self.

John, on the other hand, had no mother and probably had a sexually abusing father. Did the distortion for him begin at the peripheral/somatic level? If so, then regulating basic arousal would be an issue for John. He would be at risk of extended and dangerous lows (depression in the DMM) and intermittent, dangerous highs (intrusions of forbidden negative affect in the DMM). The intrusions could be violence, sexual abuse, cutting, etc. Treatment would need to begin with helping John to modify his arousal so as to maintain a more moderate state. Verbal treatment, at the beginning of treatment, that called for reflection and construction of new DRs to regulate behavior would be likely to fail, as would treatment aimed at procedures and images (including fantasies), because perceptual learning in the peripheral nervous system regulated his behavior.

In both examples, preverbal information would be sought and treated as informative, rather than as something bad to be gotten rid in the hope of not triggering inappropriate behavior. In the latter case, the risk would be that the avoidance procedures would fail, leaving the man where he was prior to treatment. By accepting and exploring the meaning of the information, treatment might be able to generate new meanings, new dispositions, and new, appropriate ways of meeting basic human needs.

The role of treatment and the psychotherapist

Treatment, as envisioned in the DMM, should free individuals from the constraints of their developmental history such that they gain access to the full range of human possibility. Treatment offers individuals two resources, a set of therapeutic techniques and a professional who makes them available. A great deal of attention has been focused on therapeutic techniques recently (i.e., the search for evidence-based treatments), with the unexpected outcome that techniques account for very little of the variance in treatment outcome.

The role of the therapist has been somewhat less emphasized, especially in studies using randomized, controlled tests (which almost require inter-changeability of treatment providers). From the perspective of the DMM, the relationship between client/patient and therapist is crucial to the success of psychotherapy (as opposed to counseling or educational services). The therapeutic relationship is the connection between (a) the patient's suffering and the hope that brought the patient to treatment, and (b) the therapist's image of the patient as the person he or she could become, together with the knowledge of how to relieve suffering and make change.

The DMM suggests that individuals who had problems with safety and comfort early in life, who developed distorted information processing, and who use maladaptive protective strategies are likely to have had very anxious childhood attachments and to need a corrective attachment relationship to undertake a successful therapeutic process. The role of the therapist as a transitional attachment figure is to be sensitively responsive to the needs and desires of the patient in his or her actual ZPD. This framing of the therapist's role serves several functions. As the therapist slowly comes to know the individual, including both past and current suffering, the therapist's empathy gives meaning to the suffering. That is, having a foot in both worlds, i.e., both the patient's world of danger, suffering and dread and our world of safety, comfort and hope, the therapist's compassion regarding what was experienced and what must be managed for the suffering to end becomes the bridge to the future. As a transitional attachment figure, the therapist becomes the person to whom the patient learns to turn in times of discomfort, doubt and uncertainty.

When dealing with family members, it is crucial that the therapist cares in a genuine and personal way about *all* the family members (whether they are part of the treatment or not), not supporting one in preference to the others. Keeping the perspectives and needs of several people in balance is difficult, of course, but it is the everyday task of parents. Observing the therapist manage this task is highly relevant to the real-life issues of troubled parents.

Parenting

This book is an attempt to understand why some parents endanger their own children and to suggest ways to increase family safety. Using empirical studies, case studies, clinical cases and material from attachment assessments, I have tried to construct an understanding of how men and women who love their children could harm or even kill them. I have done this within the context of a general theory of psychological functioning around self-protection and reproduction (the DMM) and applied it to severe problems in parenting.

Parenting, survival and culture

Parents play a crucial role in the survival of our species through their reproductive capacity and protection of their children. It is quite clear, however, that parents differ in how they choose mates and raise their children. These differences exist both among individuals and families and also among cultures. When the differences become substantial, especially when survival or reproduction is jeopardized, ethical standards are applied. Ethical standards are culturally variable, however, and behavior that one culture considers unethical and unacceptable another may approve of or even deem necessary and desirable. Examination of the danger in the context (both currently and historically) can often explain why different standards of parenting behavior have developed. Nevertheless, the basis of the standards in safety and reproductive opportunity is universal. Awareness of this link between historical experience in varied contexts and strategies for protection and reproduction can be helpful when considering the child-rearing practices of foreign cultures and, particularly, when evaluating the parenting of immigrant populations.

The DMM of attachment and adaptation begins with the assumption that all parents (all people) are motivated to protect themselves, to reproduce, and to protect their progeny. Moreover, the notion is that, at any point in time, a person's behavior is the most adaptive response they could produce, given their innate attributes, previous experience, and current circumstances. By framing dangerous parental behavior as misguided protective behavior regulated by implicit organizing processes, it becomes possible to understand endangering parents' behavior as a positive intention that failed to protect for reasons that the parent cannot fully understand. Acknowledging the parents' developmental process of past exposure to danger that led to their distorted information processing in the present requires that one appreciate the parents' suffering, both in the past and now. This creates both the possibility of compassion for the parents and an approach to treatment based on information processing. Further, this approach suggests that both parents whose behavior appears to be a volitional violation of ethical/legal standards (e.g., child abuse and criminal violence) and those whose behavior appears to be the nonvolitional outcome of mental illness are similar in that (a) all the parents were endangered as children, (b) all the children were harmed, (c) all the parents were distressed by what happened, and (d) the endangering behavior was generated, at least in part, by preconscious, implicit dispositional processes.

Potentially helpful changes

In the opening of this book, I said I had some 'revolutionary' ideas that the average person took for granted and that professionals said were impossible. The DMM theory regarding endangering parents and treatment lays the groundwork for six proposed changes in how we respond to endangering parents and their children. Condensed, they focus on two ideas:

1 understanding the problem of dangerous child-rearing practices in a more complexly accurate manner, both interpersonally and psychologically;
2 simplifying the response to each family by offering a transitional attachment figure who functions to address a critical cause of change.

Six ideas

1 *Define problems interpersonally* (not as individual illness or crimes). If maladaptive behavior were defined functionally as an interactive pattern among two or more people, we would have a fuller understanding of the problem and more options for entering the system that maintains the behavior. If the problem is defined as being in one individual, particularly the one with symptoms, we may be forced to treat symptom display without understanding the source of the distress and without confidence that the symptoms won't reappear in a new guise or that aggressive

symptoms won't be repeated under some intense or unimagined pressure.

2 *Combine child, adolescent and adult services as human psychological services.* Once problems within a family are defined interpersonally, it becomes clear that the division between child-and-adolescent services and adult services is both artificial and obstructive. We need to combine services across the life span. After all, parents have all been children and childhood experience affects daily parenting. In addition, children's experience is defined, in part, by their parents. In addition, services should be focused on opportunities for prevention that occur naturally in the life span, particularly the transition to adulthood and early parenthood.

3 *Assess families, not individuals.* Before a service plan is developed, the entire family should be *seen* for evaluation of information processing, strategies and relationships. After that, the problem can be formulated properly and a mixture of individual, dyadic, family and group services applied as needed to foster more accurate information processing and more adaptive use of protective information processing and strategies. The information derived from assessment can be used to identify a critical cause of change and thus to simplify and focus what otherwise would have been a multipronged, complex and potentially confusing treatment.

4 *Use the transitional attachment figure to deliver needed services*, not a case-management model with many service personnel. Structure treatment around (a) achieving safety, (b) level of awareness, (c) type and distortions of information, and (d) achieving comfort. Focus the intervention on a family-specific critical cause of change while protecting family members in areas they cannot yet manage. Mature professionals who have themselves managed some of life's problems are probably better prepared to function in this way than young and inexperienced professionals (however well educated) who cannot yet draw on life experience. Experienced professionals should do more people work than paperwork.

5 *Manage the treatment developmentally*, in the client/patient's ZPD, using the interpersonal methods that you want the parent to learn to use with their children. That is, expect parents to do with their children as the therapist does with them. If the therapist threatens, expect parents to threaten their children. If the therapist listens and adapts to what the parents say, expect parents to learn to do this with their children. Being explicit to the parent about what you are doing can facilitate this process.

6 *Fund unlimited family services* and limit expenses for out-of-home care, not the reverse. Current funding contingencies promote out-of-home care, resulting in more suffering and a pool of maladapted young adults in the next generation of parents. Daily support services, family placements in protected communities, and protected therapeutic communities for

dangerous people are all underused options for preserving families. Fostering families is a largely untried service that could help. Given the huge baby-boomer generation that is just concluding their own parenting years, we have an available grandparent generation, many of whom do not have locally living grandchildren. Couldn't professionals assist troubled families to 'rent-a-granny', especially one who came with a nice, gray-haired grandpa?

Finally, we need to carry out treatment-efficacy research in a manner that is both scientifically sound and directed toward the sorts of goals that the full range of psychotherapists find to be important. To date, outcome research suffers from (a) a narrow range of outcomes that are not accepted as important by many psychotherapists, (b) studies carried out without sufficient controls by proponents of the treatment method being tested, (c) laboratory settings and resources that are not typical of treatment as it is offered in the field, and (d) unpublished negative findings.

From survival to healing to living

This is a speculative volume that challenges current understanding and practice regarding parents whose behavior endangers their children. The DMM, like all theory, is ahead of confirmatory data. Nevertheless, the ideas that are offered are consistent with existing data and compassionate in understanding the needs of families with endangering parents. Moreover, they are often consistent with existing professional guidelines that, unfortunately, are not always implemented broadly. In proposing these changes, the DMM seeks to find our common humanity as it is experienced in different contexts and with varied developmental histories.

The DMM is a theory of hope. Development is seen as a dynamic, self-correcting process aimed toward safety and production of the next generation of children. If the sun, and moon, and stars are all in the right places, development unfolds without interruption. But life on our planet is dangerous and we have evolved to cope with danger, recover from danger, and thrive on what we learn from surviving danger. We are not a timid species, nor one without innate resources. If the miracle of safety and comfort does not occur, change – and with it, hope – are built into our species. Maturation will change the child, bringing new potential for understanding, for fitting in, and for becoming safe and comfortable. By adulthood, humans have the most elegant psychological processes of any species. With these, many misunderstandings can be corrected, lives can be reshaped, and developmental pathways redirected to increase the probability of being safe, reproducing, and guiding one's progeny to their adulthood.

When that is not possible, the mind can construct its own world, one that highlights the danger so sharply that self-protection becomes all pervasive or, conversely, one that creates a wished-for, delusionally ideal world.

Yet even when exposure to severe danger leads to an endangering parent, there is hope. What the family could not do for itself, other attachment relationships may do for it. Other people can fulfill the attachment functions of offering safety, comfort and a means of shaping the mind so it can use information to protect the self. These people can be temporary or enduring in the endangered person's life. They can be as brief as a special babysitter, as intermittent as a visiting uncle who appreciates a child, as distant as a teacher who nurtures possibility where the parent sees none, or as enduring as grandparents who themselves may have needed extra time to become the parent, for their grandchildren, that they had intended to be for their children.

Even with these naturally occurring possibilities for support, some children are not protected and comforted. For these children and their parents, there are healers. All communities of humans everywhere and for all of our history have had a tradition of healing. Priests, shamans, medicine women, elders and, most recently, professionals have filled this role. Moreover, for all our sophisticated, modern language and concepts, the tools we humans use to heal those of us who suffer are quite constant. Special procedures and belief systems for bringing order into chaotic lives. Rhythms and regularities for restoring inner peace when experience cast one down in depression or tossed one up in terror. Potions and drugs whose effects free the mind to heal itself. And most important of all, the thing without which there is nothing, unique caring relationships in which someone who knows how to find safety and comfort guides someone who fears that these are impossible goals. Healing occurs in relationships. These relationships give new meaning to old experiences and offer new possibilities for the future.

Healing comes one person at a time as a gift from a person who cares compassionately about another while providing the steadying structure that makes being calm enough to imagine possible. Healing the past begins with imagining a different future. When those who would help to heal another person's suffering can themselves find the calm mind space to imagine a better future, then they can hope. Hope is contagious; it can be borrowed and practiced until it becomes one's own.

Shared hope requires revealing oneself – and this is the scary part. Imagining a better future together means knowing well who is imagining; this is what suffering people rarely know about themselves. When rejection by family and society are how one knows oneself, one can hardly imagine a loved and valued self. It can be difficult even to look at oneself, far less to reveal oneself to another person. If we want to heal others, our understanding of each person's human potential must be expressed so personally to the hurt person that they can risk stepping almost blindly off the cliff of the past into the unknown abyss of the future – because they trust us to be with them and to know the way. Attachment, even a transitional attachment, can make finding a new pathway forward possible.

Notes

1 The notion of 'development' is used here to include both species-typical and individually unique genes, maturational unfolding of the effects of these, expected and unexpected contexts, and unique, person-specific experience.

Bibliography

Abramson, L.Y., Seligman, M.E. and Teasdale, J.D. (1978) 'Learned helplessness in humans: critique and reformulation', *Journal of Abnormal Psychology*, 87 (1): 49–74.

Ainsworth, M.D.S. (1979) 'Attachment as related to mother-infant interaction', *Advances in the Study of Behaviour*, 9: 2–52.

Ainsworth, M., Blehar, M., Waters, E. and Wall, S. (1978) *Patterns of Attachment: A Psychological Study of the Strange Situation*. Hillsdale, NJ: Erlbaum.

Ainsworth, M.D.S. and Wittig, B.A. (1969) 'Attachment and exploratory behaviour of one-year-olds in a strange situation', in B.M. Foss (ed.), *Determinants of Behaviour IV*. London: Methuen, pp. 111–36.

Altman, H., Collins, M. and Mundy, P. (1997) 'Subclinical hallucinations and delusions in nonpsychotic adolescents', *Journal of Child Psychology and Psychiatry*, 38: 413–420.

American Psychiatric Association (1994) '*Diagnostic and Statistical Manual of Mental Disorders* (4th edn). Washington, DC: Author.

Andrews, G. (2001) 'The placebo response in depression: bane of research, boon to therapy', *British Journal of Psychiatry*, 178: 192–4.

Anthony, E. (2002) *Psychoanalytic Theory: An Introduction* (2nd edn). Durham, NC: Duke University Press.

Ascher-Svanum, H., Faries, D.E., Zhu, B., Ernst, F.R., Swartz, M.S. and Swanson, J.W. (2006) 'Schizophrenia in usual care', *Journal of Clinical Psychiatry*, 67: 453–60.

Associated Press (2002, 21 February) 'Transcript of Andrea Yates confession', retrieved 5 March 2008, from http://www.chron.com/disp/story.mpl/special/drownings/1266294.html.

Aubé, M. (2002) 'Improving patient compliance to prophylactic migraine therapy', *Canadian Journal of Neurological Sciences*, 29 (Suppl. 2): S40–3.

Australian Institute of Health and Welfare (2004) *Child Protection Australia 2002–03*. Child Welfare Series no. 34. Canberra: Author.

Baddeley, A.D. and Hitch, G.J. (1974) 'Working memory', in G.A. Bower (ed.), *The Psychology of Learning and Motivation: Advances in Research and Theory*, Vol. 8. New York: Academic Press, pp. 47–89.

Bae, S.H., Joo, E. and Orlinsky, D.E. (2003) 'Psychotherapists in South Korea: professional and practice characteristics', *Psychotherapy: Theory, Research, Practice, Training*, 40 (4): 302–16.

Bandura, A. (1998) 'Health promotion from the perspective of social cognitive theory', *Psychology and Health*, 13: 623–49.

Barbaree, H.E. (1991) 'Denial and minimizations among sex offenders: assessment and treatment outcome', *Forum on Corrections Research*, 3: 30–3.

Barnes, J. and Stein, A. (2000) 'Effects of parental psychiatric and physical illness on child development', in M. Gelder, J.J. Lopez-Ibor and N. Andreasen (eds), *New Oxford Textbook of Psychiatry*. Oxford: Oxford University Press.

Bateman, A. and Fonagy, P. (2001) 'Treatment of borderline personality disorder with psychoanalytically oriented partial hospitalization: an 18-month follow-up', *American Journal of Psychiatry*, 158: 36–42.

Bateman, A. and Holmes, J. (1995) *An Introduction to Psychoanalysis: Contemporary Theory and Practice*. London: Routledge.

Bateson, G. (1972/1987) *Steps to an Ecology of Mind: Collected Essays in Anthropology, Psychiatry, Evolution, and Epistemology*. Lanham, MD: Jason Aronson.

Baumrind, D. (1971) 'Current patterns of parental authority', *Developmental Psychology*, 4 (1): 1–103.

Bearup, R.S. and Palusci, V.J. (1999) 'Improving child welfare through a children's ombudsman', *Child Abuse and Neglect*, 23 (5): 449–57.

Beck, A.T. (1976) *Cognitive Therapy and the Emotional Disorders*. New York: International Universities Press.

Beck, C.T. and Gable, R.K. (2005) 'The postpartum depression screening scale (PDSS)', in C. Henshaw and S. Elliott (eds), *Screening for Perinatal Depression*. London: Jessica Kingsley, pp. 133–40.

Beck-Sander, A. (1995) 'Childhood abuse in adult offenders: the role of control in perpetuating cycles of abuse', *Journal of Forensic Psychiatry*, 6: 486–98.

Beckett, R.C. (1994) 'Cognitive-behavioural treatment with sex offenders', in T. Morrison, M. Erooga and R.C. Beckett (eds), *Sexual Offending Against Children: Assessment and Treatment of Male Abusers*. London: Routledge, pp. 80–101.

Beckett, C., McKeigue, B. and Taylor, H. (2007) 'Coming to conclusions: social workers' perceptions of the decision-making process in care proceedings', *Child and Family Social Work*, 12: 54–63.

Beecher, H. (1946) 'Pain in men wounded in battle', *Annals of Surgery*, 123: 96–105.

Bell, L.G. and Bell, D.C. (1979) 'Triangulation: pitfall for the developing child', *Handbook of International Sociometry*, 32: 150–5.

Bellis, M.A., Hughes, K., Hughes, S. and Ashton, J.R. (2005) 'Measuring paternal discrepancy and its public health consequences', *Journal of Epidemiology and Community Health*, 59 (9): 749–54.

Belsky, J. and Draper, P. (1987) 'Reproductive strategies and radical solutions', *Transaction/Society*, 24: 20–4.

Bender, D. and Lösel, F. (2005) Riskofaktoren, Schutzfaktoren und Resilienz bei Mißhandlung und Vernachlässigung ['Risk factors, protective factors and resilience with ill-treatment and neglect'], in U.T. Egle, S.O. Hoffmann and P. Joraschky (eds), *Sexueller Mißbrauch, Mißhandlung, Vernachlässigung*. Stuttgart: Schattauer, pp. 85–115.

Benoit, D. and Parker, K. (1994) 'Stability and transmission of attachment across three generations', *Child Development*, 65 (5): 1444–56.

Berg, I.K. and Miller, S. (1992) *Working with the Problem Drinker: A Solution-Focused Approach*. New York: Norton.

Berne, E. (1964) *Games People Play: The Psychology of Human Relationships*. New York, NY: Grove Press.

Bettelheim, B. (1967) *The Empty Fortress: Infantile Autism and the Birth of the Self*. New York: Free Press.

Bianchi, S. and Spain, D. (1996) 'Women, work and family in America', *Population Bulletin*, 51: 12.

Black, S., Hardy, G., Turpin, G. and Parry, G. (2005) 'Self-reported attachment styles and therapeutic orientation of therapists and their relationship with reported general alliance quality and problems in therapy', *Psychology and Psychotherapy: Theory, Research and Practice*, 78 (3): 363–77.

Blaney, P.H. (1986) 'Affect and memory: a review', *Psychological Bulletin*, 99: 229–46.

Blumberg, M.L. (1974) 'Psychopathology of the abusing parent', *American Journal of Psychotherapy*, 28 (1): 21–9.

Bosco, G.L., Renk, K., Dinger, T.M., Epstein, M.K. and Phares, V. (2003) 'The connections between adolescents' perceptions of parents, parental psychological symptoms, and adolescent functioning', *Journal of Applied Developmental Psychology*, 24: 179–200.

Botvinick, M., Jha, A.P., Bylsma, L.M., Fabian, S., Solomon, P. and Prkachin, K. (2005) 'Viewing facial expressions of pain engages cortical areas involved in the direct experience of pain', *Neuroimaging*, 25: 312–19.

Bowen, M. (1994) *Family Therapy in Clinical Practice*. London: Jason Aronson.

Bowlby, J. (1944a) 'Forty-four juvenile thieves: their characters and home-life. I', *International Journal of Psycho-Analysis*, 25: 19–53.

Bowlby, J. (1944b) 'Forty-four juvenile thieves: their characters and home-life. II', *International Journal of Psycho-Analysis*, 25: 107–28.

Bowlby, J. (1949) 'The study and reduction of group tension in the family', *Human Relations*, 2: 123–8.

Bowlby, J. (1958) 'The nature of a child's tie to his mother', *International Journal of Psycho-Analysis*, 39: 350–73.

Bowlby, J. (1969/1983) *Attachment and Loss: Vol. 1. Attachment*. New York: Basic Books.

Bowlby, J. (1973) *Attachment and Loss: Vol. 2. Separation*. New York: Basic Books.

Bowlby, J. (1979) *The Making and Breaking of Affectional Bonds*. New York: Routledge.

Bowlby, J. (1980) *Attachment and Loss: Vol. 3. Loss, Sadness and Depression*. New York, NY: Basic Books.

Bowlby, J. (1988) *A Secure Base: Clinical Applications of Attachment Theory*. London: Routledge.

Bradley, R., Greene, J., Russ, E., Dutra, L. and Westen, D. (2005) 'A multidimensional meta-analysis of psychotherapy for PTSD', *American Journal of Psychiatry*, 162 (2): 214–27.

Breier, A., Albus, M., Pickar, D., Zahn, T.P., Wolkowitz, O.M. and Paul, S.M. (1987) 'Controllable and uncontrollable stress in humans: alterations in mood and neuroendocrine and psychophysiological function', *American Journal of Psychiatry*, 144 (11): 1419–25.

Breunlin, D.C. and Schwartz, R.C. (1986) 'Toward a common denominator of family therapy', *Family Process*, 25: 67–87.

Brodsky-Jones, N. (2003) 'Exploring decision-making: children's services workers choices', *Dissertation Abstracts International*, 64 (2-B): 1000.

Bronfenbrenner, U. (1979a) 'Contexts of child rearing: problems and prospects', *American Psychologist*, 34 (10): 844–50.

Bronfenbrenner, U. (1979b) *The Experimental Ecology of Human Development*. Cambridge, MA: Harvard University Press.

Bronstein, C. (ed.) (2001) *Kleinian Theory: A Contemporary Perspective*. London: Whurr.

Brown, C.A. (2004) 'Generational boundary dissolution in post-divorce parent–child relationships', *Dissertation Abstracts International*, 64 (8-B): 4106.

Bruner, J. (1984) 'Notes on the cognitive revolution: OISE's Centre for Applied Cognitive Science', *Source Interchange*, 15: 1–8.

Buchanan, A. (1996) *Cycles of Child Maltreatment*. Chichester: Wiley.

Budd, S. and Rushbridger, R. (eds) (2005) *Introducing Psychoanalysis: Essential Themes and Topics*. London: Routledge.

Bumpy, K. and Hansen, J.D. (1997) 'Intimacy deficits, fear of intimacy, and loneliness among sex offenders', *Criminal Justice and Behavior*, 24: 315–31.

Burke, L. (2003) 'The impact of maternal depression on familial relationships', *International Review of Psychiatry*, 15: 243–55.

Burton, L. (2007) 'Childhood adultification in economically disadvantaged families: a conceptual model', *Family Relations*, 56: 329–45.

Byng-Hall, J. (1995) *Rewriting Family Scripts: Improvization and Systems Change*. New York & London: Guilford Press.

Byng-Hall, J. (2002) 'Relieving parentified children's burdens in families with insecure attachment', *Family Process*, 41: 375–88.

Byng-Hall, J. (2008) 'The significance of children fulfilling parental roles: implications for family therapy', *Journal of Family Therapy*, 30: 147–62.

Cain, A.C. (2006) 'Parent suicide: pathways of effects into the third generation', *Psychiatry: Interpersonal and Biological Processes*, 69 (3): 204–27.

Cannon, W.B. (1914) 'The emergency function of the adrenal medulla in pain and the major emotions', *American Journal of Physiology*, 33: 356–72.

Carter, B.J. (1993) 'But you should have known: child sexual abuse and the non-offending mother', *Dissertation Abstracts International*, 53 (12-A): 4476.

Cassidy, J.P. (2002) 'The Stockholm syndrome, battered woman syndrome and the cult personality: an integrative approach', *Dissertation Abstracts International*, 62 (11-B): 5366.

Cassileth, B.R. (1998) *The Alternative Medicine Handbook: The Complete Reference Guide to Alternative and Complementary Therapies*. New York: W.W. Norton.

Chambers, J.A., Power, K.G. and Durham, R.C. (2004) 'Parental styles and long-term outcome following treatment for anxiety disorders', *Clinical Psychology and Psychotherapy*, 11: 187–98.

Chestand, L.W. and Heymann, I. (1973) 'Reducing the length of foster care', *Social Work*, 18: 88–92.

Child Welfare League of America (n.d.) *Fact Sheet: Behavioral Management and Children in Residential Care*. Retrieved 16 March 2008, from http://www.cwla. org/advocacy/secresfactsheet.htm

Child Welfare League of America (2003, 6 November) *Adoption: CWLA Testimony Submitted to the House Subcommittee on Human Resources of the Committee on Ways and Means for the Hearing to Examine Recent Failure to Protect Child Safety*. Retrieved 3 March 2008, from http://www.cwla.org/advocacy/adoption031106.htm.

Chronis, A.M., Lahey, A.M., Pelham, W.E., Kipp, H.L., Baumann, B.L. and Lee, S. (2003) 'Psychopathology and substance abuse in parents of young children with attention-deficit/hyperactivity disorder', *Journal of the American Academy of Child and Adolescent Psychiatry*, 42 (12): 1424–32.

Clark, D.C., Cavanaugh, S.V. and Gibbons, R.D. (1983) 'The core symptoms of depression in medical and psychiatric patients', *Journal of Nervous and Mental Disease*, 171: 705–13.

Cochrane, M.G., Bala, M.V., Down, K.E., Mauskopf, J. and Ben-Joseph, R.H. (2000) 'Inhaled corticosteroids for asthma therapy: patient compliance, devices, and inhalation technique', *Chest*, 117 (2): 542–50.

Corden, Z.M., Bosley, C.M., Rees, P.J. and Cochrane, G.M. (1997) 'Home nebulized therapy for patients with COPD: patient compliance with treatment and its relation to quality of life', *Chest*, 112 (5): 1278–82.

Courtney, M. and Barth, R.P. (1996) 'Pathways of older adolescents out of foster care: implications for independent living services', *Social Work*, 41: 75–83.

Courtney, M.C. and Piliavin, I. (1998) *Foster Youth Transitions to Adulthood: Outcomes 12 to 18 Months After Leaving Out-of-Home Care*. Madison, WI: Institute for Research on Poverty, University of Wisconsin-Madison.

Couzin, J. and Kaiser, J. (2007, 11 May) 'Closing the net on common disease genes: Huge data sets and lower cost analytical methods are speeding up the search for DNA variations that confer an increased risk for diabetes, heart disease, cancer, and other common ailments', *Science*, 316 (5826): 820–3.

Craig, C. (1995) '"What I need is a mom": the welfare state denies homes to thousands of foster children', *Policy Review*, 73 (40): 10.

Cremer, J.M. (1996) 'Empathy and nurturance: a study of incest offenders', *Dissertation Abstracts International*, 57 (6-B): 4024.

Crighton, D. (2006) 'Psychological research into reducing suicides', in G.J. Towl (ed.), *Psychological Research in Prisons*. Malden, MA: Blackwell.

Crighton, D. and Towl, G. (2007) 'Experimental interventions with sex offenders: a brief review of their efficacy', *Evidence-Based Mental Health*, 10: 35–7.

Crighton, D. and Towl, G. (2008) *Psychology in Prisons*. Malden, MA: Wiley-Blackwell.

Critchley, H.D., Mathias, C.J. and Dolan, R.J. (2001) 'Neuroanatomical basis for first- and second-order representation of bodily states', *Nature Neuroscience*, 4: 207–12.

Crittenden, P.M. (1979–2005) *CARE-Index: Infant Coding Manual*. Unpublished manuscript, Miami, FL. Available from the author.

Crittenden, P.M. (1981) 'Abusing, neglecting, problematic, and adequate dyads: Differentiating by patterns of interaction', *Merrill-Palmer Quarterly*, 27: 1–18.

Crittenden, P.M. (1982) Parents' Interview. University of Virginia, Charlottesville, VA. Available from the author.

Crittenden, P.M. (1983) 'Mother and infant patterns of interaction: developmental relationships', *Dissertation Abstracts International*, 45 (8-B), 2710.

Crittenden, P.M. (1985) 'Social networks, quality of child-rearing, and child development', *Child Development*, 56: 1299–313.

Crittenden, P.M. (1987) 'Non-organic failure-to-thrive: deprivation or distortion?', *Infant Mental Health Journal*, 8: 56–64.

Crittenden, P.M. (1988–2004) *Preschool Assessment of Attachment Manual*. Unpublished manuscript. Available from the author.

Crittenden, P.M. (1988a) 'Distorted patterns of relationship in maltreating families: the role of internal representational models', *Journal of Reproductive and Infant Psychology*, 6: 183–99.

Crittenden, P.M. (1988b) 'Family and dyadic patterns of functioning in maltreating families', in K. Browne, C. Davies and P. Stratton (eds), *Early Prediction and Prevention of Child Abuse*. Chichester: Wiley, pp. 161–89.

Crittenden, P.M. (1988c) 'Relationships at risk', in J. Belsky and T. Nezworski (eds), *The Clinical Implications of Attachment*. Hillsdale, NJ: Lawrence Erlbaum, pp. 136–74.

Crittenden, P.M. (1991) *Strategies for Changing Parental Behavior*. APSAC Advisor, Spring, 9.

Crittenden, P.M. (1992a) *CARE-Index: Toddlers Coding Manual*. Unpublished manuscript, Miami, FL. Available from the author.

Crittenden, P. M. (1992b) 'Children's strategies for coping with adverse home environments', *International Journal of Child Abuse and Neglect*, 16: 329–43.

Crittenden, P.M. (1992c) 'Quality of attachment in the preschool years', *Development and Psychopathology*, 4: 209–41.

Crittenden, P.M. (1992d) 'The social ecology of treatment: case study of a service system for maltreated children', *American Journal of Orthopsychiatry*, 62: 22–34.

Crittenden, P.M. (1993) 'Characteristics of neglectful parents: an information processing approach', *Criminal Justice and Behavior*, 20: 27–48.

Crittenden, P.M. (1995) 'Attachment and risk for psychopathology: The early years', *Journal of Developmental and Behavioral Pediatrics: Supplemental Issue on Developmental Delay and Psychopathology in Young Children*, 16: S12–S16.

Crittenden, P.M. (1997) 'Truth, error, omission, distortion, and deception: the application of attachment theory to the assessment and treatment of psychological disorder', in S.M.C. Dollinger and L.F. DiLalla (eds), *Assessment and Intervention Across the Lifespan*. Hillsdale, NJ: Erlbaum, pp. 35–76.

Crittenden, P.M. (1997–2005) *School-Age Assessment of Attachment Coding Manual*. Unpublished manuscript, Miami, FL. Available from the author.

Crittenden, P.M. (1998) 'Dangerous behavior and dangerous contexts: a thirty-five year perspective on research on the developmental effects of child physical abuse', in P. Trickett (ed.), *Violence to Children*. Washington, DC: American Psychological Association, pp. 11–38.

Crittenden, P.M. (1999a) *Attaccamento in etâ adulta.: L'approccio dinamico-maturativo alla adult attachment interview*. ['Attachment in adulthood: the dynamic-maturational approach to the adult attachment interview']. Edizione Italiana a cura di Graziella Fava Vizziello e Andrea Landini. Milan: Cortina.

Crittenden, P.M. (1999b) 'Child neglect: causes and contributors', in H. Dubowitz (ed.), *Neglected Children: Research, Practice, and Policy*. Thousand Oaks, CA: Sage, pp. 47–68.

Crittenden, P.M. (1999c) 'Danger and development: the organization of self-protective strategies', in J.I. Vondra and D. Barnett (eds), *Atypical Attachment in Infancy and Early Childhood Among Children at Developmental Risk*. Monographs of the Society for Research on Child Development, 64, (3, Serial No. 258), pp. 145–71.

Crittenden, P.M. (2000a) 'A dynamic-maturational exploration of the meaning of security and adaptation: empirical, cultural, and theoretical considerations', in P.M. Crittenden and A.H. Claussen (eds), *The Organization of Attachment Relationships: Maturation, Culture, and Context*. New York: Cambridge University Press, pp. 358–84.

Crittenden, P.M. (2000b) 'A dynamic-maturational model of the function, development, and organization of human relationships', in R.S.L. Mills and S. Duck (eds), *Developmental Psychology of Personal Relationships*. Chichester, UK: Wiley, pp. 199–218.

Crittenden, P.M. (2000c) 'Moldear la arcilla: El proceso de construción del self y su relación conla psicoterapia' ['Molding clay: The process of constructing the self and its relation to psychotherapy'], *Revista de Psicoterapia*, 41: 67–82.

Crittenden, P.M. (2002) 'Attachment theory, information processing, and psychiatric disorder', *World Journal of Psychiatry*, 1: 72–5.

Crittenden, P.M. (2004) 'Frühe Förderung von Hochrisiko-Kindern: Der Beitrag von Bindungstheorie und Bindungsforschung', in *It takes two to tango: Frühne Kindheit an der Schnittstelle zwischen Jungendhilfe und Entwickiungspsychologie*. Berlin, pp. 36–57.

Crittenden, P.M. (2005a) 'Der CARE-Index als Hilfsmittel für Früherkennung, Intervention und Forschung. Frühförderung interdisziplinär' ['Early inter-disciplinary intervention']. Special issue: *Bindungsorientierte Ansätze in der Praxis der Frühförderung* 24: S.99–106 (English on www.patcrittenden.com.).

Crittenden, P.M. (2005b, June) 'Kate and the cutters: a hard rock in search of balance', in P. Crittenden, *Assessing Representations of Danger: The AAI and Child, Sexual, Self, and Delusional Abuse: Using the AAI as a Case-Specific Therapeutic Tool for Assessing Representations of Danger as a Guide to Treatment*. Symposium conducted at the meeting of the International Congress on Cognitive Psychotherapy, Göteborg, Sweden.

Crittenden, P.M. (2005c) 'The origins of physical punishment: an ethological/ attachment perspective on the use of punishment by human parents', in M. Donnelly and M.A. Strauss (eds), *Corporal Punishment of Children in Theoretical Perspective*. New Haven, CT: Yale University Press, pp. 73–90.

Crittenden, P.M. (2005d) *Transition to Adulthood Attachment Interview*. Unpublished manuscript, Miami, FL. Available from the author.

Crittenden, P.M. (2006) 'A dynamic-maturational model of attachment', *Australian and New Zealand Journal of Family Therapy*, 27: 105–15.

Crittenden, P. and Ainsworth, M.D.S. (1989) 'Child maltreatment and attachment theory', in D. Cicchetti and V. Carlson (eds), *Child Maltreatment: Theory and Research on the Causes and Consequences of Child Abuse and Neglect*. New York: Cambridge University Press, pp. 432–63.

Crittenden, P.M. and Claussen, A.H. (1993) 'Severity of maltreatment: assessment and policy implications', in C.J. Hobbes and J.M. Wynne (eds), *Baillière's Clinical Paediatrics: International Practice and Research*. London: Baillière Tindall, pp. 87–100.

Crittenden, P.M. and Claussen, A.H. (eds) (2000) *The Organization of Attachment Relationships: Maturation, Culture, and Context*. New York: Cambridge University Press.

Crittenden, P.M. and DiLalla, D.L. (1988) 'Compulsive compliance: the development of an inhibitory coping strategy in infancy', *Journal of Abnormal Child Psychology*, 16: 585–99.

Crittenden, P.M., Claussen, A.H. and Kozlowska, K. (2007) 'Choosing a valid assessment of attachment for clinical use: A comparative study', *Australia New Zealand Journal of Family Therapy*, 28: 78–87.

Crittenden, P.M., Claussen, A.H. and Sugarman, D.B. (1994) 'Physical and psychological maltreatment in middle childhood and adolescence', *Development and Psychopathology*, 6: 145–64.

Crittenden, P.M. and Craig, S. (1990) 'Developmental trends in child homicide', *Journal of Interpersonal Violence*, 5: 202–16.

Crittenden, P.M. and Kulbotten, G.R. (2007) 'Familial contributions to ADHD: an attachment perspective', *Tidsskrift for Norsk Psykologorening*, 10: 1220–29.

Crittenden, P.M. and Heller, M.B. (2008) *Chronic PTSD and Attachment: A Comparison Study of Self-Protective Strategies and Unresolved Childhood Trauma*. Manuscript submitted for publication.

Crittenden, P.M. and Landini, A. (1999) *Administering the School-Age Assessment of Attachment*. Unpublished manuscript, Miami, FL. Available from the author.

Crittenden, P.M., Lang, C., Claussen, A.H. and Partridge, M.F. (2000) 'Relations among mothers' procedural, semantic, and episodic internal representational models of parenting', in P.M. Crittenden and A.H. Claussen (eds), *The Organization of Attachment Relationships: Maturation, Culture, and Context*. New York: Cambridge University Press, pp. 214–33.

Crittenden, P.M., Partridge, M.F. and Claussen, A.H. (1991) 'Family patterns of relationship in normative and dysfunctional families', *Development and Psychopathology*, 3: 491–512.

Dallos, R. and Draper, R. (2005) *An Introduction to Family Therapy: Systemic Theory and Practice*. Maidenhead: Open University Press.

Dallos, R. and Smith, J.A. (2008) 'Practice as research and research as practice: How the qualitative case study can invigorate clinical psychology', *Clinical Psychology Forum*, 182: 18–23.

Daly, M. and Wilson, M. (1996) 'Violence against stepchildren', *Current Directions in Psychological Science*, 5: 77–81.

Damasio, A.R. (1994) *Descartes' Error: Emotion, Reason, and the Human Brain*. New York: Avon Books.

Damasio, A.R. (1999) *The Feeling of What Happens: Body and Emotion in the Making of Consciousness*. Fort Worth, TX: Harcourt.

Damasio, A.R. (2003) *Looking for Espinoza, Joy, Sorrow and the Feeling Brain*. Orlando, FL: Harcourt.

Davidson, J.R.T. (2004) 'Long-term treatment and prevention of posttraumatic stress disorder', *Journal of Clinical Psychiatry*, 65: 44–8.

Davidson, M. (1983) *Uncommon Sense*. Los Angeles: J.P. Tarcher.

Dawkins, R. (1976) *The Selfish Gene*. New York: Oxford University Press.

Dawkins, R. (2008) *The God Delusion*. New York: First Mariner Books.

Denno, D.W. (2003) 'Who is Andrea Yates?: a short story about insanity', *Duke Journal of Gender Law and Policy*, 10 (1): 1–60.

DeWaal, F.B.M. (2000) 'Primates: a natural heritage of conflict resolution', *Science*, 289: 586–90.

Diatchenko, L., Nackley, A.G., Tchivileva, I.E. Shabalina, S.A. and Maixner, W. (2007) 'Genetic architecture of human pain perception', *Trends in Genetics*, 23 (12): 605–13.

Dietz, P. (2002) *Report to the Court*, 25 February 2002. Park Dietz Associates, Inc. Retrieved 17 March 2008, from http://www.parkdietzassociates.com/files/Report_of_Dr._Park_Dietz_re._Andrea_Yates__2002.pdf.

Diorio, J. and Meaney, M.J. (2007) 'Maternal programming of defensive responses through sustained effects on gene expression', *Journal of Psychiatry & Neuroscience*, 32 (4): 275–84.

Dixon, L., Hamilton-Giachritsis, C. and Browne, K. (2005) 'Attributions and behaviors of parents abused as children: a mediational analysis of the intergenerational continuity of child maltreatment', II, *Journal of Child Psychology and Psychiatry*, 46: 58–68.

Dobash, R.P., Dobash, R.E., Wilson, M. and Daly, M. (1992) 'The myth of sexual symmetry in marital violence', *Social Problems*, 39: 71–91.

Doidge, N. (2007) *The Brain That Changes Itself: Stories of Personal Triumph from the Frontiers of Brain Science*. New York: Viking.

Donnelly, D. and Fraser, J. (1998) 'Gender differences in sado-masochistic arousal among college students', *Sex Roles*, 39 (5–6): 391–407.

Duane, Y., Carr, A., Cherry, J., MacGrath, K. and O'Shea, D. (2003) 'Profiles of the parents of adolescent CSA perpetrators attending a voluntary outpatient treatment program in Ireland', *Child Abuse Review*, 12: 5–24.

Dubowitz, H. (1990) 'Costs and effectiveness of interventions in child maltreatment', *Child Abuse and Neglect*, 14: 177–86.

Duncan, B.L. and Miller, S.D. (2000) *The Heroic Client: Doing Client-Directed, Outcome-Informed Therapy*. San Francisco: Jossey-Bass.

Edelman, G. (1989) *The Remembered Present*. New York: Basic Books.

Eibl-Eibesfeldt, I. (1970) *Love and Hate: On the Natural History of Behavior Patterns*. New York: Methuen.

Eisenberger, N.I., Lieberman, M.D. and Williams, K.D. (2003) 'Does rejection hurt? An FMRI study of social exclusion', *Science*, 302: 290–92.

Elliott, D.M. and Guy, J.D (1993) 'Mental health professionals versus non-mental-health professionals: childhood trauma and adult functioning'. *Professional Psychology: Research and Practice*, 24 (1): 83–90.

Ellis, A. (1974) 'Rational-emotive theory: Albert Ellis', in A. Burton (ed.), *Operational Theories of Personality*. Oxford: Brunner/Mazel, pp. 308–44.

England National Statistics (2005) *Children Looked After by Local Authorities Year Ending 31 March 2004. Commentary and National Tables National Statistics*, Vol. 1. London: Stationery Office.

England National Statistics (2006) *Children Looked after in England (Including Adoption and Care Leavers), 2005–2006*. First Release (SFR 44/2006). London: Department for Education and Skills.

Enns, M.W., Cox, B.J. and Clara, I. (2002) 'Parental bonding and adult psychopathology: results from the US national comorbidity survey', *Psychological Medicine*, 32: 997–1008.

Erikson, E.H. (1950) *Childhood and Society*. New York: Norton.

Etherton, J., Bridge, S., Hertzell, D., Horder, J. and Parker, K. (2007) *Cohabitation: The Financial Consequences of Relationship Breakdown*. London. Retrieved 28 April 2008, from www.lawcom.gov.uk.

Eysenck, H.J. (1952) 'The effects of psychotherapy: an evaluation', *Journal of Consulting Psychology*, 16: 319–24.

Fairbairn, R.W.D. (1944) 'Endosychic structure considered in terms of object relationships', *International Journal of Psycho-Analysis*, 25: 70–93.

Fairbairn, W.R.D. (1952) *An Object-Relations Theory of the Personality*. New York: Basic Books.

Falkov, A. (1996) *Study of Working Together 'Part 8' Reports: Fatal Child Abuse and Parental Psychiatric Disorder*. London: Department of Health.

Fanshel, D., Finch, S.J. and Grundy, J.F. (1990) *Foster Children in a Life Course Perspective*. New York: Columbia University Press.

Federal Criminal Police Office/Bundeskriminalamt (2004) *Police Crime Statistics*. Wiesbaden, Germany: Author.

Feldman, H.N. (1994) 'Domestic cats and passive submission', *Animal Behaviour*, 47 (2): 457–59.

Finkelhor, D. (1984) *Child Sexual Abuse*. New York: Free Press.

Finkelhor, D., Ormrod, R., Turner, H. and Hamby, S.L. (2005) 'The victimization of children and youth: a comprehensive national survey', *Child Maltreatment*, 10 (1): 5–25.

Fischer, D.G. and McDonald, W.L. (1998) 'Characteristics of intrafamilial and extrafamilial child sexual abuse', *Child Abuse and Neglect*, 22: 915–29.

Fisher, H. (1992) *Anatomy of Love: A Natural History of Monogamy, Adultery, and Divorce*. New York: W.W. Norton.

Fisher, D., Beech, A. and Brown, K. (1998) 'Locus of control and its relationship to treatment change and abuse history in child sexual abuse', *Legal and Criminological Psychology*, 42: 141–8.

Fivush, R. and Hamond, N.R. (1990) 'Autobiographical memory across the preschool years: Toward reconceptualizing childhood amnesia', in R. Fivush and J.A. Hudson (eds), *Emory Symposia in Cognition: Vol. 3. Knowing and Remembering in Young Children*. New York: Cambridge University Press, pp. 223–48.

Fluke, J.D., Shusterman, G.R., Hollinshead, D. and Yuan, Y.T. (2005) *Rereporting and Recurrence of Child Maltreatment: Findings from NCANDS*. Washington, DC: Department of Health and Human Services.

Fombonne, E., Wostear, G., Cooper, V., Harrington, R. and Rutter, M. (2001) 'The Maudsley long-term follow-up of child and adolescent depression. I: Psychiatric outcomes in adulthood', *British Journal of Psychiatry*, 179: 210–17.

Fonagy, P. (1999) 'The transgenerational transmission of holocaust trauma: Lessons learned from the analysis of an adolescent with obsessive-compulsive disorder', *Attachment and Human Development*, 1: 92–114.

Fonagy, P., Target, M., Cottrell, D. Phillips, J. and Kurtz, Z. (2002) *What Works for Whom?: A Critical Review of Treatments for Children and Adolescents*. New York: Guilford.

Fonagy, P., Roth, A. and Higgit, A. (2005) 'Psychodynamic psychotherapies: evidence-based practice and clinical wisdom', *Bulletin of the Menninger Clinic*, 69: 1–58.

Fortner, B.V. (2000) 'The effectiveness of grief counseling and therapy: a quantitative review', *Dissertation Abstracts International*, 60 (8-B): 4221.

Foster, S., Rollefson, M., Doksum, T., Noonan, D. and Robinson, G. (2005) *School Mental Health Services in the United States, 2002–2003* (No. SMA 05-4068). Rockville, MD: Center for Mental Health Services, Substance Abuse and Mental Health Services Administration.

Freeman, D., Garety, P.A., Kuipers, E., Fowler, D., Bebbington, P.E. and Dunn, G. (2007) Acting on persecutory delusions: the importance of safety seeking', *Behaviour Research and Therapy*, 45: 89–99.

Freid, V.M., Makuc, D.M. and Rooks, R.N. (1998) 'Ambulatory health care visits by children: principal diagnosis and place of visit', *Vital Health Statistics Series*, 13 (137): 1–23. Hyattsville, MD: National Center for Health Statistics.

Frenken, J. (1994) 'Treatment of incest perpetrators: a five-phase model', *Child Abuse and Neglect*, 18 (4): 357–65.

Freundlich, M., Avery, R.J., Gerstenzang, S. and Munson, S. (2006) 'Permanency options and goals: Considering multifaceted definitions', *Child and Youth Care Forum*, 35: 355–74.

Friedrich, W. and Wheeler, K.K. (1982) 'The abusing parent revisited: a decade of psychological research', *Journal of Nervous and Mental Disease*, 170 (10): 577–87.

Garlick, Y., Marshall, W.L. and Thornton, D. (1996) 'Intimacy deficits and attribution of blame among sexual offenders', *Legal and Criminological Psychology*, 1: 251–8.

Garwood, M.M. and Close, W. (2001) 'Identifying the psychological needs of foster children', *Child Psychiatry and Human Development*, 32 (2): 125–35.

Gau, S.F. and Soong, W.T. (1999) 'Psychiatric comorbidity of adolescents with sleep terrors or sleepwalking: a case-control study', *Australian and New Zealand Journal of Psychiatry*, 33: 734–9.

Gazzaniga, M. (2005) *The Ethical Brain*. Chicago, IL: Dana Press.

Gelles, R.J. (1991) 'Physical violence, child abuse, and child homicide: a continuum of violence, or distinct behaviors?', *Human Nature*, 2 (1): 59–72.

George, C., Kaplan, N. and Main, M. (1985/1996) *The Adult Attachment Interview: Interview Protocol*. Unpublished manuscript, University of California, Berkeley.

George, C. and Solomon, J. (1999) 'Attachment and caregiving: the caregiving behavioral system', in J. Cassidy and P.R. Shaver (eds), *Handbook of Attachment: Theory, Research, and Clinical Applications*. New York: Guilford Press, pp. 649–70.

Glaser, D. (2000) 'Child abuse and neglect and the brain: a review', *Journal of Child Psychology and Psychiatry*, 41: 97–116.

Glick, I., Pham, D. and Davis, J.M. (2006) 'Concomitant medications may not improve outcome of antipsychotic monotherapy for stabilized patients with nonacute schizophrenia', *Journal of Clinical Psychiatry*, 67 (8): 1261–65.

Goddard, C.R. and Stanley, J.R. (1994) 'Viewing the abusive parent and the abused child as captor and hostage: the application of hostage theory to the effects of child abuse', *Journal of Interpersonal Violence*, 9 (2): 258–69.

Godfrey, K. (2006) 'The "developmental origins" hypothesis: epidemiology', in P.D. Gluckman and M.A. Hanson (eds), *Developmental Origins of Health and Disease*. Cambridge: Cambridge University Press, pp. 6–32.

Godinho, F., Magnin, M., Frot, M., Perchet, C. and Garcia-Larrea, L. (2006) 'Emotional modulation of pain: is it the sensation or what we recall?', *Journal of Neuroscience*, 26 (44): 11454–61.

Goglia, L.R., Jurkovic, G.J., Burt, A.M. and Burge-Callaway, K.G. (1992) 'Generational boundary distortions by adult children of alcoholics: child-as-parent and child-as-mate', *American Journal of Family Therapy*, 20 (4): 291–9.

Goldstein, K. (1934/1995) *The Organism: A Holistic Approach to Biology Derived from Pathological Data in Man*. New York: Zone Books.

Goldstein, J., Freud, A. and Solnit, A.J. (1973) *Beyond the Best Interests of the Child*. New York: Free Press.

Goldstein, J., Solnit, A.J. and Goldstein, S. (and the estate of Anna Freud) (1996) *Best Interest of the Child: The Least Detrimental Alternative*. New York: Free Press.

Goodman, L., Corcoran, C., Turner, K., Yuan, N. and Green, B. (1998) 'Assessing traumatic event exposure: general issues and preliminary findings for the stressful life events screening questionnaire', *Journal of Traumatic Stress*, 11: 521–42.

Göpfert, M., Webster, J. and Seeman, M.V. (eds) (2004) *Parental Psychiatric Disorder: Distressed Parents and Their Families* (2nd edn). New York: Cambridge University Press.

Gregory, R. (1998) 'Snapshots from the decade of the brain: brainy mind', *British Medical Journal*, 317: 1693–5.

Guerin, P.G., Fay, L., Burden, S. and Kautto, J. (1987) *The Evaluation and Treatment of Marital Conflict: A Four Stage Approach*. New York : Basic Books.

Guidano, V.F. (1991) *The Self in Process*. New York: Guilford.

Guidano, V.F. and Liotti, G. (1983) *Cognitive Processes and Emotional Disorders*. New York: Guilford.

Gunlicks, M.L. and Weissman, M.M. (2008) 'Change in child psychopathology with improvement in parental depression: a systematic review', *Journal of the American Academy of Child and Adolescent Psychiatry*, 47 (4): 379–89.

Guttmann, A., Dick, P. and To, T. (2004) 'Infant hospitalization and maternal depression, poverty, and single parenthood: a population-based study', *Child: Care, Health and Development*, 30: 67–75.

Haapasalo, J., Puupponen, M. and Crittenden, P.M. (1999) 'Victim to victimizer: the psychology of isomorphism in a case of a recidivist pedophile', *Journal of Child Sexual Abuse*, 7: 97–115.

Haley, J. (1973) *Uncommon Therapy*. New York: Norton.

Haley, J. (1976a) 'Development of a theory: a history of a research project', in C.E. Sluzki and D.C. Ransom (eds), *Double Bind: The Foundation of the Communicational Approach to the Family*. New York: Grune and Stratton.

Haley, J. (1976b) *Problem Solving Therapy*. San Francisco: Jossey-Bass.

Haley, J. (1980) *Leaving Home: The Therapy of Disturbed Young People*. New York: Basic Books.

Hall, G.C.N. and Hirschman, R. (1992) 'Sexual agression against children', *Criminal Justice and Behavior*, 19 (1): 8–23.

Hanson, D.R. and Gottesman, I.I. (2007) 'Choreographing genetic, epigenetic, and stochastic steps in the dances of developmental psychopathology', in A. Masten (ed.), *The Minnesota Symposium on Child Psychology: Vol. 34. Multilevel Dynamics in Developmental Psychopathology: Pathways to the Future*. Mahwah, NJ: Lawrence Erlbaum, pp. 27–44.

Havez, J.Y. (1992) 'Prise en charge de l'abuseur, après abus sexuel sur mineur d'âge: Un point de vue systémique' ['Management of the abuser after child sexual abuse: A systemic viewpoint']. *Thérapie Familiale*, 13 (4): 363–75.

Hawes, V. and Cottrell, D. (1999) 'Disruption of children's lives by maternal psychiatric admission', *Psychiatric Bulletin*, 23: 153–56.

Hay, D.F. and Pawlby, S. (2003) 'Prosocial development in relation to children's and mothers' psychological problems', *Child Development*, 74: 1314–27.

Haynes, R.B., Montague, P., Oliver, T., McKibbon, K.A., Brouwers, M.C. and Kanani, R. (2000) 'Interventions for helping patients follow prescriptions for medicines', *Cochrane Database Systematic Reviews*, 2: CD 000011.

Heide, K.M. (1992) *Why Kids Kill Parents: Child Abuse and Adolescent Homicide*. Columbus, OH: Ohio State University Press.

Hendry, S. (1999) 'Pain', in R.A. Wilson and F. Keil (eds), *The MIT Encyclopedia of the Cognitive Sciences (MITECS)*. Cambridge, MA: Mit Press. Retrieved on 22 March 2008, from http://rm-f.net/%7Epennywis/MITECS/Entry/hendry.

Herman, J.L. (1992) *Trauma and Recovery*. New York: Basic Books.

Hermans, C. (2002) *The Smallest Momentum Possible*. Retrieved 30 March 2008, from http://www.du.ahk.nl/mijnsite/papers/reactiontime.htm.

Hien, D.A. and Miele, G.M. (2003) 'Emotion-focused coping as a mediator of maternal cocaine use and anti-social behavior', *Psychology of Addictive Behaviors*, 17: 49–55.

Higgins, D. (2005) 'Differentiating between child maltreatment experiences', *Family Matters*, 69: 50–55.

Hinde, R. (1982) *Ethology: Its Nature and Relations with Other Sciences*. New York: Oxford University Press.

Hochman, J. (2002) '"Where is the body?": revisiting Ahsen's triple code ISM model and dynamic imagery', *Journal of Mental Imagery*, 26 (1–2): 54–60.

Hochman, J. (2007) 'Introduction', *Journal of Mental Imagery*, 31 (1–2): 15–22.

Hoffmeyer, J. (1995) 'The semiotic body-mind', in N. Tasca (ed.), *Essays in Honour of Thomas Sebeok. Cruzeiro Semiótico* (special issue), 22/25: 367–83.

Holden, G.W. and Zambarano, R.J. (1992) 'Passing the rod: similarities between parents and their children in orientations toward physical punishment', in I.E. Sigel, A.V. McGillicuddy-DeLisi and J.J. Goognow (eds), *Parental Belief Systems: The Psychological Consequences for Children* (2nd edn). Hillsdale, NJ: Erlbaum, pp. 143–72.

Holmes, J. (1997) 'Editorial. Mental health of doctors', *Advances in Psychiatric Treatment*, 3: 251–3.

Honoré, C. (2008) *Under Pressure: Rescuing Childhood from the Culture of Hyper-parenting*. Ontario: Knopf Canada.

Horwitz, S.M., Balestracci, K.M.B. and Simms, M.D. (2001) 'Foster care placement improves children's functioning. *Archives of Pediatrics and Adolescent Medicine*, 155: 1255 60.

Howard, L. (2000) 'Psychotic disorders and parenting – the relevance of patients' children for general adult psychiatric services', *Psychiatric Bulletin*, 24: 324–6.

Howard, L.M. and Simon, H. (2003) 'Sudden infant death syndrome and psychiatric disorders', *British Journal of Psychiatry*, 182 (5): 379–80.

Hubble, M.A., Duncan, B.L. and Miller, S.D. (1999) *The Heart and Soul of Change: What Works in Therapy*. Washington, DC: American Psychological Association.

Hughes, S.M., Harrison, M.A. and Gallup, G.G. (2007) 'Sex differences in romantic kissing among college students: an evolutionary perspective', *Evolutionary Psychology*, 5: 612–31.

Hunter, J.A., Figueredo, A.J., Malamuth, N.M. and Becker, J.V. (2003) 'Juvenile sex offenders: toward the development of a typology', *Sexual Abuse: Journal of Research and Treatment*, 15: 27–48.

Impett, E.A. and Peplau, L.A. (2003) 'Sexual compliance: gender, motivational, and relationship perspectives', *Journal of Sex Research*, 40 (1): 87–100.

Issa, F.A. and Edwards, D.H. (2006) 'Ritualized submission and the reduction of aggression in an invertebrate', *Current Biology*, 16: 2217–21.

Jacobvitz, D., Riggs, S. and Johnson, E. (1999) 'Cross-sex and same-sex family alliances: immediate and long-term effects on sons and daughters', in N.D. Chase (ed.), *Burdened Children: Theory, Research, and Treatment of Parentification*. Thousand Oaks, CA: Sage pp. 34–55.

Jasny, B.R. (2008, 7 March) 'Human genetics: an autism association', *Science*, 319: 1311.

Jean-Gilles, M. and Crittenden, P.M. (1990) 'Maltreating families: a look at siblings', *Family Relations*, 39: 323–9.

Jensen, P.S., Arnold, L.E., Swanson, J.M. *et al.* (2007) '3-year follow-up of the NIMH MTA study', *Journal of the American Academy of Child and Adolescent Psychiatry*, 46: 989–1002.

Johnson, J.G., Cohen, P., Kasen, S., Smailes, E. and Brook, S.D. (2001) 'Association of maladaptive parental behavior with psychiatric disorder among parents and their offspring', *Archives of General Psychiatry*, 58: 453–60.

Joseph, J. (2000) 'Not in their genes: a critical view of the genetics of attention-deficit hyperactivity disorder', *Developmental Review*, 20 (4): 539–67.

Josephson, A.M. and AACAP Work Group on Quality Issues (2007) 'Practice parameter for the assessment of the family: AACAP official action', *Journal of the American Academy of Child & Adolescent Psychiatry*, 46 (7): 922–37.

Kan, P., Popendikyte, V., Kaminsky, Z.A.,Yolken, R.H. and Petronis, A. (2004) 'Epigenetic studies of genomic retroelements in major psychosis', *Schizophrenia Research*, 67 (1): 95–106.

Kanemasa, Y. (2007) 'Intergenerational transmission of late-adolescent adult attachment styles: does attachment recur?', *Japanese Journal of Psychology*, 78 (4): 398–406.

Karterud, S. and Urnes, Ø. (2004) 'Short-term day treatment programmes for patients with personality disorders: what is the optimal composition?', *Nordic Journal of Psychiatry*, 58: 243–9.

Karterud, S. and Wilberg, T. (2007) 'From general day hospital treatment to specialized treatment programmes', *International Review of Psychiatry*, 19: 39–9.

Kaufman, J. and Zigler, E. (1987) 'Do abused children become abusive parents?', *American Journal of Orthopsychiatry*, 57 (2): 186–92.

Kazdin, A.E. (2000) *Psychotherapy for Children and Adolescents: Directions for Research and Practice*. New York: Oxford University Press.

Kazdin, A.E. (2005) *Parent Management Training: Treatment for Oppositional, Aggressive, and Antisocial Behavior in Children and Adolescents*. New York: Oxford University Press.

Kazdin, A.E. and Wassell, G. (1998) 'Treatment completion and therapeutic change among children referred for outpatient therapy', *Professional Psychology: Research and Practice*, 29 (4): 332–40.

Kazdin, A.E. and Wassel, G. (2000) 'Predictors of barriers to treatment and therapeutic change in outpatient therapy for antisocial children and their families', *Mental Health Services Research*, 2 (1): 27–40.

Kazui, M., Endo, T., Tanaka, A., Skagami, H. and Suganuma, M. (2000) 'Intergenerational transmission of attachment: Japanese mother–child dyads', *Japanese Journal of Educational Psychology*, 48 (3): 323–32.

Keller, T.E., Cusick, G.R. and Courtney, M.E. (2007) 'Approaching the transition to adulthood: Distinctive profiles of adolescents aging out of the child welfare system', *Social Service Review*, 81 (3): 453–84.

Kelley, S.J. (1996) 'Ritualistic abuse of children', in J. Briere, L. Berliner, J. Bulkley, C. Jenny and T. Reid (eds), The *APSAC Handbook on Child Maltreatment*. Thousand Oaks, CA: Sage, pp. 90–9.

Kelly, G.A. (1955) *The Psychology of Personal Constructs*. New York: Norton.

Kenardy, J. (2000) 'The current status of psychological debriefing', *British Medical Journal*, 321: 1032–33.

Kendell, R. and Jablensky, A. (2003) 'Distinguishing between the validity and utility of psychiatric diagnoses', *American Journal of Psychiatry*, 160: 4–12.

Kerig, P.K., Cowan, P.A. and Cowan, C.P. (1993) 'Marital quality and gender differences in parent–child interaction', *Developmental Psychology*, 29 (6): 931–9.

Kernberg, O.F. (1972) 'Early ego integration and object relations', *Annals of the New York Academy of Sciences*, 193: 233–47.

Kerr, M. and Bowen, M. (1988) *Family Evaluation*. New York: Norton.

Kessler, R.C., Sonnega, A., Bromet, E., Hughes, M. and Nelson, C.B. (1995) 'Posttraumatic stress disorder in the national comorbidity survey', *Archives of General Psychiatry*, 52 (12): 1048–60.

Khashan, A.S., Abel, K.M., McNamee, R. *et al.* (2008) 'Higher risk of offspring schizophrenia following antenatal maternal exposure to severe adverse life events', *Archives of General Psychiatry*, 65: 146–52.

Kihyun, K., Noll, J.G., Trickett, P.K. and Putnam, F.W. (2007) 'Psychosocial characteristics among non-offending mothers of sexually abused girls: findings from a prospective, multigenerational study', *Child Maltreatment*, 12: 338–51.

Klaus, M.H., Jerauld, R., Kreger, M.C., McAlpine, W., Steffa, M. and Kennell, J.H. (1972) 'Maternal attachment: importance of the first post-partum days', *New England Journal of Medicine*, 286: 460–3.

Klaus, M.H. and Kennell, J.H. (1976) *Maternal–infant Bonding*. St. Louis, MO: Mosby.

Klaus, M.H. and Kennell, J.H. (1982) *Parent–Infant bonding* (2nd edn). St. Louis, MO: Mosby.

Klein, D.C., Fencil-Morse, E. and Seligman, M.E. (1976) 'Learned helplessness, depression, and the attribution of failure', *Journal of Personality and Social Psychology*, 33 (5): 508–16.

Kohut, H. (1971) *The Analysis of the Self*. New York: International Universities Press.

Kohut, H. (1977) *The Restoration of the Self*. New York: International Universities Press.

Kolko, D.J. (1996) 'Child physical abuse', in J.N. Briere, L. Berliner, J. Bulkley, C., Jenny and T.A. Reid (eds), *The APSAC Handbook on Child Maltreatment*. Thousand Oaks, CA: Sage, pp. 21–50.

Kozlowska, K., Foley, S. and Crittenden, P.M. (2006) 'Factitious illness by proxy: Understanding underlying psychological processes and motivations', *Australia and New Zealand Journal of Family Therapy*, 27: 92–104.

Kozlowska, K., Nunn, K.P., Rose, D. Morris, A., Ouvrier, R.A. and Varghese, J. (2007) 'Conversion disorder in Australian pediatric practice', *Journal of the American Academy of Child and Adolescent Psychiatry*, 46 (1): 68–75.

Kreppner, J.M., O'Connor, T.G., Rutter, M. and the English and Romanian Adoptees Study Team (2001) 'Can inattention/overactivity be an institutional deprivation syndrome?', *Journal of Abnormal Child Psychology*, 29: 513–28.

Krug, E.G., Dahlberg, L.L., Mercy, J.A., Zwi, A.B. and Lozano, R. (2002) *World Report on Violence and Health*. Geneva: World Health Organization.

Kuleshnyk, I. (1984) 'The Stockholm syndrome: toward an understanding', *Social Action and the Law*, 10 (2): 37.

Kupper, K.A. (1995) 'Sudden infant and chronic illness in young children: effects on parental grief and family functioning', *Dissertation Abstracts International*, 56 (1-B): 0528.

Laing, R.D. and Esterson, A. (1964) *Sanity, Madness and the Family*. London: Tavistock.

Lambert, M.J. and Ogles, B.M. (2004) 'The efficacy and effectiveness of psychotherapy', in M. Lambert (ed.), *Bergin and Garfield's Handbook of Psychotherapy and Behavior Change*. New York: Wiley, pp. 139–93.

Laming, L. (2003, July) *The Victoria Climbié Inquiry*. Paper presented to Parliament by the Secretary of State for Health and the Secretary of State for the Home Department. London: Crown Copyright.

Larrance, D.T. and Twentyman, C.T. (1983) 'Maternal attributions and child abuse', *Journal of Abnormal Psychology*, 92 (4): 449–57.

Laws, D.R., Hanson, R.K., Osborn, C.A. and Greenbaum, P.E. (2000) 'Classification of child molesters by plethysmographic assessment of sexual arousal and a self-report measure of sexual preference', *Journal of Interpersonal Violence*, 15: 1297–1312.

LeDoux, J.E. (1994, June) 'Emotion, memory, and the brain', *Scientific American*, 270 (6): 50–8.

LeDoux, J.E. (1995) 'In search of an emotional system in the brain: leaping from fear to emotion and consciousness', in M. Gazzaniga (ed.), *The Cognitive Neurosciences*. Boston: MIT Press, pp. 1049–61.

Lehar, S. (2003) 'Gestalt isomorphism and the primacy of subjective conscious experience: a Gestalt bubble model', *Behavioral and Brain Sciences*, 26 (4): 375–444.

Leonard, L.M. (2003) 'Retreat, a treatment model for abusive families and their children ages birth through five', *Dissertation Abstracts International*, 63 (8-B): 3925.

Levant, M. and Bass, B. (1991) 'Parental identification of rapists and pedophiles', *Psychological Reports*, 69: 463–6.

Levine, P.A. (1997) *Waking the Tiger: Healing Trauma*. Berkeley, CA: North Atlantic Books.

Lewontin, R.C. (2001) 'Gene, organism and environment: a new introduction', in S. Oyama, P.E. Griffiths and R.D. Gray (eds), *Cycles of Contingency: Developmental Systems and Evolution*. Cambridge, MA: MIT Press, pp. 55–7.

Lieberman, M.D., Eisenberger, N.I., Crockett, M.J., Tom, S.M., Pfeifer, J.M. and Way, B.M. (2007) 'Putting feelings into words: Affect labeling disrupts amygdala activity in response to affective stimuli', *Psychological Science*, 18: 421–8.

Lilienfeld, S.O. (2007) 'Psychological treatments that cause harm', *Perspectives on Psychological Science*, 2: 53–70.

Linehan, M. (1993) *Cognitive-Behavioral Treatment of Borderline Personality Disorder*. New York: Guilford Press.

Linehan, M.M. and Dimeff, L. (2001) 'Dialectical behavior therapy in a nutshell', *California Psychologist*, 34: 10–13.

Linehan, M.M., Dimeff, L.A. and Koerner, K. (2007) *Dialectical Behavior Therapy in Clinical Practice: Applications Across Disorders and Settings*. New York: Guilford Press.

Lipton, B.H. (2005) *The Biology of Belief: Unleashing the Power of Consciousness, Matter, and Miracles*. Santa Rosa, CA: Elite Books.

Lohr, J.M., Devilly, G.J., Lilienfeld, S.O. and Olatunji, B.O. (2006) 'First do no harm, and then do some good: Science and professional responsibility in the response to disaster and trauma', *Behavior Therapist*, 29: 131–5.

Luthar, S.S., Suchman, N.E. and Altomare, M. (2007) 'Relational psychotherapy mothers' group: a randomized clinical trial for substance abusing mothers', *Development and Psychopathology*, 19: 243–61.

MacLean, P.D. (1990) *The Triune Brain in Evolution: Role in Paleocerebral Functions*. New York: Plenum Press.

Mahler, M., Fine, F. and Bergman, A. (1975) *The Psychological Birth of the Human Infant: Symbiosis and Individuation*. New York: Basic Books.

Main, M. and Goldwyn, R. (1984) 'Predicting rejection of her infant from mother's representation of her own experience: implications for the abused–abusing intergenerational cycle', *Child Abuse and Neglect. Special Issue: Infant Mental Health – from Theory to Intervention*, 8 (2): 203–17.

Maletzky, B.M. (1991) *Treating the Sexual Offender*. Newbury Park, CA: Sage.

Marano, H.E. (2008) *A Nation of Wimps: The High Cost of Invasive Parenting*. New York: Broadway Books.

Marks, I. (1987) 'The development of normal fear: a review', *Journal of Child Psychology and Psychiatry*, 28: 667–97.

Marmorstein, N.R. and Ianono, W.G. (2004) 'Major depression and conduct disorder in youth: associations with parental psychopathology and parent–child conflict', *Journal of Child Psychology and Psychiatry and Allied Disciplines*, 45: 377–86.

Marsa, F., O'Reilly, G., Carr, A. *et al.* (2004) 'Attachment styles and psychological profiles of child sex offenders in Ireland', *Journal of Interpersonal Violence*, 19: 228–51.

Marshall, W.L. and Barbaree, H.E. (1990) 'Outcome of comprehensive cognitive-behavioral treatment programs', in W.L. Marshall, D.R. Laws and H.E. Barbaree (eds), *Handbook of Sexual Assault*. New York: Plenum Press, pp. 363–85.

Marshall, W.L. and Hucker, S.J. (2006) 'Issues in the diagnosis of sexual sadism', in *Sexual Offender Treatment*, 1 (2). Retrieved 12 March 2008, from http://www.sexual-offender-treatment.org/40.0.html.

Maslow, A.H. (1954/1987) *Motivation and Personality* (3rd edn). New York: HarperCollins.

Maslow, A.H. (1969) *Psychology of Science: A Reconnaissance*. Chicago: Henry Regnery Pub.

Maslow, A.H. (1943/2006) 'A theory of human motivation', *Psychological Review*, 50: 370–96.

Matthias, R. (2005) 'Effective treatment of eating disorders in Europe: treatment outcome and its predictors', *European Eating Disorders Review*, 13 (3): 169–79.

Maturana, H.R. and Varela, F.J. (1980) *Autopoiesis and Cognition: The Realization of Living*. Boston: D. Reidel.

Maturana, H.R. and Varela, F.J. (1987) *The Tree of Knowledge: The Biological Roots of Human Understanding*. Boston: New Science Library/Shambhala Publications.

McDougall, W. (1936) 'Dynamics of the Gestalt psychology', *Character and Personality: A Quarterly for Psychodiagnostic and Allied Studies*, 4: 232–44.

McGuire, A.L., Cho, M.K., McGuire, S.E. and Caulfield, T. (2007, 21 September) 'The future of personal genomics', *Science*, 317: 1687.

McLellan, F. (2006, 2 December) 'Mental health and justice: the case of Andrea Yates', *The Lancet*, 368 (9551): 1951–5.

Meaney, M.J. (April, 2008) 'The contribution of epigenetics to psychotherapy'. Address given at the conference on Psicopatología y Apego: Desde las Neurociencias Basicás a la Psicología Clínica. Santiago, Chile, 25 April 2008.

Mee, S., Bunney, B.G., Reist, C., Potkin, S.G. and Bunney, W.E. (2006) 'Psychological pain: a review of evidence', *Journal of Psychiatric Research*, 40 (8): 680–90.

Meltzer, H., Gatward, R., Goodman, R. and Ford, T. (2000) *The Mental Health of Children and Adolescents in Great Britain: Summary Report*. London: Stationery Office.

Melzack, R., Coderre, T.J., Katz, J. and Vaccarino, A.L. (2001) 'The role of neural plasticity in chemical intolerance', *Annals of the New York Academy of Sciences*, 933 (1): 157–74.

Meyer, C.L., Oberman, M., White, K., Rone, M., Batra P. and Proano, T.C. (2001) 'Purposeful killing: neither "mad nor bad"', in *Mothers Who Kill their Children: Understanding the Acts of Moms from Susan Smith to the 'Prom Mom'*. New York: New York University Press, pp. 68–94).

Meyers, M., Diamond, R., Kezur, D., Scharf, C., Weinshel, M. and Rait, D. (1995) 'An infertility primer for family therapists. I. Medical, social, and psychological dimensions', *Family Process*, 34 (2): 219–29.

Migliano, A.B., Vinicius, L. and Lahr, M.M. (2007) 'Life history trade-offs explain the evolution of human pygmies', *Proceedings of the National Academy of Science of the United States of America*, 104: 20216–19.

Milgrom, J. and Beatrice, G. (2003) 'Coping with the stress of motherhood: cognitive and defence style of women with postnatal depression', *Stress and Health: Journal of the International Society for the Investigation of Stress*, 19 (5): 281–7.

Mill, J. and Petronis, A. (2007) 'Molecular studies of major depressive disorder: the epigenetic perspective', *Molecular Psychiatry*, 12 (9): 799–814.

Miller, J. (1987) 'Neither fish nor fowl nor good red herring', *Winnicott Studies: The Journal of the Squiggle Foundation*, 2: 4–18. London: Karnac Books.

Minuchin, S. (1974) *Families and Family Therapy*. Cambridge. MA: Harvard University Press.

Molina, B.S.G., Flory, K., Hinshaw, S.P. *et al.* (2007) 'Delinquent behavior and emerging substance use in the MTA at 36 months: Prevalence, course, and treatment effects', *Journal of the American Academy of Child and Adolescent Psychiatry*, 46 (8): 1028–40.

Molton, I.R., Graham, C., Stoelb, B.L. and Jensen, M.P. (2007) 'Current psychological approaches to the management of chronic pain', *Current Opinion in Anesthesiology*, 20 (5): 485–9.

Monaghan-Blout, S.M. (1999) 'A different kind of parent: Resisting the intergenerational legacy of maltreatment', *Dissertation Abstracts International*, 60 (2-B): 0838.

Mongillo, G., Barak, O. and Tsodyks, M.V. (2008) 'Synaptic theory of working memory', *Science*, 319: 1543–46.

Murphy, W.D. and Smith, T.A. (1996) 'Sex offenders against children: empirical and clinical issues', in J.N. Briere, L. Berliner, J. Bulkley, C.A. Jenny and T.A. Reid (eds), *The APSAC Handbook on Child Maltreatment*. Thousand Oaks, CA: Sage, pp. 175–92.

Murray, L. and Cooper, P. (2003) 'Intergenerational transmission of affective and cognitive processes associated with depression: infancy and the preschool years', in I. Goodyer (ed.), *Unipolar Depression: A Lifespan Perspective*. Oxford: Oxford University Press, pp. 17–46.

National Institute of Health (1998, 16–18 November) *Consensus Statement: Diagnosis and Treatment of Attention Deficit Hyperactivity Disorder*, 16 (2): 1–37.

Neimeyer, R.A. and Mahoney, M.J. (eds) (1995) *Constructivism in Psychotherapy*. Washington, DC: American Psychological Association.

Nelson, G. (1989) 'Life strains, coping and emotional well being: a longitudinal study of recently separated and married women', *American Journal of Community Psychology*, 17: 451–83.

Nesmith, A.A. (2002) 'Predictors of running away from foster care', *Dissertation Abstracts International*, 63 (4): 1559-A.

Noll, J.G., Horowitz, L.A., Bonanno, G., Trickett, P.K. and Putnam, F.W. (2003) 'Revictimization and self-harm in adolescent and young adult females who experienced childhood sexual abuse', *Journal of Interpersonal Violence*, 18 (12): 1452–71.

Noll, J.G., Trickett, P.K. and Putnam, F.W. (2003) 'A prospective investigation of the impact of childhood sexual abuse on the development of sexuality', *Journal of Consulting and Clinical Psychology*, 71 (3): 575–86.

Noll, J.G., Trickett, P.K., Harris, W.W. and Putnam, F.W. (2008, in press) 'The cumulative burden borne by offspring whose mothers were abused as children: descriptive results from a multigenerational study', *Journal of Interpersonal Violence*, 24.

O'Connor, R. (1991) *Child Sexual Abuse: Treatment, Prevention and Detection*. West Heidelberg, Australia: Centre for Health Program Evaluation.

O'Connor, T.G., Marvin, R.S., Rutter, M., Olrick, J.T. and Britner, P.A. (2003) 'Child–parent attachment following early institutional deprivation', *Development and Psychopathology*, 15 (1): 19–38.

Ogren, M.P. and Lombroso, P.J. (2008) 'Epigenetics: behavioral influences on gene function. I. Maternal behavior permanently affects adult behavior in offspring', *Journal of the American Academy of Child and Adolescent Psychiatry*, 47 (3): 240–4.

O'Halloran, M., Carr, A., O'Reilly, G. *et al.* (2002) 'Psychological profiles of sexually abusive adolescents in Ireland', *Child Abuse and Neglect*, 26: 349–70.

Oliver, J.E. (1993) 'Intergenerational transmission of child abuse: rates, research and clinical implications', *American Journal of Psychiatry*, 150: 1315–24.

O'Malley, S. (2004) *'Are You There Alone?': The Unspeakable Crime of Andrea Yates*. New York: Simon & Schuster.

Ornstein, R. and Thompson, R. (1984) *The Amazing Brain*. Boston, MA: Houghton.

Pavlov, I.P. (1928) *Lectures on Conditioned Reflexes*. New York: International Publishers.

Pecora, P.J., Kessler, R.C., O'Brien, K. *et al.* (2006) 'Educational and employment outcomes of adults formerly placed in foster care: results from the Northwest Foster Care Alumni Study', *Children and Youth Services Review*, 28 (12): 1459–81.

Pepe, M.V. and Byrne, T.J. (1991) 'Women's perceptions of immediate and long-term effects of failed infertility treatment on marital and sexual satisfaction', *Family Relations*, 40 (3): 303–9.

Peplau, L.A. (2003) 'Human sexuality: how do men and women differ?', *Current Directions in Psychological Science*, 12 (2): 37–40.

Perls, F.S. (1961) *Gestalt Therapy Verbatim*. Lafayette, CA: Real People Press.

Perls, F.S., Hefferline, R.E. and Goodman, P. (1951) *Gestalt Therapy*. New York: Delta.

Perry, B.D., Conroy, L. and Ravitz, A. (1991) 'Persisting psychophysiological effects of traumatic stress: the memory of "states"', *Violence Update*, 1: 1–11.

Peterson, C., Maier, S.F. and Seligman, M.E.P. (1993) *Learned Helplessness: A Theory for the Age of Personal Control*. New York: Oxford University Press.

Petronis, A. (2004) 'The origin of schizophrenia: genetic thesis, epigenetic antithesis, and resolving synthesis', *Biological Psychiatry*, 55: 965–70.

Peyron, R., García-Larrea, L., Grégoire, M. *et al.* (1999) 'Haemodynamic brain responses to acute pain in humans: sensory and attentional networks', *Brain: A Journal of Neurology*, 122: 1765–79.

Pope, K.S. and Feldman-Summers, S. (1992) 'National survey of psychologists' sexual and physical abuse history and their evaluation of training and competence in these areas', *Professional Psychology: Research and Practice*, 25: 247–58.

Pope, K.S. and Tabachnick, B.G. (1994) 'Therapists as patients: a national survey of psychologists' experiences, problems and beliefs', *Professional Psychology: Research and Practice*, 25: 247–58.

Post, R.M. and Weiss, S.R.B. (1997) 'Emergent properties of neural systems: how focal molecular neurobiological alterations can affect behavior', *Development and Psychopathology*, 9: 907–29.

Post, R.M., Weiss, S.R.B., Li, H. *et al.* (1998) 'Neural plasticity and emotional memory', *Development and Psychopathology: Special Issue: Risk, Trauma, and Memory*, 10: 829–55.

Procter, H. (1981) 'Family construct psychology', in S. Walrond-Skinner (ed.), *Family Therapy and Approaches*. London: RKP, pp. 350–66.

Radeke, J.T. (1998) 'Comparing the personal lives of psychotherapists and research psychologists', *Dissertations Abstracts International*, 58: 6267.

Rafter, N.H. and Stanley, D.L. (1999) *Prisons in America: A Reference Handbook*. Santa Barbara, CA: ABC-CLIO.

Rahman, A., Lovel, H., Bunn, J., Iqbal, Z. and Harrington, R. (2004) 'Mothers' mental health and infant growth: a case-control study from Rawalpindi, Pakistan', *Child: Care, Health and Development*, 30: 21–7.

Read, J. (1998) 'Child abuse and severity of disturbance among adult psychiatric inpatient', *Child Abuse and Neglect*, 22: 359–68.

Rekers, G. (1996) *Susan Smith: Victim or Murderer?* Lakewood, CO: Glenbridge.

Rhudy, J.L. and Meagher, M.W. (2001) 'The role of emotion in pain modulation', *Current Opinion in Psychiatry*, 14: 241–5.

Rieber, R.W. and Carlton, A.S. (eds) (1987) *The Collected Works of L.S. Vygotsky* (N. Minick, trans.). New York: Plenum Press.

Ringel, Y., Drossman, D.A., Leserman, J.L. *et al.* (2008) 'Effect of abuse history on pain reports and brain responses to aversive visceral stimulation: an FMRI study', *Gastroenterology*, 134: 396–404.

Ringer, F. and Crittenden, P.M. (2007) 'Eating disorders and attachment: the effects of hidden family processes on eating disorders', *European Eating Disorders Review*, 15 (2): 119–30.

Roberts, A.R. and Everly, G.S. Jr. (2006) 'A meta-analysis of 36 crisis intervention studies', *Brief Treatment and Crisis Intervention*, 6 (1): 10–21.

Rolls, C. (2007, December) 'Brief treatment of a type C child using the SAA', *DMM News: International Association for the Study of Attachment (IASA)*, 2: 4. Retrieved 28 March 2008, from www.iasa-dmm.org/dmm_news_dec07.pdf.

Ronnestad, M. and Skovholt, T.M. (2003) 'The journey of the counselor and therapist: research findings and perspectives on professional development', *Journal of Career Development*, 30 (1): 5–44.

Rozin, P. and Fallon, A.E. (1987) 'A perspective on disgust', *Psychological Review*, 94: 23–41.

Russel, D.E.H. (1986) *The Secret Trauma: Incest in the Lives of Girls and Women*. New York: Basic Books.

Rutter, M. (1966) *Children of Sick Parents: An Environmental and Psychiatric Study*. Maudsley Monographs. London: Oxford University Press.

Rutter, M. (2002) 'Family influences on behavior and development: challenges for the future', in J.P. McHale and W.S. Grolnick (eds), *Retrospect and Prospect in the Psychological Study of Families*. Mahwah, NJ: Lawrence Erlbaum, pp. 321–51.

Rutter, M. (2004) 'Intergenerational continuities and discontinuities in psychological problems', in P.L. Chase-Lansdale, K. Kiernan and R.J. Friedman (eds), *Human Development Across Lives and Generations: The Potential for Change. Jacobs Foundation Series on Adolescence*. New York: Cambridge University Press, pp. 239–77.

Rutter, M. (2005) 'Genetic influences and autism', in F.R.Volkmar, R. Paul, A. Klin and D. Cohen (eds), *Handbook of Autism and Pervasive Developmental Disorders: Vol. 1. Diagnosis, Development, Neurobiology, and Behavior* (3rd edn). Hoboken, NJ: Wiley, pp. 425–52.

Rutter, M. (2006a) *Genes and Behaviour: Nature/Nurture Interplay Explained*. Malden, MA: Blackwell.

Rutter, M. (2006b) 'Implications of resilience concepts for scientific understanding', in B.M. Lester, A. Masten and B. McEwen (eds), *Annals of the New York Academy of Sciences. Resilience in Children*. Malden, MA: Blackwell, pp. 1–12.

Rutter, M. (2006c) 'The promotion of resilience in the face of adversity', in A. Clarke-Stewart and J. Dunn (eds), *Families Count: Effects on Child and Adolescent Development. Jacobs Foundation Series on Adolescence*. New York: Cambridge University Press, pp. 26–52.

Rutter, M. (2006d) 'The psychological effects of early institutional rearing', in P.J. Marshall and N.A. Fox (eds), *Series in Affective Science. The Development of Social Engagement: Neurobiological Perspectives*. New York: Oxford University Press, pp. 355–91.

Rutter, M. (2007) 'Gene–environment interdependence', *Developmental Science*, 10: 12–18.

Rutter, M., Andersen-Wood, L., Beckett, C. *et al.* (1999) 'Quasi-autistic patterns following severe early global privation', *Journal of Child Psychology and Psychiatry*, 40: 537–49.

Rutter, M., Moffitt, T.E. and Caspi, A. (2006) 'Gene environment interplay and psychopathology: multiple varieties but real effects', *Journal of Child Psychiatry and Psychology Annual Review*, 47: 226–61.

Rutter, M. and Rutter, M. (1993) *Developing Minds: Challenge and Continuity Across the Life-Span*. Harmondsworth: Penguin.

Ryle, A. and Kerr, I.B. (2002) *Introducing Cognitive Analytic Therapy: Principles and Practice*. Chichester: Wiley.

Sajatovic, M., Bauer, M. S., Kilbourne, A.M., Vertrees, J.E. and Williford, W. (2006) 'Self-reported medication treatment adherence among veterans with bipolar disorder', *Psychiatric Services*, 57: 56–62.

Salmon, M., Abel, K., Cordingley, L., Friedman, T. and Appleby, L. (2003) 'Clinical and parenting skills outcomes following joint mother-baby psychiatric admission', *Australian and New Zealand Journal of Psychiatry*, 37: 556–62.

Salter, D., McMillan, D., Richards, M. *et al.* (2003) 'Development of sexually abusive behavior in sexually victimized males: a longitudinal study', *Lancet*, 361: 471–6.

Sameroff, A.J. (1983) 'Developmental systems: contexts and evolution', in P.H. Mussen (series ed.) and W. Kessen (vol. ed.), *Handbook of Child Psychology: Vol. 1. History, Theory, and Methods*. New York: Wiley, pp. 237–94.

Sameroff, A.J. (2000) 'Developmental systems and psychopathology', *Development and Psychopathology*, 12 (3): 297–312.

Sameroff, A.J. and Chandler, M.J. (1975) 'Reproductive risk and the continuum of caretaker casualty', in F.D. Horowitz, M. Hetherington, S. Scarr-Salapatek and G. Siegel (eds), *Review of Child Development Research*, vol. 4. Chicago: University of Chicago Press, pp. 187–242.

Scaer, R. (2001) 'The neurophysiology of dissociation and chronic disease', *Applied Psychophysiology and Biofeedback*, 26: 73–91.

Scavo, R. and Buchanan, B.D. (1989) 'Group therapy for male adolescent sex offenders: a model for residential treatment', *Residential Treatment for Children and Youth*, 7 (2): 59–74.

Schachar, R.J. and Wachsmuth, R. (1991) 'Family dysfunction and psychosocial adversity: comparison of attention deficit disorder, conduct disorder, normal and clinical controls', *Canadian Journal of Behavioural Science/Revue canadienne des Sciences du comportement*, 23 (3): 332–48.

Schacter, D.L. (1996) *Searching for Memory: The Brain, the Mind, and the Past*. New York: Basic Books.

Schacter D.L. and Tulving, E. (eds) (1994) *Memory Systems*. Cambridge, MA: The MIT Press.

Schauenburg, H., Dinger, U. and Strack, M. (2005) 'Zur Bedeutung der Einzeltherapeuten für das Therapie-ergebnis in der stationären Psychotherapie – Eine Pilotstudie' ['Individual therapists in inpatient psychotherapy – A pilot study on their importance for therapeutic outcome'], *Psychotherapie Psychosomatik Medizinische Psychologiel*, 55 (7): 339–46.

Schmahmann, J.D. (ed.) (1997) *The Cerebellum and Cognition*. San Diego, CA: Academic Press.

Schore, A.N. (1994) *Affect Regulation and the Origin of Self: The Neurobiology of Emotional Development*. Hillsdale, NJ: Erlbaum.

Schore, A.N. (2000) 'The self-organization of the right brain and the neurobiology of emotional development', in N. Eisenberg, R.N. Emde, W.W. Hartup, L.W. Hoffman, F.J. Manks, R.D. Parke, M. Rutter, C. Shantz and C. Zahn-Waxler (series eds) and M.D. Lewis and I. Granic (vol. eds), *Emotion, Development, and Self-Organization: Dynamic Systems Approaches to Emotional Development. Cambridge Studies in Social and Emotional Development*. Cambridge: Cambridge University Press, pp. 155–85.

Schore, A.N. (2002) 'Dysregulation of the right brain: a fundamental mechanism of traumatic attachment and the psychopathogenesis of posttraumatic stress disorder', *Australian and New Zealand Journal of Psychiatry*, 36: 9–30.

Schore, A.N. (2003) *Affect Dysregulation and Disorders of the Self*. New York: W. W. Norton.

Schultz, D. and Shaw, D.S. (2003) 'Boys' maladaptive social information processing, family emotional climate, and pathways to early conduct problems', *Social Development*, 12 (3): 440–60.

Schwab, R. (1997) 'Parental mourning and children's development', *Journal of Counseling and Development*, 75 (4): 258–65.

Schwartz, M. and Masters, W. (1994) 'Integration of trauma-based, cognitive behavioral, systemic and addiction approaches for treatment of hypersexual pair-bonding disorder', *Sexual Addiction and Compulsivity*, 1 (1): 57–76.

Seefeldt, L.J. (1997) *Models of Parenting in Maltreating and Non-Maltreating Mothers*. Dissertation presented to the Graduate School of Nursing, University of Wisconsin at Milwaukee.

Segal, H. (1964) *Introduction to the Work of Melanie Klein*. New York: Basic Books.

Seligman, M.P.E. (1975) *Helplessness: On Depression, Development, and Death*. New York: W. H. Freeman.

Selvini-Palazzoli, M., Boscolo, L., Cecchin, G. and Prata, G. (1980) 'Hypothesizing-circularity-neutrality: three guidelines for the conductor of the session', *Family Process*, 19: 3–12.

Selye, H. (1976) *The Stress of Life*. New York: McGraw-Hill.

Shang, C.-Y., Gau, S.S-F., Soong, W.-T. (2006) 'Association between childhood sleep problems and perinatal factors, parental mental distress and behavioral problems', *Journal of Sleep Research*, 15: 63–73.

Shaw, P., Eckstrand, K., Sharp, W. *et al.* (2007) 'Attention-deficit/hyperactivity disorder is characterized by a delay in cortical maturation', *Proceedings of the National Academy of Sciences of the United States*, 104 (49): 19649–54.

Shine, J., McCloskey, H. and Newton, M. (2002) 'Self-esteem and sex offending', *Journal of Sexual Aggression*, 8 (1): 51–8.

Siegel, D.J. (1999) *The Developing Mind: Toward a Neurobiology of Interpersonal Experience*. New York: Guilford Press.

Siegel, D.J. (2001) 'Memory: An overview, with emphasis on developmental, interpersonal, and neurobiological aspects', *Journal of the American Academy of Child and Adolescent Psychiatry*, 40 (9): 997–1011.

Singer, T., Seymour, B., O'Doherty, J., Kaube, H., Dolan, R.J. and Frith, C.D. (2004) 'Empathy for pain involves the affective but not sensory components of pain', *Science*, 303: 1157–62.

Skinner, B.F. (1938) *The Behavior of Organisms: An Experimental Analysis*. Oxford: Appleton-Century.

Skinner, B.F. (1950) 'Are learning theories necessary?', *Psychological Review*, 57: 193–216.

Skinner, B.F. (1953) *Science and Human Behavior*. New York: Macmillan.

Smallbone, S. and Dadds, M. (1998) 'Childhood attachment and adult attachment in incarcerated adult male sex offenders', *Journal of Interpersonal Violence*, 13: 555–73.

Smallbone, S. and Dadds, M. (2000) 'Attachment and coercive sexual behavior', *Sexual Abuse: A Journal of Research and Treatment*, 12: 3–15.

Smith, D. (with Calef, C.) (1995) *Beyond All Reason: My Life with Susan Smith*. New York: Kensington Books.

Smith, S. (1994) 'The Susan Smith trial: nine days in Union: Susan Smith's handwritten confession', *Herald-Journal*. Retrieved 5 March 2008, from http://www.teleplex.net/shj/smith/ninedays/ssconf.html.

Snyder, H. and Sickmund, M. (2006) *Juvenile Offenders and Victims: 2006 National Report*. Washington, DC: US Department of Justice.

Sowell, E.R., Peterson, B.S., Thompson, P.M., Welcome, S.E., Henkenius, A.L. and Toga, A.W. (2003) 'Mapping cortical change across the human life span', *Nature Neuroscience*, 6: 309–15.

Sroufe, A., Carlson, E., Levy, A. and Egeland, B. (1999) 'Implications of attachment theory for developmental psychopathology', *Development and Psychopathology*, 11: 1–13.

Sroufe, L.A. and Ward, J.J. (1980) 'Seductive behavior of mothers of toddlers: occurrence, correlates, and family origins', *Child Development*, 51: 1222–9.

Stanger, C., Higgins, S.T., Bickel, W.K. *et al.* (1999) 'Behavioral and emotional problems among children of cocaine and opiate dependent parents', *Journal of the American Academy of Child and Adolescent Psychiatry*, 38: 421–8.

Starzyk, K.B. and Marshall, W.L. (2003) 'Childhood family and personological risk factors for sexual offending', *Aggression and Violent Behavior*, 8: 93–105.

Stein, T.J., Gambrill, E.D. and Wiltse, K.T. (1977) 'Contracts and outcomes in foster care', *Social Work*, 22: 148–9.

Stern, D. (1985) *The Interpersonal World of the Infant: A View from Psychoanalysis and Developmental Psychology*. New York: Basic Books.

Strathearn, L. (2008, October) 'Does attachment shape a mother's brain? Exploring the neurobiology of attachment.' Keynote address at the First Biennial Conference of the International Association for the Study of Attachment, Bertinoro, Italy.

Stratton, P. (2003) 'Causal attributions during therapy. I. Responsibility and blame', *Journal of Family Therapy*, 25: 134–58.

Stroebe, W., Schut, H. and Stroebe, M.S. (2005) 'Grief work, disclosure and counseling: do they help the bereaved?', *Clinical Psychology Review*, 25: 395–414.

Sudak, D.M. (2006) *Cognitive Behavioral Therapy for Clinicians: Psychotherapy in Clinical Practice*. Philadelphia: Lippincott Williams & Wilkins.

Swanson, J.M., Elliott, G.R., Greenhill, L.L. *et al.* (2007) 'Effects of stimulant medication on growth rates across 3 years in the MTA follow-up', *Journal of American Academy of Child and Adolescent Psychiatry*, 26 (8): 1015–27.

Swanson, J.M., Hinshaw, S.P., Arnold, L.E. *et al.* (2007) 'Secondary evaluations of MTA 36-month outcomes: propensity score and growth mixture model analyses', *Journal of the American Academy of Child and Adolescent Psychiatry*, 46 (8): 1003–14.

Szasz, T.S. (1960) 'The myth of mental illness', *American Psychologist*, 15: 113–18.

Szasz, T.S. (1961) *The Myth of Mental Illness: Foundations of a Theory of Personal Conduct*. New York: Hoeber-Harper.

Taumoepeau, M. and Ruffman, T. (2006) 'Mother and infant talk about mental states relates to desire language and emotion understanding', *Child Development*, 77: 465–81.

Taussig, H.N., Clyman, R.B. and Landsverk, J. (2001) 'Children who return home from foster care: A 6-year prospective study of behavioral health outcomes in adolescence', *Pediatrics*, 108 (1): 170.

Thomas-Peter, B.A. (2006) 'The needs of offenders and the process of changing them', in G. Towl (ed.), *Psychological Research in Prisons*. Malden, MA: Blackwell, pp. 40–53.

Thompson, R.F. (1991) 'Are memory traces localized or distributed?', *Neuropsychologia*, 29: 571–82.

Tinbergen, N. (1951) *The Study of Instinct*. Oxford: Oxford University Press.

Trickett, P.K., Noll, J.G., Reiffman, A. and Putnam, F.W. (2001) 'Variants of intrafamilial sexual abuse experience: implications for long term development', *Journal of Development and Psychopathology*, 13 (4): 1001–19.

Tsankova, N. , Renthal, W., Kumar, A. and Nestler, E.J. (2007) 'Epigenetic regulation in psychiatric disorders', *Nature*, 8: 355–67.

Tulving, E. (1979) 'Memory research: what kind of progress?', in L.G. Nilsson (ed.), *Perspectives on Memory Research: Essays in Honor of Uppsala University's 500th Anniversary*. Hillsdale, NJ: Erlbaum, pp. 19–34.

Tulving, E. (1987) 'Multiple memory systems and consciousness', *Human Neurobiology*, 6 (2): 67–80.

Üçok, A. and Bikmaz, S. (2007) 'The effects of childhood trauma in patients with first-episode schizophrenia', *Acta Psychiatrica Scandinavica*, 116: 371–7.

UK Home Office (2001) *Making Punishments Work: Report of a Review of the Sentencing Framework for England and Wales*. Retrieved 24 March 2008, from http://www.homeoffice.gov.uk/documents/halliday-report-sppu/?version=1.

US Census Bureau (2007) *Annual Estimates of the Population by Selected Age Groups and Sex for the United States* (NC-EST2006-01). Washington, DC: Author.

US Department of Health and Human Services (2005) *The AFCARS Report: Preliminary FY 2003*. Washington, DC: US Government Printing Office.

US Department of Health and Human Services (2006a) *Child Maltreatment 2004*. Washington, DC: US Government Printing Office.

US Department of Health and Human Services (2006b) *The AFCARS Children's Bureau Preliminary Estimates for FY 2005*. Washington, DC: US Government Printing Office.

US Department of Health and Human Services (2007) *Child Maltreatment 2005*. Washington, DC: US Government Printing Office.

US Department of Health and Human Services and Faller, K.C. (1993) *Child Sexual Abuse: Intervention and Treatment Issues*. Washington, DC: Child Welfare Information Gateway.

Valenstein, M., Ganoczy, D., McCarthy, J.F. *et al.* (2006) 'Antipsychotic adherence over time among patients receiving treatment for schizophrenia: a retrospective review', *Journal of Clinical Psychiatry*, 67, 1542–50.

Vandivere, S., Chalk, R. and Moore, K.A. (2003) 'Children in foster homes: how are they faring?', *Child Trends Research Brief*, 23.

Van Ijzendoorn, M. (1995) 'Adult attachment representations, parental responsiveness, and infant attachment: a meta-analysis on the predictive validity of the adult attachment interview', *Psychological Bulletin*, 117: 387–403.

Veneziano, C. and Veneziano, L. (2002) 'Adolescent sex offenders: a review of the literature', *Trauma Violence and Abuse*, 3: 246–60.

Vogt, B.A. (2005) 'Pain and emotion interactions in subregions of the cingulate gyrus', *Nature Reviews Neuroscience*, 6: 533–44.

Von Bertalanffy, L. (1968) *General System Theory: Foundations, Development, Applications*. New York: George Braziller.

Vygotsky, L.S. (1978) *Mind and Society: The Development of Higher Psychological Processes*. Cambridge, MA: Harvard University Press.

Wager, T.D., Rilling, J.K., Smith, E.E. *et al.* (2004) 'Placebo-induced changes in FMRI in the anticipation and experience of pain', *Science*, 303: 1162–7.

Wajnryb, R. (2001) *The Silence: How Tragedy Shapes Talk*. Crows Nest, Australia: Allen & Unwin.

Walsh, F. (1979) 'Breaching of family generation boundaries by schizophrenics, disturbed, and normals', *International Journal of Family Therapy*, 1 (3): 254–75.

Walsh, F. and McGoldrick, M. (eds) (2004) *Living Beyond Loss: Death in the Family* (2nd edn). New York: W.W. Norton.

Walter, J. and Peller, J. (1992) *Becoming Solution-Focused in Brief Therapy*. New York: Brunner/Mazel.

Ward, T. and Beech, A. (2006) 'An integrated theory of sexual offending', *Aggression and Violent Behavior*, 11: 44–63.

Ward, T., Polaschek, L.L. and Beech, A.R. (2006) *Theories of Sexual Offending*. Wiley Series in Forensic Clinical Psychology. Chichester: Wiley-Blackwell.

Watanabe, N., Hunot, V., Omori, I.M., Churchill, R. and Furukama, T.A. (2007) 'Psychotherapy for depression among children and adolescents: a systematic review', *Acta Psychiatrica Scandinavica*, 116 (2): 84–95.

Waterman, J., Kelley, R.J., McCord, J. and Oliveri, M.K. (eds) (1993) *Behind Playground Walls: Sexual Abuse in Day Care*. New York: Guilford.

Weakland, J., Fisch, R., Watzlawick, P. and Bodin, A. (1974) 'Brief therapy: focused problem resolution', *Family Process*, 13: 141–68.Weaver, S.A., Diorio, J. and Meaney, M.J. (2007) 'Maternal separation leads to persistent reductions in pain sensitivity in female rats', *Journal of Pain*, 8 (12): 962–9.

Weaver, I.C.G., Meaney, M.J. and Szyf, M. (2006) 'Maternal care effects on the hippocampal transcriptome and anxiety-mediated behaviors in the offspring that are reversible in adulthood', *Proceedings of the National Academy of Sciences of the United States of America*, 103 (9): 3480–5.

Weiss, L.A., Shen, Y., Korn, J.M. *et al.* (2008) 'Association between microdeletion and microduplication at 16p11.2 and autism', *New England Journal of Medicine*, 358: 667–75.

Wente, M. (2004, 6 July) 'Thirteen years of abuse, nine months in prison: the Blackstock secret: Anger greets sentence for couple who caged two boys', *The Globe and Mail*, p. A1.

Wertheimer, M. (1938) 'Laws of organization in perceptual forms', in W. Ellis (ed.), *A Source Book of Gestalt Psychology*. London: Routledge & Kegan Paul, pp. 71–88.

Wertheimer, M. (1959) *Productive Thinking*. New York: Harper & Row.

White, M. and Epston, D. (1990) *Narrative Means to a Therapeutic End*. New York: Norton.

Whitfield, C., Dube, S.R., Felitti, V.J. and Anda, R.F. (2005) 'Adverse childhood experiences and hallucinations', *Child Abuse and Neglect*, 29 (7): 797–810.

Wickramasekera, I. (2008) 'Review of current psychological approaches to the management of chronic pain', *American Journal of Clinical Hypnosis*, 50 (3): 289.

Widom, C.S. (1989) 'Child abuse, neglect, and violent criminal behaviour', *Criminology*, 27: 251–71.

Wilkinson, S.R. (2003) *Coping and Complaining: Attachment and the Language of Disease*. New York: Brunner-Routledge.

Wilson, C.A. and Hill, W.L. (2007, November) 'Oxytocin and cortisol changes after kissing in adult human heterosexual pairs'. Paper presented at the 37th Annual Meeting of the Society for Neuroscience, San Diego, CA.

Wilson, C.A. and Oswald, A.J. (2005) 'How does marriage affect physical and psychological health: a survey of the longitudinal evidence', *IZA Discussion Papers, 1619*. Bonn: Institute for the Study of Labor (IZA).

Wilson, M. and Daly, M. (1992) 'The man who mistook his wife for a chattel', in J.H. Barkow, L. Cosmides and J. Tooby (eds), *The Adapted Mind: Evolutionary Psychology and the Generation of Culture*. London: Oxford University Press, pp. 289–322.

Winnicott, D. (1956) 'On transference', *International Journal of Psycho-Analysis*, 37: 386–8.

Winnicott, D.W. (1957) *Mother and Child: A Primer of First Relationships*. New York: Basic Books.

Winnicott, D.W. (1986) 'The theory of the parent-infant relationship', in P. Buckley (ed.), *Essential Papers on Object Relations. Essential Papers in Psychoanalysis*. New York: University Press, pp. 233–53.

Wolfe, D.A. (1985) 'Child abusive parents: an empirical review and analysis', *Psychological Bulletin*, 97 (3): 462–82.

Wolpe, D.A. (1948) *An Approach to the Problem of Neurosis Based on the Conditioned Response*. Unpublished M.D. thesis. University of Witwatersrand, Johannesburg, South Africa.

Wolpe, J. (1958) *Pyschotheraphy by Reciprocal Inhibition*. Stanford, CA: Stanford University Press.

World Health Organization (1993) *The ICD-10 Classification of Mental and Behavioural Disorders: Diagnostic Criteria for Research*. Geneva: Author.

World Health Organization (2002) 'Child abuse and neglect by parents and other caregivers', in *World Report on Violence and Health* (chap. 3). Geneva: Author.

Yeomans, F.E., Clarkin, J.F. and Kernberg, O.F. (2002) *A Primer of Transference-Focused Psychotherapy for the Borderline Patient*. Northvale, NJ: Jason Aronson.

Yerkes, R.M. and Dodson, J.D. (1908) 'The relation of strength of stimulus to rapidity of habit-formation', *Journal of Comparative Neurology and Psychology*, 18: 459–82.

Young, J., Klosko, J. and Weishar, M.E. (2003) *Schema Therapy: A Practitioner's Guide*. New York: Guilford Press.

Young, W.C., Sachs, R.G., Braun, B.G. and Watkins, R.T. (1991) 'Patients reporting ritual abuse in childhood: a clinical syndrome: report of 37 cases', *Child Abuse and Neglect*, 15: 181–9.

Zhang, L.X., Xing, G.Q., Levine, S., Post, R.M. and Smith, M.A. (1997) 'Maternal deprivation induces neuronal death', *Society for Neuroscience Abstracts*, 23: 1113.

Zigler, E. and Aber, J.L. (1981) 'Developmental considerations in the definition of child maltreatment', *New Directions for Child Development*, 11: 1–29.

Index